Math for the Pharmacy Technician: Concepts and Calculations

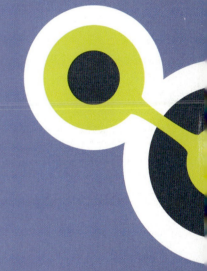

Math for the Pharmacy Technician: Concepts and Calculations

Lynn M. Egler, RMA, AHI, CPhT

Dorsey Schools, Madison Heights, Michigan

Kathryn A. Booth, RN-BSN, MS, RMA, RPT, CPhT

Total Care Programming, Palm Coast, Florida

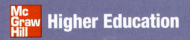
McGraw-Hill Higher Education

Boston   Burr Ridge, IL   Dubuque, IA   New York   San Francisco   St. Louis
Bangkok   Bogotá   Caracas   Kuala Lumpur   Lisbon   London   Madrid   Mexico City
Milan   Montreal   New Delhi   Santiago   Seoul   Singapore   Sydney   Taipei   Toronto

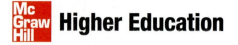

Higher Education

MATH FOR THE PHARMACY TECHNICIAN: CONCEPTS AND CALCULATIONS

Published by McGraw-Hill, a business unit of The McGraw-Hill Companies, Inc., 1221 Avenue of the Americas, New York, NY, 10020. Copyright 2010 by The McGraw-Hill Companies, Inc. All rights reserved. No part of this publication may be reproduced or distributed in any form or by any means, or stored in a database or retrieval system, without the prior written consent of The McGraw-Hill Companies, Inc., including, but not limited to, in any network or other electronic storage or transmission, or broadcast for distance learning.

Some ancillaries, including electronic and print components, may not be available to customers outside the United States.

This book is printed on acid-free paper.
Printed in China
3 4 5 6 7 8 9 0 CTP/CTP 12 11

ISBN 978-0-07-337396-6
MHID 0-07-337396-6

Vice president/Editor in chief: *Elizabeth Haefele*
Vice president/Director of marketing: *John E. Biernat*
Senior sponsoring editor: *Debbie Fitzgerald*
Developmental editor: *Connie Kuhl*
Executive marketing manager: *Roxan Kinsey*
Lead media producer: *Damian Moshak*
Media producer: *Marc Mattson*
Director, Editing/Design/Production: *Jess Ann Kosic*
Project manager: *Christine M. Demma*

Senior production supervisor: *Janean A. Utley*
Senior designer: *Srdjan Savanovic*
Senior photo research coordinator: *Lori Hancock*
Media project manager: *Mark A. S. Dierker*
Interior design: *Ellen Pettengell*
Typeface: *10.5/13 New Aster*
Compositor: *Macmillan Publishing Solutions*
Printer: *CTPS*
Cover Credit: © *Ryan McVay/Getty Images*

Credits: The credits section for this book begins on page 362 and is considered an extension of the copyright page.
Photo credits: Chapter Openers 1,2: © Total Care Programming, Inc; Chapter Opener 3: © Getty RF; 3 1: © The McGraw-Hill Companies, Inc./Stephen Frisch, photographer; Chapter Openers 4-7: © Total Care Programming, Inc.; 7.1: © Getty RF; 7.2: © Alamy RF; 7 3(both): © Total Care Programming, Inc.;7.4: © Creatas/Punchstock RF; 7.5: © Digital Vision/Superstock; Chapter Opener 8: © Total Care Programming, Inc.; Chapter Opener 9: © Corbis RF; Chapter Opener 10: © Bananastock/PictureQuest RF; Chapter Opener 11: © Stockbyte/Punchstock.

Library of Congress Cataloging-in-Publication Data

Egler, Lynn M.
  Math for the pharmacy technician : concepts and calculations / Lynn M. Egler, Kathryn A. Booth.
      p. ; cm.
  Includes index.
  ISBN-13: 978-0-07-337396-6 (alk. paper)
  ISBN-10: 0-07-337396-6 (alk. paper)
  1. Pharmaceutical arithmetic—Examinations, questions, etc. 2. Pharmacy technicians—Examinations, questions, etc. I. Booth, Kathryn A., 1957- II. Title.
  [DNLM: 1. Drug Dosage Calculations—Examination Questions. 2. Mathematics—Examination Questions. 3. Pharmacists' Aides—education—Examination Questions.
QV 18.2 E31m 2010]
RS57.E35 2010
615'.1401513076—dc22

                                                    2008045883

WARNING NOTICE: The clinical procedures, medicines, dosages, and other matters described in this publication are based upon research of current literature and consultation with knowledgeable persons in the field. The procedures and matters described in this text reflect currently accepted clinical practice. However, this information cannot and should not be relied upon as necessarily applicable to a given individual's case. Accordingly, each person must be separately diagnosed to discern the patient's unique circumstances. Likewise, the manufacturer's package insert for current drug production information should be consulted before administering any drug. Publisher disclaims all liability for any inaccuracies, omissions, misuse, or misunderstanding of the information contained in this publication. Publisher cautions that this publication is not intended as a substitute for the professional judgment of trained medical personnel.

www.mhhe.com

Dedication

Lynn Egler: *To all the "teachers" I have learned from and all the students I have been able to share that knowledge with.*

To my family members and friends who have supported me in this effort, and have realized what a precious opportunity it was for me. Especially my niece, Jennifer Jiminey, thank you for your administrative assistance on this project. I love you.

To Carol Buchanan for her unwavering support and friendship, if it were not for her, this opportunity would have never come to be.

To Andy Tysinger for encouraging my best interests regardless of the consequences.

To my loving retired Navy husband, Scott, who stood the watch at home during this project. Without his love and support I never could have achieved this dream.

Kathryn Booth: *To the future pharmacy technicians who use this program, congratulations on your selection of this profession. Your skills and training are greatly needed.*

To my youngest son, Jack for his love and everlasting faithfulness and my dear husband for his enduring support.

About the Authors

Lynn M. Egler, RMA, AHI, CPhT, has worked in the health care and education fields across the country for the past 25 years. She served in the United States Navy as a hospital corpsman and emergency medical technician during Operations Desert Shield and Desert Storm. Mrs. Egler's health care experience includes; emergency department, endoscopy, anesthesia and recovery, hospital pediatrics and maternal health, hospital laboratory, family practice, and retail pharmacy.

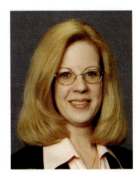

As a dedicated educator, she has held the positions of Medical Assistant and Medical Office Specialist Program Director, Medical Assistant Education Chair, Allied Health instructor, externship coordinator, and American Heart Association CPR instructor and training center faculty. Mrs. Egler developed and standardized multiple curricula for eight college campuses across four states, including medical assisting, medical office administration, dental assisting, surgical technician, and pharmacy technician programs. Mrs. Egler is currently employed with Dorsey Schools in Madison Heights, Michigan, as an Allied Health instructor.

Kathryn A. Booth, RN–BSN, MS, **RMA, RPT, CPhT,** is an author, consultant, vice president, and owner of Total Care Programming, a multimedia software development company. Her background includes a bachelor's degree in nursing and a master's degree in education. Her 29 years of teaching, nursing, and health care experience span five states. She has authored and developed multimedia CD-ROM software and health occupations educational textbooks and educational materials for Total Care Programming Inc., Glencoe/McGraw-Hill, Mosby Lifeline, Lippincott, Williams, and Wilkins, and McGraw-Hill Higher Education. Her most recent textbook is *Medical Assisting: Administrative and Clinical Competencies*, 3rd ed., published by McGraw-Hill Higher Education. Mrs. Booth has presented at numerous state and national conferences since 1994. Her current focus is to develop additional health care materials that will assist health care educators and promote the health care profession.

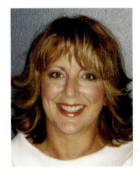

Brief Table of Contents

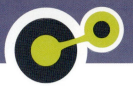

Contents

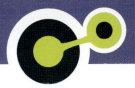

Feature List

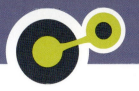

TABLES

"Critical Thinking in the Pharmacy"

Tech Check

Caution!

Review and Practice

Chapter Review Questions

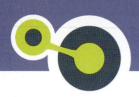

Preface

Recognizing the enormous need for well-trained pharmacy technicians as well as the serious need to decrease medication errors, we have developed *Math for Pharmacy Technicians: Concepts and Calculations.* This textbook is organized from simple to complex and walks the student through the necessary information to pass the math portion of the Pharmacy Technician Certification Board (PTCB) exam. More important, we have created pharmacy technician–specific information that is nonthreatening and will help the student learn to safely practice as a pharmacy technician. This text is organized into 11 chapters, along with a pretest and a comprehensive evaluation, or posttest.

The **Pretest** gives students an opportunity to review the basic math skills they will need as they continue within the book. The content of the Pretest parallels much of the content of Chapters 1 and 2.

- **Chapter 1, Numbering Systems and Mathematical Review,** provides a comprehensive review of fractions and decimals. These are the basic building blocks for all that follows.
- **Chapter 2, Working with Percents, Ratios, and Proportions**, continues the math review by introducing percents, ratios, and proportions as well cross-multiplication and means and extremes. The concepts of ratio strengths and strengths of mixtures are also introduced.
- **Chapter 3, Systems of Measurement and Weight**, reviews weights and measures. It introduces the metric system as well as apothecary and household systems. Time and temperature conversions are included. Special attention is given to conversion factors, and the procedures for ratio proportion, fraction proportion, and dimensional analysis methods are introduced as building blocks for later chapters.
- **Chapter 4, Drug Orders**, begins with the seven rights of medication administration, abbreviations, and controlled substances. This chapter shows the various ways in which drug orders may be written and how to interpret physicians' orders and prescriptions. It emphasizes safety and shows how drug orders and prescriptions can easily be misread, giving added detail to detecting errors and forged or altered prescriptions.
- **Chapter 5, Drug Labels, Package Inserts, and References**, teaches students how to find a wide range of information common to all drug labels and package inserts, then specifically how to find information about oral and parenteral medications and medications administered by other routes.
- **Chapter 6, Dosage Calculations**, teaches the techniques for calculating doses. Building on information from earlier chapters, students

are taught how to calculate the amount to dispense, using all four methods of dosage calculations: ratio proportion, fraction proportion, dimensional analysis, and formula. Students will also learn to calculate estimated days supply.

- **Chapter 7, Oral Medications and Parenteral Dosages,** discusses tablets and capsules in depth and gives information about breaking or crushing them. Liquid oral medications are also discussed. Chapter 7 applies techniques learned in Chapter 6 to calculations of parenteral dosages, emphasizing injectable medications. The chapter concludes with a look at other medication routes such as eye and ear drops, inhalants, rectal and vaginal medications, transdermal systems, and topical medications.
- **Chapter 8, Intravenous Calculations,** presents information and calculations unique to administering intravenous (IV) medications. After introducing IV solutions, attention is turned to calculating flow rates. Students also learn calculations for intermittent IV infusions, infusion times, and infusion volumes.
- **Chapter 9, Special Preparations and Calculations**, presents information and calculations unique to compounds, alligations, preparation of a dilution from a concentrate, and special considerations for insulin calculations.
- **Chapter 10, Pediatric and Geriatric Considerations,** includes drug orders based upon body weight. It introduces body surface area (BSA) calculations. Discussions of special concerns for pediatric and geriatric patients are also presented.
- **Chapter 11, Operational Calculations**, presents information and calculations related to business operations in the pharmacy. This chapter also discusses inventory and reimbursement considerations and calculating correct costs and correct change.

A **Comprehensive Evaluation,** or posttest, covers calculations from all 11 chapters.

Textbook

Math for Pharmacy Technicians: Concepts and Calculations has the following unique features to stimulate the learning process.

PTCB correlations—For students and programs of study to document the coverage of necessary content

Actual Medication Labels—real up-to-date medication labels that will be seen in a job setting give a realistic view of on the job training.

Tables—Summarizes important information at a glance

Caution—Draws attention to mistakes that can occur in pharmacy practice

Memory Tip—Introduces students to techniques to help them remember key information

Marginal Key Terms—Provide easy reference to the important terms within each chapter

Critical Thinking in the Pharmacy/Chapter Scenario—Improves thinking skills of students and provides discussion opportunities in the classroom and online

Super Tech CD-ROM Reference—Provides review and lots of additional practice problems

Tech Check—Provides immediate check of students' understanding of content covered; prior to end of chapter review in order to ensure understanding

Review and Practice—Provides concepts as multiple problems of all types in the chapter for students to review and practice

Chapter Review—Reinforces the chapter outcomes to help retain what was learned

Internet Activity Boxes—Direct the student to factual content and resources and stimulate the use of the Internet as a professional tool.

Special Features of *Math for Pharmacy Technician: Concepts and Calculations*

- Back-of-the-book **p**ocket cards for handy reference during clinical training, externship, or work experience.
- Student **CD-ROM** with **references** throughout the **textbook** that direct the student to exercises and provide for independent review, reinforcement, and evaluation.
- Individual or classroom **games** for pharmacy technicians on the student CD-ROM include Math Challenge, Spin the Wheel, and Key Term Concentration.
- Up-to-date g**lossary** with **pronunciations** on the student CD-ROM.
- Online Learning Center at www.mhhe.com/EglerMathPharmacyTech with q**uick links** to the Internet activities presented in the textbook
- **Companion textbook** (*Pharmacy Technician Practice and Procedures*) with similar features to make the complete pharmacy technician learning and teaching process easier.
- **Instructor's manual** with complete answer keys and solutions, correlations to ASHP and PTCB content, additional practice problems for each chapter, teaching outlines and the Instructor Productivity Center CD-ROM.
- Instructor Productivity Center CD-ROM includes:
  - Ready to use **PowerPoint** presentations with Apply Your Knowledge Questions.
  - Electronic **instructor manual** documents and other teaching resources.
  - **Test banks** for every chapter that include labels and EZ Test Bank Editor.

Acknowledgments

Lynn Egler: Special thanks to Jennifer Jiminey for her administrative assistance and to Kathy Booth for mentoring me on this project. Additional thanks to the McGraw-Hill team for all of their hard work, guidance, and support.

Kathy Booth: Special thanks to Gary Glisson and his employees at Ward Pharmacy in Nashville, North Carolina, for providing us the opportunity to take photographs at their facility. Additional thanks goes to Carla May, Pharmacy Technician Program Coordinator at Vance-Granville Community College, for her time and consultation.

Reviewer Acknowledgments

Robert W. Aanonsen, C.Ph.T.
Platt College

Julette Barta, C.Ph.T., B.S.I.T.
Redlands Regional Occupational Program

Nina Beaman, M.S., B.A., A.A.S.
Bryant and Stratton College

Elizabeth S. Bock
Platt College

Mandy Chapple, B.A.
Salt Lake Tooele Applied Technology College

Christina Rauberts Conklin, A.A., R.M.A., C.D.E.
Keiser University

Chris P. Crigger, C.Ph.T.
San Antonio College

Karen Davis, C.Ph.T.
Consultant

William S. Duzansky, C.Ph.T.
Kaplan Career Institute

Donna Fresnilla, B.A.
Community College of Rhode Island

Coelle Lynette Harper Deaton, B.S.E.
Career Centers of Texas

Linda Hart
High-Tech Institute

Michael M. Hayter, Pharm. D., M.B.A.
Virginia Highlands Community College

Eddy van Hunnik, Ph.D.
Gibbs College of Boston

Dr. Dianne M. Jedlicka, Ph.D, M.S.
DeVry University

Cathy Kelley-Arney, B.S.H.S., A.S.
National College

Mindy Koppel
Pennsylvania Institute of Technology

Rosie Koehler, B.S.
Salt Lake Tooele Applied Technology College

David L. London, C.Ph.T.
Pennsylvania Institute of Technology

Marcy May, M.Ed., C.Ph.T.
Virginia College at Austin

Michelle C. McCranie, C.Ph.T.
Ogeechee Technical College

Nancy L. Needham, M.Ed., C.Ph.T.
American Career College

Hieu T. Nguyen, M.Ed., B.S.
Western Career College

Jean A. Oldham, M.S., B.S., A.B.D. for E.D.D.
St. Catharine College

Jason M. Pankey, C.Ph.T.
National College of Business & Technology

David R. Reiter, C.Ph.T.
Pueblo Community College

Patricia Rowe
Columbus State Community College

Philip Rushing, B.S.
Consultant

Pat Schommer, M.A., C.Ph.T.
National American University

Cardiece Sylvan
MedVance Institute of Baton Rouge

Janet E. Teeguarden
Ivy Tech Community College of Indiana

Joseph A. Tinervia, C.Ph.T., M.B.A.
Tulsa Community College and Tulsa Job Corps Pharmacy Technican

Lisa R. Thompson
MedVance Institute of Fort Lauderdale

Sandi Tschritter, B.A., C.Ph.T.
Spokane Community College

Pedro A. Valentin, C.Ph.T., B.B.A.
Columbus Technical College

Marvin L. Walker Jr., A.A.S.
Austin Community College

Marsha L. Wilson, M.A., B.S., M.Ed.
Clarian Health

Hwa H. Yeon, A.A.
Everest College

Susan K. Zolvinski, B.S., M.B.A.
Brown Mackie College

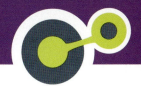

Visual Guide to Math for Pharmacy Technicians

Learning Outcomes and **Key Terms** at the beginning of each chapter introduce you to the chapter and prepare you for the information that will be presented.

PTCB Correlations list the content that will be covered in the chapter to help you prepare for the examination.

Critical Thinking in the Pharmacy introduces the chapter and improves your thinking skills. Discussion about these situations will prepare you to understand the content in the chapter.

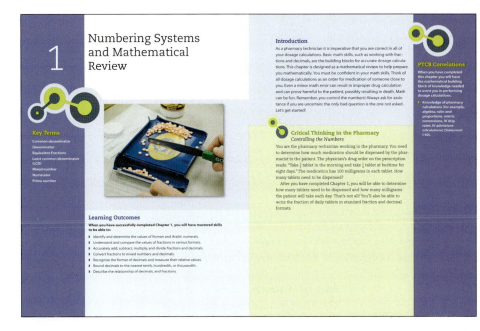

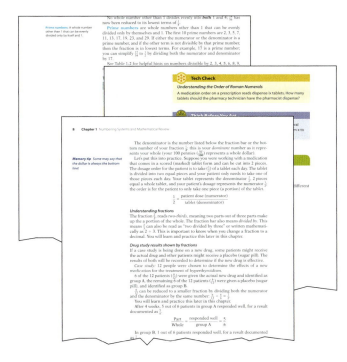

"*I especially like the breakdown and organizational features of the mathematical process. The steps followed on the table of contents are the building blocks of math. By following the table of contents chapter by chapter, the instructor can teach more constructively. This enables the student to more fully understand the process of building a foundation where math is concerned.*"

Christina Conklin, *Keiser University; A.A., R.M.A., C.D.E.*

Marginal key terms provide a quick definition of the important words that you should be familiar with throughout each chapter.

Tech Check boxes are exercises that help you *check* your understanding of the content that was just presented.

Memory Tips provide a novel technique to help you remember key information.

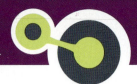

Tables within each chapter summarize important information for you.

Up-to-date full color medication labels provide the real-world connection to labels that you will see on the job.

Caution boxes draw your attention to possible mistakes that can occur within the pharmacy practice.

"The language is such that a student can read and understand. The generous use of tables, charts, prescription examples, and the very thorough practical exercises make this book very useful. Wish I had it in my class right now!"

Michael M. Hayter, *Pharm. D., M.B.A., Virginia Highlands Community College*

Super Tech CD-ROM references direct you to CD exercises to help reinforce the concepts just learned.

Review and Practice follows each major section, giving you the opportunity to apply new concepts.

Pocket conversion cards provide a handy reference to use while working as a pharmacy technician.

Chapter review reinforces the chapter outcomes to help you retain what was just learned.

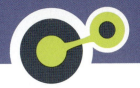

The following test covers basic mathematical concepts that you will need to understand and calculate dosages. This test will help you determine which concepts you need to review before continuing. You should already be able to perform basic operations—addition, subtraction, multiplication, and division— with whole numbers. The test covers fractions, decimals, percents, ratios, and proportions.

Take 90 minutes to answer the following 50 questions.

1. Convert $\frac{14}{3}$ to a mixed number.

2. Convert $3\frac{7}{8}$ to a fraction.

Find the missing numerator in the following equations.

3. $\frac{2}{7} = \frac{?}{21}$

4. $1\frac{1}{8} = \frac{?}{16}$

5. Reduce $\frac{40}{100}$ to lowest terms.

6. Which fraction has the greater value, $\frac{3}{8}$ or $\frac{2}{6}$?

Calculate the following. Reduce fractions to lowest terms and rewrite any fractions as mixed numbers.

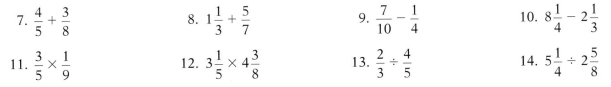

7. $\frac{4}{5} + \frac{3}{8}$

8. $1\frac{1}{3} + \frac{5}{7}$

9. $\frac{7}{10} - \frac{1}{4}$

10. $8\frac{1}{4} - 2\frac{1}{3}$

11. $\frac{3}{5} \times \frac{1}{9}$

12. $3\frac{1}{5} \times 4\frac{3}{8}$

13. $\frac{2}{3} \div \frac{4}{5}$

14. $5\frac{1}{4} \div 2\frac{5}{8}$

15. Which number has the lesser value, 1.01 or 1.009?

16. Round 14.42 to the nearest whole number.

17. Round 6.05 to the nearest tenth.

18. Round 19.197 to the nearest hundredth.

19. Convert $3\frac{4}{5}$ to a decimal number. If necessary, round to the nearest hundredth.

20. Convert 0.045 to a fraction or a mixed number. Reduce to lowest terms.

Calculate the following.

21. 7.289 + 8.011

22. 0.012 + 0.9 + 4.2

23. 19.1 − 4.4

24. 100.03 − 0.6

25. 0.07 × 3.2

26. 0.4 ÷ 0.02

27. Convert 0.8 percent to a decimal number.

28. Convert 0.99 to a percent.

29. Convert 260 percent to a fraction or mixed number.

30. Convert $1\frac{1}{8}$ to a percent.

31. Convert $7:12$ to a fraction.

32. Convert $\frac{10}{50}$ to a ratio. Reduce to lowest terms.

33. Convert $1:12$ to a decimal. Round to the nearest hundredth, if necessary.

34. Convert 0.4 to a ratio. Reduce to lowest terms.

35. Convert $3:8$ to a percent. Round to the nearest percent, if necessary.

36. Convert 0.5 percent to a ratio. Reduce to lowest terms.

Find the missing value in the following proportions.

37. $8:16::?:8$ 38. $\frac{5}{9} = \frac{?}{27}$ 39. $8:12::?:9$ 40. $\frac{2}{7} = \frac{?}{28}$

41. The prescription reads to take $1\frac{1}{2}$ teaspoons of cough syrup 4 times a day. How many teaspoons of cough syrup will the patient take each day?

42. A pharmacy technician tries to keep the equivalent of 12 bottles of a medication on hand. The hospital's first floor has $1\frac{1}{2}$ bottles, the second floor has $1\frac{3}{4}$ bottles, the third floor has $3\frac{1}{4}$ bottles, and the supply closet has 3 bottles. Is there enough medication on hand? If not, how much should the technician order?

43. A bottle contains 75 milliliters (mL) of a liquid medication. Since the bottle was opened, one patient has received 3 doses of 2.5 mL. A second patient has received 4 doses of 2.2 mL. How much medication remains in the bottle?

44. A tablet contains 0.125 milligram (mg) of medication. A patient receives 3 tablets a day for 5 days. How many milligrams of medication does the patient receive over the 5 days?

45. An IV bag contained 1000 mL of a liquid. The liquid was administered to a patient, and now there is 400 mL left in the bag after 3 hours. How much IV fluid did the patient receive each hour?

46. The patient is taking 0.5 mg of medication 4 times a day. How many milligrams would the patient receive after $1\frac{1}{2}$ days?

47. The patient took 0.88 microgram (mcg) every morning and 1.2 mcg each evening for 4 days. What was the total amount of medication taken?

48. Write a ratio that represents that 500 mL of solution contains 5 mg of drug.

49. Write a ratio that represents that every tablet in a bottle contains 25 mg of drug.

50. Write a ratio that represents that 3 mL of solution contains 125 mg of drug.

1

Numbering Systems and Mathematical Review

Key Terms

Common denominator

Denominator

Equivalent Fractions

Least common denominator (LCD)

Mixed number

Numerator

Prime number

Learning Outcomes

When you have successfully completed Chapter 1, you will have mastered skills to be able to:

- Identify and determine the values of Roman and Arabic numerals.
- Understand and compare the values of fractions in various formats.
- Accurately add, subtract, multiply, and divide fractions and decimals.
- Convert fractions to mixed numbers and decimals.
- Recognize the format of decimals and measure their relative values.
- Round decimals to the nearest tenth, hundredth, or thousandth.
- Describe the relationship of decimals, and fractions.

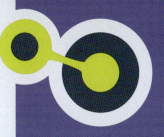

Introduction

As a pharmacy technician it is imperative that you are correct in all of your dosage calculations. Basic math skills, such as working with fractions and decimals, are the building blocks for accurate dosage calculations. This chapter is designed as a mathematical review to help prepare you mathematically. You must be confident in your math skills. Think of all dosage calculations as an order for medication of someone close to you. Even a minor math error can result in improper drug calculation and can prove harmful to the patient, possibly resulting in death. Math can be fun. Remember, you control the numbers! Always ask for assistance if you are uncertain; the only bad question is the one not asked. Let's get started!

Critical Thinking in the Pharmacy
Controlling the Numbers

You are the pharmacy technician working in the pharmacy. You need to determine how much medication should be dispensed by the pharmacist to the patient. The physician's drug order on the prescription reads: "Take $\frac{1}{2}$ tablet in the morning and take $\frac{1}{4}$ tablet at bedtime for eight days." The medication has 100 milligrams in each tablet. How many tablets need to be dispensed?

After you have completed Chapter 1, you will be able to determine how many tablets need to be dispensed and how many milligrams the patient will take each day. That's not all! You'll also be able to write the fraction of daily tablets in standard fraction and decimal formats.

PTCB Correlations

When you have completed this chapter you will have the mathematical building block of knowledge needed to assist you in performing dosage calculations.

▶ Knowledge of pharmacy calculations (for example, algebra, ratio and proportions, metric conversions, IV drip rates, IV admixture calculations) (Statement I-50).

Arabic Numbers and Roman Numerals

Arabic Numbers

Arabic numbers include all numbers used today. Numbers are written using the 10 digits of 0, 1, 2, 3, 4, 5, 6, 7, 8, and 9. You can write any number such as whole numbers, decimals, and fractions by simply combining digits.

EXAMPLE ▶ The Arabic digits 2 and 5 are combined to write different numbers such as the whole number 25, the decimal 2.5, and the fraction $\frac{2}{5}$.

Note that the same two digits are used in each of the above Arabic numbers; however, they have different values.

Let's compare it to the value of a dollar. The whole number 25 is the same as the value of $25.00. The decimal 2.5 is the same as the value of $2.50 and the fraction $\frac{2}{5}$ has the value of 0.40 cents. This is why it is so important that, as a pharmacy technician, you calculate all dosages correctly. You will learn how to work with all of these values in this chapter.

Roman Numerals

Roman numerals are still sometimes used in drug orders, including prescriptions and physician's drug orders. You should know how to identify the value of Roman numerals and convert them to Arabic numbers to perform dosage calculations.

In the Roman numeral system, letters are used to represent numbers.

Roman numerals can be written in either uppercase or lowercase letters or symbols. If lowercase letters are used, it is common practice to write a line above the lowercase letters.

EXAMPLE ▶ The number "one" can be written as an uppercase I, a lowercase i, or a lowercase ī with a line placed over the i and under the dot of the i̇.

$$1 = \text{I, i, and i̇}$$

The Roman numerals from 1 to 30 are the ones you are most likely to see in physicians' orders. Let's look at the most commonly used Roman numerals on prescription orders.

ss = the value of 1/2	I = the value of 1
V = the value of 5	X = the value of 10

Table 1-1 lists the most commonly used Roman numerals in physicians' orders from numbers 1 to 30 and shows the conversion to Arabic numbers.

Table 1-1   Converting Roman Numerals

Roman Numeral*	Arabic Number	Roman Numeral	Arabic Number	Roman Numeral	Arabic Number
SS, $\overline{ss}$	$\frac{1}{2}$				
I, i	1	XI, xi	11	XXI, xxi	21
II, ii	2	XII, xii	12	XXII, xxii	22
III, iii	3	XIII, xiii	13	XXIII, xxiii	23
IV, iv	4	XIV, xiv	14	XXIV, xxiv	24
V, v	5	XV, xv	15	XXV, xxv	25
VI, vi	6	XVI, xvi	16	XXVI, xxvi	26
VII, vii	7	XVII, xvii	17	XXVII, xxvii	27
VIII, viii	8	XVIII, xviii	18	XXVIII, xxviii	28
IX, ix	9	XIX, xix	19	XXIX, xxix	29
X, x	10	XX, xx	20	XXX, xxx	30

*Roman numerals written with small letters are also correctly written with a line over the top; for example, iv and $\overline{iv}$ are both correct.

Combining Roman Numerals

There are more Roman numerals than I, V, and X. You need to learn how to combine the letters of the Roman numeral system and then convert them to Arabic numbers. Recall how Arabic digits are combined to the write numbers. Roman numerals are written by combining the letters that indicate the appropriate number value.

Once you have written the Roman numeral correctly you can then convert it to an Arabic number.

When you read a Roman numeral containing more than one letter, always read left to right and follow these three simple rules:

1. If any letter with a smaller value is written to the **left** of a letter with a larger value, subtract the smaller value (left) from the larger value (right).

Memory tip Left is less

IV is the same as 5 − 1

2. If the letter value to the left is equal to or greater than the number on the right, add values of the letters.

XV is the same as 10 + 5

3. If you have three or more letters and one is between two letters of higher value, subtract the smaller value from the letter to its right, then add the number to the left.

XIV is the same 10 + 5 − 1 = 14

EXAMPLE 1 ▶
   a. IX = 10 − 1 = 9
   b. iv = 5 − 1 = 4
   c. xix = 10 + (10 − 1) = 19

EXAMPLE 2 ▶
   a. XV = 10 + 5 = 15
   b. VII = 5 + 1 + 1 = 7
   c. xxv = 10 + 10 + 5 = 25

EXAMPLE 3 ▶
   a. XIV = 10 + (5 − 1) = 14
   b. ixss = 10 − 1 + $\frac{1}{2}$ = 9$\frac{1}{2}$
   c. xiii = 10 + 3 = 13

Super Tech . . .

Open the CD-ROM that accompanies your textbook and select Chapter 1, Exercise 1-1. Review the animation and example problems, and then complete the practice problems.

Tech Check

Understanding the Order of Roman Numerals

A medication order on a prescription reads dispense ix tablets. How many tablets should the pharmacy technician have the pharmacist dispense?

Think Before You Act

The numeral with the smaller value is written to the left of the numeral with the larger value. The pharmacy technician should subtract i from x to calculate the correct number of 9 tablets to dispense.

✓ Review and Practice 1-1 Arabic Numbers and Roman Numerals

Practice Writing Numbers Using Arabic Digits

Write a whole number, a decimal, and fraction for each of the combinations of digits.
(Reminder: the same two digits are used in each of the Arabic numbers, however they will have different values).

1. Digits 1 and 7:

   Whole number _____   Decimal _____   Fraction _____

2. Digits 3 and 5:

   Whole number _____   Decimal _____   Fraction _____

3. Digits 2 and 3:

   Whole number _____   Decimal _____   Fraction _____

4. Digits 5 and 6:

Whole number _____   Decimal _____   Fraction _____

Convert the following Roman numerals to Arabic numbers.

5. VI = _____   11. vss = _____

6. XII = _____   12. ixss = _____

7. IX = _____   13. xiss = _____

8. XIV = _____   14. xxv = _____

9. xxiv = _____   15. xix = _____

10. xviii = _____   16. viiiss = _____

Write the answers to the following exercises as Arabic numbers.

17. IV + XVII _____   21. XXIII − VII _____

18. xii + xiv _____   22. xvi − ix _____

19. VIII + III _____   23. XXI − III _____

20. V + V _____   24. XXX − V _____

Fractions and Mixed Numbers

Fractions measure a portion or part of a whole number. They are written as common fractions or as decimals. As a pharmacy technician, you must often convert from one type of fraction to another.

Common Fractions

A common fraction represents the parts of a whole, and has a numerator that is less than the denominator. This is also referred to as a proper fraction. It consists of two numbers separated by a fraction bar, and is written in the following format.

$$\frac{1}{2}$$

Numerator: The number on the top of the fraction bar; represents parts of the whole.

Denominator: The number listed below the fraction bar or the bottom number of your fraction; represents the whole.

The **numerator** is top number in a fraction and represents part of the whole. The **denominator** is the bottom number in a fraction and represents the whole.

$$\frac{\text{Numerator} \rightarrow 1}{\text{Denominator} \rightarrow 2}$$

EXAMPLE ▶

When you have a whole dollar, it is worth 100 pennies, but in the fraction of $\frac{50}{100}$ which is worth 50 pennies, you only have a half ($\frac{1}{2}$) of a dollar.

Let's break it down into all the elements of the mathematical properties. The numerator is the number on the top of the fraction bar $\frac{1}{2}$.

The numerator represents only a **portion or part** of the whole (remember in the example of $\frac{50}{100}$ you only have 50 pennies, or a half ($\frac{1}{2}$) of a dollar).

The denominator is the number listed below the fraction bar or the bottom number of your fraction $\frac{1}{2}$; this is your *dominant* number as it represents your whole (your 100 pennies ($\frac{50}{100}$) represents a whole dollar).

Let's put this into practice. Suppose you were working with a medication that comes in a scored (marked) tablet form and can be cut into 2 pieces. The dosage order for the patient is to take ($\frac{1}{2}$) of a tablet each day. The tablet is divided into two equal pieces and your patient only needs to take one of those pieces each day. Your tablet represents the denominator $\frac{1}{2}$, 2 pieces equal a whole tablet, and your patient's dosage represents the numerator $\frac{1}{2}$; the order is for the patient to only take one piece (a portion) of the tablet.

$$\frac{1}{2} = \frac{\text{patient dose (numerator)}}{\text{tablet (denominator)}}$$

Understanding fractions

The fraction $\frac{2}{3}$, reads *two-thirds,* meaning two parts out of three parts make up the a portion of the whole. The fraction bar also means *divided by*. This means $\frac{2}{3}$ can also be read as "two divided by three" or written mathematically as $2 \div 3$. This is important to know when you change a fraction to a decimal. You will learn and practice this later in this chapter.

Drug study results shown by fractions

If a case study is being done on a new drug, some patients might receive the actual drug and other patients might receive a placebo (sugar pill). The results of both will be recorded to determine if the new drug is effective.

Case study: 12 people were chosen to determine the effects of a new medication for the treatment of hyperthyroidism.

6 of the 12 patients ($\frac{6}{12}$) were given the actual new drug and identified as group A, the remaining 6 of the 12 patients ($\frac{6}{12}$) were given a placebo (sugar pill), and identified as group B.

$\frac{6}{12}$ can be reduced to a smaller fraction by dividing both the numerator and the denominator by the same number: $\frac{6}{12} \div \frac{6}{6} = \frac{1}{2}$.

You will learn and practice this later in this chapter.

After 4 weeks, 5 out of 6 patients in group A responded well, for a result documented as $\frac{5}{6}$.

$$\frac{\text{Part}}{\text{Whole}} = \frac{\text{responded well}}{\text{group A}} = \frac{5}{6}$$

In group B, 1 out of 6 patients responded well, for a result documented as $\frac{1}{6}$.

$$\frac{\text{Part}}{\text{Whole}} = \frac{\text{responded well}}{\text{group B}} = \frac{1}{6}$$

Rules used in fractions

When the denominator is 1, the fraction will always equal the numerator because any number divided by 1 yields the number itself.

EXAMPLE ▶ $\frac{4}{1} = 4$ $\frac{100}{1} = 100$

Check these equations by writing each fraction as a division problem.

$$4 \div 1 = 4 \qquad 100 \div 1 = 100$$

Practice

Solve the following fractions by writing them as division problems.

1. $\frac{6}{1}$ _____.

2. $\frac{200}{1}$ _____.

3. $\frac{45}{1}$ _____.

4. $\frac{72}{1}$ _____.

1. When the numerator of the fraction is less than the denominator, the fraction has a value less than (<) 1

EXAMPLE ▶ The fraction $\frac{8}{9}$ is less than 1 because the numerator (8) is less than the denominator (9). This can be written $\frac{8}{9} < 1$

2. When the numerator of the fraction is the same as (equals) the denominator, the fraction is equal to (=) 1

EXAMPLE ▶ $\frac{12}{12}$ is equal to 1 because the numerator (12) is the same as (equal to) the denominator (12). This can be written as $\frac{12}{12} = 1$

3. When the numerator of the fraction is greater than the denominator, the fraction has a value greater than (>) 1. Fractions with a value greater than 1 are also called improper fractions and can be written as a mixed number.

EXAMPLE ▶ $\frac{8}{5}$ is greater than 1 because the numerator (8) is greater than the denominator (5). This can be written $\frac{8}{5} > 1$

Memory tip *When you use the symbols for less than (<) or greater than (>), the symbols always point to the smaller number.*

Practice

Write the proper symbol (<, >, or =) to show the true value for each statement.

1. $\frac{3}{4}$ _____ 1

2. $\frac{9}{7}$ _____ 1

3. $\frac{6}{6}$ _____ 1

4. $\frac{11}{4}$ _____ 1

5. $\frac{3}{1}$ _____ 1

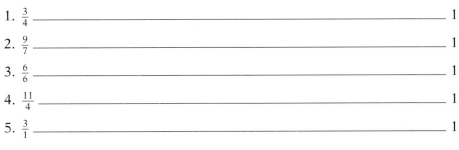

Super Tech . . .

Open the CD-ROM that accompanies your textbook and select Chapter 1, Exercise 1-2. Review the animation and example problems and then complete the practice problems.

Mixed Numbers

Mixed Number: A fraction that is greater than 1 and written as a whole number and a fraction.

Fractions with a value greater than 1 can be written as a mixed number. A **mixed number** is a fraction that is greater than one and written as a whole number and a fraction. Examples include $2\frac{2}{3}$ (two and two-thirds), $1\frac{7}{8}$ (one and seven-eighths), and $12\frac{31}{32}$ (twelve and thirty-one thirty-seconds). When the numerator is greater than the denominator the fraction can be converted to a mixed number. The fraction $\frac{11}{4}$ is more properly written as the mixed number $2\frac{3}{4}$.

To convert the fraction $\frac{11}{4}$ to a mixed number, simply divide the numerator by the denominator, the result will be a whole number plus a remainder.

$$11 \div 4 = 2\frac{3}{4}$$

$$11 \div 4 = 2 \text{ with a remainder of } 3$$

In a nonfractional equation, the remainder is written as R3.

EXAMPLE ▶ $11 \div 4 = 2 \text{ R3}$

In a fractional equation the remainder is written as the numerator over the original denominator.

EXAMPLE ▶ $\dfrac{\text{Remainder}}{\text{Denominator}} = \dfrac{3}{4}$

Combine the whole number and the fractional remainder. This mixed number equals the original fraction.

EXAMPLE ▶ $2 + \dfrac{3}{4} = 2\dfrac{3}{4}$

The mixed number $2\frac{3}{4}$ equals the original fraction $\frac{11}{4}$.

You can check your work by multiplying your denominator by 2 then adding your numerator. Write the answer over your original denominator of 4.

2×4 (original denominator) $= 8$, $8 + 3$ (remainder numerator) $= 11$; write the answer over the original denominator: $\frac{11}{4}$.

Practice
Convert the following fractions to mixed numbers:

1. $\frac{27}{12} =$ _____

2. $\frac{5}{4} =$ _____

3. $\frac{90}{60} =$ _____

4. $\frac{7}{3} =$ _____

5. $\frac{12}{6} =$ _____

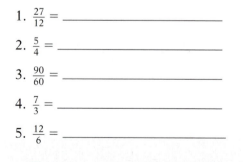

Super Tech . . .

Open the CD-ROM that accompanies your textbook and select Chapter 1, Exercise 1-3. Review the animation and example problems, and then complete the practice problems.

You can also convert a mixed number to an improper fraction. This is often necessary before you use a number in a calculation; $10\frac{7}{8}$ converts to $\frac{87}{8}$ (eighty seven-eighths).

Math terms used in converting mixed number to fractions are product, quotient, sum, and difference.

A product is the answer to a multiplication problem.
A quotient is the answer to a division problem.
A sum is the answer to an addition problem.
The difference is the answer to a subtraction problem.

To convert the **mixed number** $10\frac{7}{8}$ to an improper fraction:

$$10 \text{ (whole number)} + \frac{7 \text{ (numerator)}}{8 \text{ (denominator)}} = \frac{87}{8}$$

10 is the whole number, 7 is the numerator, and 8 is the denominator.

1. Multiply the whole number by the denominator in the fraction.

$$10 \times 8 \text{ (denominator)} = 80 \text{ (product)}$$

2. Add the product from step one to the numerator of the fraction.

$$80 + 7 \text{ (numerator)} = 87 \text{ (sum)}$$

3. Write the sum from step 2 over the original denominator.

$$\frac{87}{8} \text{ (original denominator)}$$

Practice
Convert the following mixed numbers to improper fractions:

1. $5\frac{1}{3} = $ _____

2. $8\frac{3}{5} = $ _____

3. $\frac{94}{9} = $ _____

4. $10\frac{2}{3} = $ _____

5. $1\frac{1}{2} = $ _____

Super Tech . . .

Open the CD-ROM that accompanies your textbook and select Chapter 1, Exercise 1-4. Review the animation and example problems, and then complete the practice problems.

Review and Practice 1-2 Fractions and Mixed Numbers

1. What is the numerator in $\frac{17}{100}$?

2. Circle the numerator in $\frac{8}{3}$.

3. Circle the denominator in $\frac{4}{100}$.

4. Circle the denominator in $\frac{60}{1}$.

5. Write this expression as a fraction: $3 \div 16$

6. Write this expression as a fraction: $4 \div 15$

7. Write this expression as a fraction: $3 \div 4$

8. Insert $<$, $>$, or $=$ to make a true statement, where $<$ means less than, $>$ means greater than, and $=$ means equal to.

   a. $\frac{14}{14}$ 1   b. $\frac{24}{32}$ 1   c. $\frac{125}{100}$ 1

Convert the following fractions to mixed or whole numbers.

9. $\dfrac{43}{6}$ 10. $\dfrac{17}{3}$ 11. $\dfrac{100}{20}$ 12. $\dfrac{8}{5}$

Convert the following mixed numbers to improper fractions.

13. $2\dfrac{6}{7}$ 14. $8\dfrac{8}{9}$ 15. $1\dfrac{1}{10}$ 16. $4\dfrac{1}{8}$

Reducing Fractions to Lowest Terms

Reduced fractions are easier to use when you are performing a calculation. It is considered proper form to write your final answer in a fraction that is reduced to its lowest terms. To reduce a fraction to its lowest terms, find the largest whole number that divides evenly into both the numerator and the denominator. When no whole number except 1 divides evenly into them, the fraction is reduced to its lowest terms.

EXAMPLE 1 ▶ Reduce $\frac{2}{4}$ to its lowest terms.

Both 2 and 4 are divisible by 2

$$\frac{2 \div 2}{4 \div 2} = \frac{1}{2}$$

No whole number other than 1 divides evenly into ***both*** 1 and 2; $\frac{2}{4}$ has now been reduced to its lowest terms of $\frac{1}{2}$.

EXAMPLE 2 ▶ Reduce $\frac{15}{20}$ to its lowest terms.

Both 15 and 20 are divisible by 5

$$\frac{15 \div 5}{20 \div 5} = \frac{3}{4}$$

No whole number other than 1 divides evenly into ***both*** 3 and 4; $\frac{15}{20}$ has now been reduced to its lowest terms of $\frac{3}{4}$.

> ⚠️ **Caution!**
>
> It is extremely important to be certain you have reduced your fraction to absolute lowest terms; you may actually have to reduce some fractions more than once. Remember a fraction is reduced to its lowest terms only when both the numerator and denominator can not be evenly divided by any number except the number 1.

EXAMPLE ▶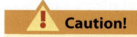

To reduce this, since both numbers are even numbers, you can divide by 2

$$\frac{14 \div 2}{56 \div 2} = \frac{7}{28}$$

This is a reduced fraction, but it is not in its lowest terms.
Both 7 and 28 can be divided again by the number 7

$$\frac{7 \div 7}{28 \div 7} = \frac{1}{4}$$

No whole number other than 1 divides evenly into **both** 1 and 4; $\frac{14}{56}$ has now been reduced to its lowest terms of $\frac{1}{4}$.

Prime numbers are whole numbers other than 1 that can be evenly divided only by themselves and 1. The first 10 prime numbers are 2, 3, 5, 7, 11, 13, 17, 19, 23, and 29. If either the numerator or the denominator is a prime number, and if the other term is not divisible by that prime number, then the fraction is in lowest terms. For example, 17 is a prime number; you can simplify $\frac{17}{34}$ to $\frac{1}{2}$ by dividing both the numerator and denominator by 17.

See Table 1-2 for helpful hints on numbers divisible by 2, 3, 4, 5, 6, 8, 9, or 10.

Prime numbers: A whole number other than 1 that can be evenly divided only by itself and 1.

Table 1-2   Is a Number Divisible by 2, 3, 4, 5, 6, 8, 9, or 10?

Number	Hint	Example
2	Even numbers (numbers ending with 2, 4, 6, 8, or 0) are divisible by 2.	112; 734; 2936; 10,118; 356, 920
3	If the sum of the digits of a number is divisible by 3, then the number is divisible by 3.	37,887 The sum of the digits is 3 + 7 + 8 + 8 + 7 = 33. 33 is divisible by 3.
4	If the last two digits of a number are divisible by 4, the entire number is divisible by 4.	126,936 The last two digits form a number, 36, that is divisible by 4.
5	Any number that ends with 5 or 0 is divisible by 5.	735 12,290
6	Combine the rules for 2 and 3. If a number is even *and* the sum of its digits is divisible by 3, then the number is divisible by 6.	582 The number is even. The sum of its digits, 5 + 8 + 2 = 15, is divisible by 3.
8	If the last three digits are divisible by 8, then the entire number is divisible by 8.	42,376 Here, 376 is divisible by 8.
9	If the sum of the digits is a multiple of 9, the number is divisible by 9.	42,705 4 + 2 + 7 + 0 + 5 = 18, which is divisible by 9.
10	If a number ends with 0, then the number is divisible by 10.	640

Super Tech . . .

Open the CD-ROM that accompanies your textbook and select Chapter 1, Exercise 1-5. Review the animation and example problems, and then complete the practice problems.

✓ Review and Practice 1-3 Reducing Fractions to Lowest Terms

Reduce the following fractions to their lowest terms.

1. $\dfrac{10}{12}$

2. $\dfrac{3}{6}$

3. $\dfrac{27}{81}$

4. $\dfrac{11}{22}$

5. $\dfrac{10}{100}$

6. $\dfrac{55}{100}$

7. $\dfrac{4}{5}$

8. $\dfrac{6}{17}$

9. $\dfrac{21}{27}$

10. $\dfrac{35}{50}$

Equivalent Fractions

Equivalent fractions: Two fractions written differently that have the same value.

Two fractions written differently that have the same value are known as **equivalent fractions.** Suppose you and a friend are sharing a pizza equally, dividing it in half. (See Figure 1-1) If you cut the pizza into eight slices, you will each get four pieces, or $\frac{4}{8}$ of the whole pizza.

If you cut the pizza into six slices, you will each get three pieces, or $\frac{3}{6}$ And if you cut the pizza into four slices, you will each get two slices, or $\frac{2}{4}$ Whether you get $\frac{4}{8}$, $\frac{3}{6}$, or $\frac{2}{4}$ of the pizza, you still have the same amount: one-half or $\frac{1}{2}$ of the pizza.

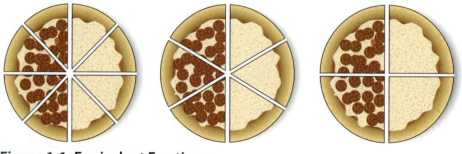

Figure 1-1 Equivalent Fractions

These four fractions are equivalent fractions $\frac{1}{2}$, $\frac{2}{4}$, $\frac{3}{6}$, and $\frac{4}{8}$.

To find an equivalent fraction, multiply or divide both the numerator and denominator by the same number. *Exception:* The numerator and denominator cannot be multiplied or divided by zero.

EXAMPLE 1 ▶   Find equivalent fractions for $\frac{2}{4}$.

$$\frac{2 \times 2}{4 \times 2} = \frac{4}{8} \qquad \frac{2 \times 3}{4 \times 3} = \frac{6}{12} \qquad \frac{2 \div 2}{4 \div 2} = \frac{1}{2} \qquad \frac{2 \times 10}{4 \times 10} = \frac{20}{40}$$

Thus, $\frac{2}{4} = \frac{4}{8} = \frac{6}{12} = \frac{1}{2} = \frac{20}{40}$. These are equivalent fractions.

EXAMPLE 2 ▶ Find equivalent fractions for 4.

To find equivalent fractions for a whole number, first write the whole number as a fraction.

Then proceed as before.

$$4 = \frac{4}{1}$$

$$\frac{4 \times 2}{1 \times 2} = \frac{8}{2} \qquad \frac{4 \times 3}{1 \times 3} = \frac{12}{3} \qquad \frac{4 \times 4}{1 \times 4} = \frac{16}{4} \qquad \frac{4 \times 5}{1 \times 5} = \frac{20}{5}$$

Thus, $4 = \frac{4}{1} = \frac{8}{2} = \frac{12}{3} = \frac{16}{4} = \frac{20}{5}$. These are equivalent fractions.

EXAMPLE 3 ▶ Find some equivalent fractions for $1\frac{4}{6}$.

To find equivalent fractions for a mixed number, first convert the mixed number to an improper fraction.

1. $1 \times 6 = 6$
2. $6 + 4 = 10$
3. $1\frac{4}{6} = \frac{10}{6}$

Now follow the same steps as in examples 1 and 2

$$\frac{10 \times 2}{6 \times 2} = \frac{20}{12} \qquad \frac{10 \times 3}{6 \times 3} = \frac{30}{18} \qquad \frac{10 \div 2}{6 \div 2} = \frac{5}{3} \qquad \frac{10 \times 10}{6 \times 10} = \frac{100}{60}$$

Thus, $1\frac{4}{6} = \frac{10}{6} = \frac{30}{18} = \frac{5}{3} = \frac{100}{60}$. These are some equivalent fractions.

Super Tech . . .

Open the CD-ROM that accompanies your textbook and select Chapter 1, Exercise 1-6. Review the animation and example problems, and then complete the practice problems.

Finding Common Denominators

Common denominator: Any number that is a common multiple of all the denominators in the fractions of your expression.

Least common denominator (LCD): This is the smallest number that is a common multiple of the denominators in a group of fractions.

Before you can add and subtract fractions with different denominators, you must first convert them to equivalent fractions with a common denominator. A **common denominator** is any number that is a common multiple of all the denominators in the fractions of your expression.

The **least common denominator (LCD)** is the smallest number that is a common multiple of the denominators in a group of fractions. You will use your recently acquired skills of finding the missing numerator once you find the least common denominator. First list the multiples of each denominator and compare the lists. The smallest number that appears on all the lists is the LCD. Once you have found the LCD, you can convert each fraction to an equivalent fraction with the LCD as the denominator.

See, you really do control the numbers; let's get started!

EXAMPLE 1 ▶ Find the least common denominator of $\frac{1}{3}$ and $\frac{1}{2}$.

1. The number 3 divides evenly into 3, **6**, 9, **12**, 15, **18**, and 21
   The number 2 divides evenly into 2, 4, **6**, 8, 10, **12**, 14, 16, and **18**
2. The numbers 6, 12, and 18 are common denominators.
3. The smallest number that appears on both lists is 6. It is the least common denominator. It is divisible by both 3 and 2.

Now convert $\frac{1}{3}$ and $\frac{1}{2}$ to equivalent fractions so that $\frac{1}{3} = \frac{?}{6}$, and $\frac{1}{2} = \frac{?}{6}$
After you determine what your least common denominator is, you need to find the missing numerator, and then convert to equivalent fractions!

4. To convert $\frac{1}{3}$ to the equivalent fraction $\frac{?}{6}$:
   a. $6 \div 3 = 2$
   b. $\frac{1}{3} = \frac{1 \times 2}{3 \times 2} = \frac{2}{6}$ and ? (*missing numerator*) = 2
   The equivalent fractions are $\frac{1}{3} = \frac{?}{6}$
5. To convert $\frac{1}{2}$ to the equivalent fraction $\frac{?}{6}$:
   a. $6 \div 2 = 3$
   b. $\frac{1}{2} = \frac{1 \times 3}{2 \times 3} = \frac{3}{6}$ and ? (*missing numerator*) = 3
   The equivalent fractions are $\frac{1}{2} = \frac{3}{6}$.

To "sum" things up, you have now found your LCD and converted your original fractions to equivalent fraction and can now add them in a fractional equation.

$$\frac{1}{3} + \frac{1}{2} = \frac{2}{6} + \frac{3}{6} = \frac{5}{6} \text{ (this is your "sum")}$$

You will learn how to add and subtract fractions in the next section.

EXAMPLE 2 ▶ Find the least common denominator of $\frac{1}{4}$, $\frac{1}{6}$, and $\frac{1}{8}$ Then convert each to an equivalent fraction with the LCD.

1. The number 4 divides evenly into 4, 8, 12, 16, 20, and **24**
   The number 6 divides evenly into 6, 12, 18, and **24**
   The number 8 divides evenly into 8, 16, and **24**
2. The number 24 is a common denominator.
3. In this case, 24 is the LCD.
4. To convert $\frac{1}{4}$ to the equivalent fraction $\frac{6}{24}$.
   a. $24 \div 4 = 6$
   b. $\frac{1}{4} = \frac{1}{4} \times \frac{6}{6} = \frac{6}{24}$ and ? (*missing numerator*) = 6
   The equivalent fractions are $\frac{1}{4} = \frac{6}{24}$.
5. To convert $\frac{1}{6}$ to the equivalent fraction $\frac{?}{24}$.
   a. $24 \div 6 = 4$
   b. $\frac{1}{6} = \frac{1}{6} \times \frac{4}{4} = \frac{4}{24}$ and ? (*missing numerator*) = 4
   The equivalent fractions are $\frac{1}{6} = \frac{4}{24}$.

To find common denominators of fractions with large denominators, you simply multiply by the individual denominators to find the common denominator.

To convert fractions with large denominators to equivalent fractions with a common denominator:

1. List the denominators of all the fractions.
2. Multiply the denominators.
3. Convert to equivalent fractions.

EXAMPLE 1 ❯   Convert $\frac{1}{9}$ and $\frac{1}{17}$ to equivalent fractions with a common denominator.

1. The denominators are 9 and 17
2. Multiply 9×17. The common denominator is 153
3. $\frac{1}{9} = \frac{1}{9} \times \frac{17}{17} = \frac{17}{153}$ and $\frac{1}{17} = \frac{1}{17} \times \frac{9}{9} = \frac{9}{153}$

The equivalent fractions are $\frac{17}{153}$ and $\frac{9}{153}$.

Super Tech . . .

Open the CD-ROM that accompanies your textbook and select Chapter 1, Exercise 1-7. Review the animation and example problems, and then complete the practice problems.

✔ Review and Practice 1-4 Finding Common Denominators

For each set of fractions, find the least common denominator. Then convert each fraction to an equivalent fraction with the LCD.

1. $\frac{1}{3}$ and $\frac{1}{7}$

2. $\frac{1}{5}$ and $\frac{1}{8}$

3. $\frac{1}{25}$ and $\frac{1}{40}$

4. $\frac{1}{24}$ and $\frac{1}{36}$

5. $\frac{1}{2}$ and $\frac{1}{12}$

Adding Fractions

As a pharmacy technician you will have to calculate how much medication needs to be dispensed based on the physician's prescription or drug order. If the prescription reads: "Take 1/2 tablet with breakfast, and 1/4 tablet at bed time, for 10 days," you need to add the fractions of tablets together and then multiple the answer by 10 days to determine how many tablets the pharmacist needs to dispense to the patient. Remember, to add or subtract fractions you need to have a common denominator. Then simply add the numerators *only* and write the sum of the numerators over the common denominator.

$$\frac{1}{2} + \frac{1}{4} = \frac{1}{2} \times \frac{2}{2} + \frac{1}{4} = \frac{2}{4} + \frac{1}{4} = \frac{3}{4}$$

When you add a whole number and a fraction simply put them together and write the mixed number as your answer: $3 + \frac{1}{2} = 3\frac{1}{2}$ (sum).

Reminder: Answers should be written in the proper form. If the answer has a value greater than 1, convert it to a mixed number. Whenever possible reduce the fraction to lower terms.

EXAMPLE 1 ▶ Add $\frac{1}{4} + \frac{2}{4}$

1. The fractions already have a common denominator of 4
2. Add the numerators only: $\frac{1}{4} + \frac{2}{4} = \frac{1+2}{4} = \frac{3}{4}$
3. Write your numerator sum over the common denominator $\frac{3}{4}$. The answer is $\frac{3}{4}$ It is already in the proper form.

EXAMPLE 2 ▶ Add $3\frac{3}{4} + \frac{1}{2}$

1. Write fractions with common denominators of 4

$$3\frac{3}{4} + \frac{1}{2} = 3\frac{3}{4} + \left(\frac{1}{2} \times \frac{2}{2}\right) = 3\frac{3}{4} + \frac{2}{4}$$

2. Add the fractional parts and the whole parts.

$$3\frac{3}{4} + \frac{2}{4} = 3\frac{3+2}{4} = 3\frac{5}{4}$$

The answer is $3\frac{5}{4}$ The proper form for this answer is $4\frac{1}{4}$, because $5 \div 4 = \mathbf{1}$ with a remainder of 1 or $\frac{1}{4}$. Add $3 + 1\frac{1}{4} = 4\frac{1}{4}$.

Look at the math from start to finish:

$$3\frac{3}{4} + \left(\frac{1}{2} \times \frac{2}{2}\right) = 3\frac{3}{4} + \frac{2}{4} = 3\frac{3+2}{4} = 3\frac{5}{4} = 4\frac{1}{4}$$

Super Tech . . .

Open the CD-ROM that accompanies your textbook and select Chapter 1, Exercise 1-8. Review the animation and example problems, and then complete the practice problems.

✓ **Review and Practice 1-5** Adding Fractions

Find the following sums. (Rewrite answers in the proper form.)

1. $\frac{1}{8} + \frac{3}{8}$

2. $\frac{1}{7} + \frac{3}{7}$

3. $\frac{1}{7} + \frac{2}{14}$

4. $\frac{2}{5} + \frac{4}{15}$

5. $\frac{1}{6} + \frac{3}{8}$

6. $\frac{4}{10} + \frac{2}{25}$

7. $\frac{5}{8} + \frac{7}{12}$

8. $\frac{5}{6} + \frac{7}{9}$

9. $2 + \frac{4}{5}$

10. $\frac{8}{11} + 3$

Subtracting Fractions

The procedure for subtracting fractions is similar to the procedure for adding fractions. When you have fractions with the same denominators, you subtract the numerators rather than adding them. Subtract the numerators *only* and write the difference of the numerators over the common denominator.

Reminder: Answers should be reported in the proper form. If the answer has a value greater than 1, convert it to a mixed number. Whenever possible reduce the fraction to lower terms.

EXAMPLE 1 ▶   Subtract $\frac{6}{8} - \frac{3}{8}$.

    1. The fractions already have a common denominator of 8
    2. Subtract the numerators only: $6 - 1 = 5$ (difference).
    3. Write your numerator difference over the common denominator $\frac{5}{8}$
       The answer is $\frac{5}{8}$ It is already in the proper form.

EXAMPLE 2 ▶   Subtract $5 - 1\frac{1}{3}$.

    1. Rewrite any whole or mixed numbers as fractions.

$$5 \times \frac{1}{1} = \frac{5}{1} \qquad\qquad 1\frac{1}{3} = \frac{(1 \times 3) + 1}{3} = \frac{4}{3}$$

       The equation is now written $\frac{5}{1} - \frac{4}{3}$.

    2. Write the fractions with common denominators.

       To convert $\frac{5}{1}$ to the fraction $\frac{?}{3}$:

       a. $3 \div 1 = 3$
       b. $\frac{5}{1} = \frac{5}{1} \times \frac{3}{3} = \frac{15}{3}$

    3. Subtract the numerators only.

$$\frac{15}{3} - \frac{4}{3} = \frac{11}{3}$$

  The difference of the numerators is 11
  The answer is $\frac{11}{3}$.
  The proper form for the answer is $3\frac{2}{3}$, because $11 \div 3 = 9$ with a remainder of 2

Super Tech . . .

Open the CD-ROM that accompanies your textbook and select Chapter 1, Exercise 1-9. Review the animation and example problems, and then complete the practice problems.

✓ Review and Practice 1-6 Subtracting Fractions

Find the following differences.

1. $\dfrac{7}{15} - \dfrac{4}{15}$

2. $\dfrac{7}{25} - \dfrac{2}{25}$

3. $\dfrac{11}{3} - \dfrac{2}{6}$

4. $\dfrac{4}{7} - \dfrac{3}{21}$

5. $\dfrac{5}{6} - \dfrac{4}{9}$

6. $\dfrac{3}{4} - \dfrac{1}{6}$

7. $1\dfrac{7}{8} - \dfrac{1}{4}$

8. $2\dfrac{5}{8} - \dfrac{1}{2}$

9. $6\dfrac{1}{3} - \dfrac{5}{6}$

10. $4\dfrac{1}{2} - \dfrac{3}{4}$

Multiplying Fractions

Multiplying fractions is basic multiplication of the numerators and the denominators. You will multiply the numerators and denominators separately, then write the answers (products) as a new fraction. You will see that **both** multiplication and division are often used to work an equation. Remember when you solve a problem you always have to write the answer in its proper form and in lowest terms. To multiply fractions, you do not need to have a common denominator. To multiply fractions, you need to convert any mixed or whole numbers to improper fractions. Then multiply the numerators and multiply the denominators. Lastly, be sure to reduce the product to its lowest term.

EXAMPLE 1 ▶ Multiply $\frac{1}{6} \times \frac{3}{4}$.

1. There are no mixed or whole numbers.
2. Multiply the numerators $1 \times 3 = 3$; the product of the numerators is 3
3. Multiply the denominators $6 \times 4 = 24$; the product of the denominators is 24

$$\frac{1}{6} \times \frac{3}{4} = \frac{1 \times 3}{6 \times 4} = \frac{3}{24}$$

4. Reduce the product to lowest terms.
   $\frac{3}{24}$ can be reduced to $\frac{1}{8}$ by dividing the fraction by 3.

$$\frac{3}{24} \div \frac{3}{3} = \frac{1}{8}$$

EXAMPLE 2 ▶ Multiply $\frac{1}{2} \times \frac{7}{3} \times \frac{4}{9}$.

The only difference from Example 1 is that now you are multiplying three numerators and three denominators.

1. There are no mixed or whole numbers.
2. Multiply the numerators.
3. Multiply the denominators.

$$\frac{1}{2} \times \frac{7}{3} \times \frac{4}{9} = \frac{1 \times 7 \times 4}{2 \times 3 \times 9} = \frac{28}{54}$$

4. Reduce the product to its lowest terms.

$\frac{28}{54}$ can be reduced to $\frac{14}{27}$ by dividing the fraction by 2

EXAMPLE 3 ▶   Multiply $1\frac{4}{7} \times 2\frac{3}{5}$.

1. First convert the mixed numbers to improper fractions.

$$1\frac{4}{7} = \frac{11}{7} \quad \text{and} \quad 2\frac{3}{5} = \frac{13}{5}$$

2. Now multiply the numerators and denominators.

$$1\frac{4}{7} \times 2\frac{3}{5} = \frac{11}{7} \times \frac{13}{5} = \frac{11 \times 13}{7 \times 5} = \frac{143}{35}$$

3. $\frac{143}{35}$ converts to $4\frac{3}{35}$

Super Tech . . .

Open the CD-ROM that accompanies your textbook and select Chapter 1, Exercise 1-10. Review the animation and example problems, and then complete the practice problems.

Canceling Terms

Now that you know how to multiply fractions, let's look at a time- and error-saving method for multiplying fractions. Think of this as a shortcut that makes it easier to multiply fractions. It is called *canceling terms*.

Recall how to reduce a single fraction to its lowest terms. Canceling terms is the same principle and is used when you have a fractional multiplication problem with two or more fractions. Canceling terms helps to reduce your equation to smaller numbers, which makes it easier to solve and reduces potential mathematical errors.

To cancel terms you divide both a numerator and a denominator by the same number. You can cancel terms only if both a numerator and a denominator are evenly divisible by the same number.

The numerator and denominator can be either in the same fraction of the equation or in the numerator of one fraction and the denominator of another fraction. Remember they must be evenly divisible by the same number.

The following multiplication problem can be solved by the conventional method of fractional multiplication and also by canceling terms, then multiplying. You will work the problem both ways. Once you have mastered both methods, you will see that you really do control the numbers!

To multiply the equation $\frac{8}{21} \times \frac{7}{16}$ multiply the numerators and the denominators:

$$\frac{8 \times 7}{21 \times 16} = \frac{56}{336}$$

$\frac{56}{336}$ reduces to $\frac{1}{6}$ by dividing the denominator of 336 by the numerator of 56.

To cancel terms to solve $\frac{8}{21} \times \frac{7}{16}$ look for terms that are evenly divisible by the same number. You may cancel terms only if both a numerator and a denominator can be divided evenly.

Both the numerator 8 and the denominator 16 can be divided evenly by 8. You can now write the problem as $\frac{\overset{1}{\cancel{8}}}{21} \times \frac{7}{\underset{2}{\cancel{16}}}$ which is equivalent to $\frac{1}{21} \times \frac{7}{2}$.

The slash marks indicate that 8 and 16 were canceled. In this case, they were divided by 8, reducing 8 and 16 to 1 and 2, respectively. Both the numerator 7 and the denominator 21 are divisible by 7.

When you cancel again, you can rewrite the problem as $\frac{1}{\underset{3}{\cancel{21}}} \times \frac{\overset{1}{\cancel{7}}}{2}$, which is equivalent to $\frac{1}{3} \times \frac{1}{2}$.

Now when you solve, the answer will already be in lowest terms.

$$\frac{8}{21} \times \frac{7}{16} = \frac{1}{3} \times \frac{1}{2} = \frac{1}{6}$$

EXAMPLE ▶ $\frac{27}{36} \times \frac{4}{5}$

In this problem, one of the fractions has not been reduced to lowest terms. Both 27 and 36 are divisible by 9

$$\frac{\overset{3}{\cancel{27}}}{\underset{4}{\cancel{36}}} \times \frac{4}{5} \quad \text{becomes} \quad \frac{3}{4} \times \frac{4}{5}$$

You can also cancel 4 from the numerator 4 and what had begun as the denominator 36. The problem now becomes:

$$\frac{\overset{3}{\cancel{27}}}{\underset{4}{\cancel{36}}} \times \frac{4}{5} = \frac{3}{\underset{1}{\cancel{4}}} \times \frac{\overset{1}{\cancel{4}}}{5} = \frac{3}{1} \times \frac{1}{5} = \frac{3}{5}$$

The answer $\frac{3}{5}$ is already reduced to lowest terms.

If you are not sure what numbers will divide evenly into both the numerator and the denominator, review Table 1-2.

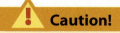

Super Tech . . .

Open the CD-ROM that accompanies your textbook and select Chapter 1, Exercise 1-11. Review the animation and example problems, and then complete the practice problems.

⚠ Caution!

You can cancel only one numerator for one denominator. In other words, you have to cancel evenly. You can not cancel one numerator and two denominators, even if two denominators are divisible by the same number. This is called a 1 to 1 ratio (1:1).

✓ Review and Practice 1-7 Multiplying Fractions

Find the following products. (Rewrite answers in the proper form.)

1. $\dfrac{1}{6} \times \dfrac{1}{8}$

2. $\dfrac{2}{7} \times \dfrac{3}{5}$

3. $\dfrac{1}{2} \times \dfrac{6}{8}$

4. $\dfrac{6}{9} \times \dfrac{1}{6}$

5. $\dfrac{3}{8} \times \dfrac{4}{9}$

6. $\dfrac{5}{12} \times \dfrac{6}{15}$

7. $\dfrac{10}{14} \times \dfrac{7}{5}$

8. $\dfrac{5}{7} \times \dfrac{3}{10} \times \dfrac{3}{4}$

9. $\dfrac{12}{25} \times \dfrac{8}{9} \times \dfrac{15}{16}$

10. $\dfrac{7}{16} \times \dfrac{4}{3} \times \dfrac{1}{2}$

Dividing Fractions

You have already learned most of the steps needed to divide fractions. In division problems you have new terms. The dividend is the number being divided. The divisor is the number that you are dividing by. The reciprocal of a fraction is the fraction inverted, the numerator becomes the denominator and vice versa. The quotient is your answer to the division. To divide, you multiply the dividend by the reciprocal of the divisor.

In pharmacy terms, the dividend = the drug stock container, the divisor = the drug order, the reciprocal = the divisor is inverted, which is, simply put, flipped upside down, and the quotient = your answer, or how much to dispense.

As a pharmacy technician you will be using division often to determine how many doses are in pill form, liquid medications, drops, creams, and lotions. Suppose you have $\frac{3}{4}$ bottle of liquid medication available in your stock container (dividend). The drug order is for $\frac{1}{16}$ bottle (divisor).

You want to know how many doses remain in the bottle. You solve this problem by dividing the fraction representing the amount in the bottle by the fraction representing the amount ordered. Your equation is written $\frac{3}{4} \div \frac{1}{16}$ and reads "three-quarters divided by one-sixteenth." You want to find out how many times $\frac{1}{16}$ goes into $\frac{3}{4}$, or more simply put, how many one-sixteenths are in three-quarters.

To divide fractions you need to flip the divisor to find the reciprocal, which is switching the numerator and the denominator. So the reciprocal of $\frac{1}{16}$ is $\frac{16}{1}$.

Now you will multiply the dividend by the reciprocal, so by flipping your divisor you turned your division problem into a multiplication problem.

$$\frac{3}{4} \div \frac{1}{16} = \frac{3}{4} \times \frac{16}{1}$$

You now solve this as a multiplication problem.

$$\frac{3}{\overset{}{\underset{1}{4}}} \times \frac{\overset{4}{16}}{1} = \frac{3}{1} \times \frac{4}{1} = \frac{12}{1} = 12$$

The bottle has 12 doses remaining.

EXAMPLE 1 ▶ Divide $\frac{1}{2} \div \frac{1}{4}$

1. The problem has no mixed or whole numbers.
2. Invert (flip) the divisor $\frac{1}{4}$ to find its reciprocal $\frac{4}{1}$.
3. Multiply the dividend by the reciprocal of the divisor.

$$\frac{1}{2} \div \frac{1}{4} = \frac{1}{2} \times \frac{4}{1} = \frac{1}{\cancel{2}_1} \times \frac{\cancel{4}^2}{1} = \frac{2}{1} = 2$$

Super Tech . . .

Open the CD-ROM that accompanies your textbook and select Chapter 1, Exercise 1-12. Review the animation and example problems, and then complete the practice problems.

Tech Check

Accuracy Counts

If the physician's drug order reads "Take $2\frac{1}{2}$ tablets with breakfast and $1\frac{1}{4}$ tablets with dinner," how many tablets will the patient take each day?

Follow through all steps of the problem

Remember that you have to convert any mixed numbers to fractions, find the LCD, and reduce to lowest terms.

$$2\frac{1}{2} = \frac{(2 \times 2) + 1}{2} = \frac{5}{2} \quad \text{and} \quad 1\frac{1}{4} = \frac{(1 \times 4) + 1}{4} = \frac{5}{4}$$

$$\frac{5}{2} \times \frac{2}{2} = \frac{10}{4}$$

$$\frac{10}{4} + \frac{5}{4} = \frac{15}{4}$$

$$15 \div 4 = 3\frac{3}{4}$$

The patient will take $3\frac{3}{4}$ tablets a day.

✓ Review and Practice 1-8 Dividing Fractions

Find the following quotients. (Rewrite the answers in proper form.)

1. $\frac{4}{9} \div \frac{5}{7}$

2. $\frac{3}{11} \div \frac{4}{5}$

3. $\frac{3}{8} \div \frac{1}{2}$

4. $\frac{1}{6} \div \frac{3}{4}$

5. $\frac{3}{5} \div \frac{2}{8}$

6. $\frac{6}{9} \div \frac{5}{11}$

7. $\dfrac{9}{10} \div \dfrac{3}{5}$

8. $\dfrac{7}{12} \div \dfrac{21}{36}$

9. $1\dfrac{3}{4} \div \dfrac{2}{3}$

10. $\dfrac{7}{8} \div 1\dfrac{3}{4}$

Decimals

The decimal system provides another way to represent whole numbers and their fractional parts. Pharmacy technicians use decimals in their daily work. The metric system, which is decimal-based, is used in dosage calculations. You must be able to work with decimals and convert fractions and mixed numbers to decimals. As a pharmacy technician you must be very careful to always write your decimal point in the correct place.

Working with Decimals

In the decimal system, the location of a digit relative to the decimal point determines its value. The decimal point separates the whole number from the decimal fraction; a good example is one dollar. One dollar is written as $1.00, and one and a half dollars is written $1.50. The whole dollar is written before the decimal point and the fraction part is written after the decimal point. The fraction $1\frac{1}{2}$ is written as 1.5 in decimal format.

Writing Decimals

Each position in a decimal number has a place value. The places to the left of a decimal point represent whole numbers. The places to the right of a decimal point represent decimal fractions. Decimal fractions are equivalent to fractions that have denominators of 10, 100, 1000 and so on. The first number or place to the right of the decimal point is valued in tenths, the second place is valued in hundredths, and the third place is valued in thousandths. Always write zero to the left of the decimal in place of a whole number when writing a decimal fraction. The decimal fraction 0.125 represents 1 tenth, 2 hundredths, and 5 thousandths.

The number 1542.567 is read "one thousand five hundred forty-two *and* five hundred sixty-seven thousandths." When you are reading or writing decimal numbers you are using words as if you were speaking the decimal number; the word *and* replaces the decimal point. See Table 1-3.

When you are working with decimals it is important to compare the numbers in order to add, subtract, multiply or divide. To compare decimals the amounts are lined up using the decimal point. Zeros are added to each number so that all numbers in the problem have the same number of decimals places. Zeros added to the right of the decimal do not change the value. For example to add 0.175, 0.92 and 2.110 you need to align the numbers and add zeros.

$$
\begin{array}{r}
0.175 \\
0.920 \\
+\ 2.110 \\
\hline
3.205
\end{array}
$$

Table 1-3 Decimal Place Values

The number 1542.567 can be represented as follows:

Whole Number				Decimal Point	Decimal Fraction		
Thousands	Hundreds	Tens	Ones	.	Tenths	Hundredths	Thousandths
1	5	4	2	.	5	6	7

When you write a decimal number,

1. Write the whole-number part to the left of the decimal point.
2. Write the decimal fraction part to the right of the decimal point.
3. Write zero to the left of the decimal point in place of a whole number when writing decimal fractions.

EXAMPLE 1 ▶

Decimal	Description	Mixed Number
1.5	One and five tenths	$1\frac{5}{10}$
0.33	Thirty-three hundredths	$\frac{33}{100}$
1.125	One and one hundred twenty-five thousandths	$1\frac{125}{1000}$

EXAMPLE 2 ▶ Write $3\frac{4}{10}$ in decimal form.

3 is the whole number, which will be written to the left of the decimal point, and $\frac{4}{10}$ is the fraction portion and will be written to the right of the decimal point.

To find your decimal fraction you simply divide the numerator of the fraction by the denominator of the fraction.

$$4 \div 10 = 0.4$$

Next, add your fractional decimal of 0.4 to your whole decimal of 3.0

$$\begin{array}{r} 0.4 \\ + 3.0 \\ \hline 3.4 \end{array}$$

3 ones and 4 tenths is written in decimal form as 3.4

$$3\frac{4}{10} = 3.4$$

EXAMPLE 3 ▶ Write $\frac{25}{1000}$ in decimal form.

To write this properly you need to know the value place of the denominator. The denominator is 1000, so your answer must be written to reflect the thousandths place which is 3 decimal places to the right of the decimal.

Divide the numerator of the fraction by the denominator of the fraction:

$$25 \div 1000 = 0.025$$

Remember to write a zero to the left of your decimal point in place of a whole number.

The fractional decimal 0.025 is read as "twenty-five thousandths."

$$\frac{25}{1000} = 0.025$$

Super Tech . . .

Open the CD-ROM that accompanies your textbook and select Chapter 1, Exercise 1-13. Review the animation and example problems, and then complete the practice problems.

✓ Review and Practice 1-9 Decimals

Write the following fractions in decimal form.

1. $\frac{2}{10}$ = _____

2. $\frac{17}{100}$ = _____

3. $6\frac{5}{10}$ = _____

4. $7\frac{19}{100}$ = _____

5. $\frac{3}{1000}$ = _____

Place > or < between each pair of decimals to make a true statement.

6. 4.27 _____ 4.02

7. 12.25 _____ 12.18

8. 0.4 _____ 0.6

9. 2.22 _____ 2.20

10. 0.0170 _____ 0.0172

11. 0.3001 _____ 0.2998

12. 5.41 _____ 5.34

13. 34.58 _____ 34.85

14. 0.7 _____ 0.9

15. 0.67 _____ 0.53

Rounding Decimals

In the pharmacy, you will usually round decimals to the nearest tenth or hundredth. If you use a calculator, the answer you get may contain many more decimal places than you need, and you must round the answer. For example, $10 \div 6 = 1.6666666 \ldots$. In some circumstances you will be asked to round to the nearest tenth, which is 1.7. In other situations you may need to round to the nearest hundredth, which is 1.67.

When rounding with 9s to the tenths decimal, if you have to round up, the value of ones to the left of the decimal will round up one. 0.$\underline{9}$7 will round to 1.0 which is equal to 1.

To round decimals:

1. Underline the target place value to which you want to round.
2. Look at the digit to the right of this target place value. If this digit is 4 or less, do not change the digit in the target place value. If this digit is 5 or more, round the digit in the target place value up one.
3. Drop all digits to the right of the target place value.

EXAMPLE 1 ▶ Round 2.42 to the nearest tenth.

1. Underline the tenths place (the target place value): 2.4̲2
2. The digit to the right of the tenths place is 2. Do not change the digit in the tenths place.
3. Drop the digits to the right of the tenths place. The number 2.42 rounded to the nearest tenth equals 2.4

EXAMPLE 2 ▶ Round 0.035 to the nearest hundredth.

1. Underline the digit in the hundredths place: 0.03̲5
2. The digit to the right of the hundredths place is 5. Round the digit in the hundredths place up one unit: 0.04
3. The number 0.035 rounded to the nearest hundredth equals 0.04

EXAMPLE 3 ▶ Round 3.99 to the nearest tenth.

1. 3.99
2. The digit to the right of the tenths value place is 9. Round the digit in the tenths value place up one unit. When 9 is rounded up, it becomes 10. Place the 0 in the tenths place, and carry the 1 to the ones place. When 1 is added to the ones place, 3 + 1 = 4. The rounded number becomes 4
3. The number 3.99 rounded to the nearest tenth equals 4

Super Tech . . .

Open the CD-ROM that accompanies your textbook and select Chapter 1, Exercise 1-14. Review the animation and example problems, and then complete the practice problems.

Review and Practice 1-10 Rounding Decimals

Round to the nearest tenth.

1. 14.34 _____

2. 3.45 _____

3. 0.86 _____

4. 0.19 _____

Round to the nearest hundredth.

5. 9.293 _____

6. 55.168 _____

7. 4.0060 _____

8. 2.2081 _____

Round to the nearest whole number.

9. 11.493 _____

10. 19.98 _____

11. 2.099 _____

12. 50.505 _____

Tech Check

Rounding Errors with 9

A pharmacy technician is calculating how much water is needed to add to a powder to reconstitute a medication. He needs to add 4.95 mL, but the syringe being used is calibrated (marked) in tenths. The pharmacy technician must round the calculation to the nearest tenth. How much water will the pharmacy technician need to add to the powder?

The pharmacy technician looks at the 5 in the hundredths place and rounds the tenths place up from 9 to 0. However, he neglects to carry the unit to the ones place and draws 4.0 mL of medication into the syringe.

Think Before You Act

Because the pharmacy technician forgets to carry a unit from the tenths place into the ones place, an error results. The patient does not receive a full dose of medication. With correct rounding, the patient should receive 5.0 mL, not 4.0 mL.

Adding and Subtracting Decimals

To add or subtract decimals, you align them by their place value by lining up the decimal points. Then simply do the math, just as you do to add or subtract whole numbers. Always be sure to align your equation perfectly. Add zeros when the numbers have different numbers of digits after the decimal so that all of the decimal fractions are of equal length; this will reduce the risk of making a math error.

To add or subtract decimals:

1. Write the problem vertically, as you would with whole numbers. Align the decimal points.
2. Add or subtract, starting from the right. Include the decimal point in your answer.

EXAMPLE 1 ▶ Add 1.87 + .92

1. Write the problem vertically, aligning the decimal points and adding zeros where needed to have an even equation.

$$
\begin{array}{r}
1.87 \\
+\ 0.92 \\
\end{array}
$$

2. Add.

$$
\begin{array}{r}
1.87 \\
+\ 0.92 \\
\hline
2.79 \\
\end{array}
$$

EXAMPLE 2 ❭ Add 12 + 2.75 + .375

Write the problem vertically, aligning the decimal points and adding zeros where needed to have an even equation. Then add.

$$
\begin{array}{r}
12.000 \\
2.750 \\
+\ 0.375 \\
\hline
15.125
\end{array}
$$

EXAMPLE 3 ❭ Subtract 64.31 − 42.17

Write the problem vertically, aligning the decimal points and adding zeros where needed. Then subtract.

$$
\begin{array}{r}
{}^{2\,1\,1}\ \\
64.3\,1 \\
-\ 42.17 \\
\hline
22.14
\end{array}
$$

EXAMPLE 4 ❭ Subtract 18.2 − 3.143

Write the problem vertically, aligning the decimal points and adding zeros where needed. Then subtract.

$$
\begin{array}{r}
{}^{1\,9\,10}\ \\
18.2\,0\,0 \\
-03.143 \\
\hline
15.057
\end{array}
$$

Super Tech . . .

Open the CD-ROM that accompanies your textbook and select Chapter 1, Exercise 1-15. Review the animation and example problems, and then complete the practice problems.

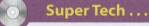

✓ Review and Practice 1-11 Adding and Subtracting Decimals

Add or subtract the following pairs of numbers.

1. 7.58 + 3.24
2. 143.05 + 22.07
3. 13.561 + 0.099
4. 24.102 + 2.410

5. 2.01 + 0.5
6. 5.66 − 0.09
7. 14.7 − 0.9

8. 1.22 − 0.4
9. 31.64 − 17.39
10. 16.250 − 1.625

Converting Decimals into Fractions

Pharmacy technicians may need to convert between decimals and fractions when interpreting prescriptions and physician drug orders. When you work with decimals, the number to the left of the decimal point is a whole number and the number to the right of the decimal point is a fraction. To convert the decimal 12.5 to a fraction, write the number to the left of the decimal point as the whole number. The numerator is always the number to the right of the decimal point, the numerator is 5. To find the denominator you need to determine the place value of the number farthest to the right of the decimal point. For example, in 12.5 the place value of 5 is the tenths place, so the denominator is 10; the fraction is 5/10. Always write your answer in lowest terms. The fraction 5/10 can be reduced to 1/2.

$$12.5 = 12\frac{5}{10} = 12\frac{1}{2}$$

EXAMPLE 1 ▶   **Convert** 3.75 to a mixed number.

1. Write the number to the left of the decimal point, 3, as the whole number.
2. Write the number to the right of the decimal point, 75, as the numerator of the fraction.
3. The digit farthest to the right of the decimal point, 5, is in the hundredths place.
    Thus, the denominator is 100. The mixed number is $3\frac{75}{100}$
4. Reduce to lowest terms: $3\frac{75}{100} = 3\frac{3}{4}$

EXAMPLE 2 ▶   **Convert** 0.010 to a fraction.

1. The number to the left of the decimal point is 0, so 0.010 has no whole number.
2. The number 010 is to the right of the decimal point. Write 10 as the numerator of the fraction.
3. The digit farthest to the right of the decimal point is 0, in the thousandths place. The denominator is 1000. The fraction is $\frac{10}{1000}$.
4. Reduce to lowest terms: $\frac{10}{1000} = \frac{1}{100}$

Super Tech . . .

Open the CD-ROM that accompanies your textbook and select Chapter 1, Exercise 1-16. Review the animation and example problems, and then complete the practice problems.

✓ Review and Practice 1-12 Converting Decimals into Fractions

Convert the following decimals to fractions or mixed numbers. Reduce the answer to its lowest terms.

1. 1.2 = _____

2. 98.6 = _____

3. 0.3 = _____

4. 0.442 = _____

5. 5.03 = _____

Converting Fractions into Decimals

Conversions between fractions and decimals are important in the pharmacy. For example, you may receive a drug order in fractions, and the medication is measured in decimals.

When you convert proper fractions, the equivalent decimals are less than 1. When you convert fractions to decimals, think of the fractions as division problems. To convert a fraction to a decimal, divide the numerator by the denominator.

Write $\frac{1}{4}$ as $1 \div 4$ and solve the equation by dividing the numerator by the denominator.

EXAMPLE ▶

$$
\begin{array}{r}
0.25 \\
4\overline{)1.00} \\
\underline{8} \\
20 \\
\underline{20}
\end{array}
\qquad \text{so } \frac{1}{4} = 1 \div 4
$$

EXAMPLE 1 ▶ Convert $\frac{3}{4}$ to a decimal. $\frac{3}{4} = 3 \div 4$

Divide the numerator by the denominator.

$$
\begin{array}{r}
0.75 \\
4\overline{)3.00} \\
\underline{2\ 8} \\
20 \\
\underline{20}
\end{array}
\qquad \text{so } \frac{3}{4} = 0.75
$$

EXAMPLE 2 ▶ Convert $\frac{2}{3}$ to a decimal. $\frac{2}{3} = 2 \div 3$

Divide the numerator by the denominator.

$$
\begin{array}{r}
0.666 \\
3\overline{)2.000} \\
\underline{1\ 8} \\
20 \\
\underline{18} \\
20 \\
\underline{18} \\
2\ldots
\end{array}
$$

Sometimes the decimal repeats rather than terminates, as with $\frac{2}{3}$. In such cases, you round to the nearest hundredth. For example,

$$
\frac{2}{3} \cong 0.67
$$

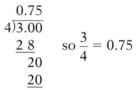

Super Tech . . .

Open the CD-ROM that accompanies your textbook and select Chapter 1, Exercise 1-17. Review the animation and example problems, and then complete the practice problems.

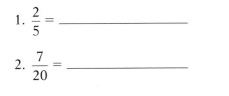 **Review and Practice 1-13** Converting Fractions into Decimals

Convert the following numbers into decimals. Where necessary, round to the nearest thousandth.

1. $\dfrac{2}{5}$ = _____

3. $\dfrac{9}{12}$ = _____

5. $\dfrac{1}{3}$ = _____

2. $\dfrac{7}{20}$ = _____

4. $\dfrac{12}{24}$ = _____

Multiplying Decimals

Multiplying decimals is the same as multiplying whole numbers, with one extra step of placing your decimal point in the answer. When you are multiplying, the decimal points *do not* need to line up as they do for adding and subtracting.

To multiply decimals, simply work the problem as if it were written in whole numbers and do the multiplication. Next count how many decimal places are to the right of the decimal point in all numbers in the equation. To place the decimal point in the answer, start at its right end. Move the decimal point to the left the same number of places as the sum of the number of digits to the right of the point you counted in the numbers of the problem.

EXAMPLE 1 ▶   Multiply 3.42 × 2.5

1. First multiply without considering the decimal points.

$$
\begin{array}{r}
3.42 \\
\times\ 2.5 \\
\hline
1710 \\
684\ \ \\
\hline
8550
\end{array}
$$

2. Count the total number of decimal places (to the right of the decimal point) in the numbers. The number 3.42 has two decimal places; 2.5 has one decimal place. The numbers have a total of three decimal places.
3. Place the decimal point in the answer. Start at the right of the answer, 8550 Move the decimal point three places to the left: 8.550. *After* placing the decimal point, you can drop the final zero so that the answer is 8.55.

EXAMPLE 2 ▶   Multiply 0.001 × 0.02

1. Multiply.

$$
\begin{array}{r}
0.001 \\
\times\ \ 0.02 \\
\hline
0.00002
\end{array}
$$

(0.54321) *Five decimal places*

←

2. The number 0.001 has three decimal places, which is the thousandths place, and 0.02 has two decimal places, which is the hundredths place. When they are multiplied together your answer is in the hundred-thousandths place, which is 5 decimal places to the right of decimal.

3. Start to the right of the answer 2. Move the decimal point five places to the left. Insert zeros to the left of 2 in order to correctly place the decimal point. The correct answer is 0.00002.

Super Tech . . .

Open the CD-ROM that accompanies your textbook and select Chapter 1, Exercise 1-18. Review the animation and example problems, and then complete the practice problems.

Tech Check

Placing Decimals Correctly

A pharmacy technician was instructed to calculate 0.25 gram (g) of medication for every 1.0 kilogram (kg) of body weight. The baby needing the medication weighed 6.25 kg. She set up this calculation:

$$
\begin{array}{r}
6.25 \\
\times\ 0.25 \\
\hline
3125 \\
1250 \quad \\
\hline
156.20
\end{array}
$$

Think Before You Act

The Technician got confused when placing the decimal in the answer. She followed the rule for addition rather than that for multiplication of decimals. The result, had the error not been caught, would have been a disastrous overdose. The baby should have received 1.5625 g of medication, which rounds to 1.56 g.

Review and Practice 1-14 Multiplying Decimals

Multiply the following numbers.

1. 7.4×8.2
2. 8.21×1.1
3. 4.2×0.3
4. 3.04×0.04
5. 0.55×0.5
6. 0.027×0.4

Dividing Decimals

The key to dividing decimals correctly is to place the decimal point properly. Remember that the dividend is the number that will be divided into and the divisor is the number you are dividing by and the answer to a division problem is the quotient. To divide decimals write the problem as a fraction; you already know how to divide fractions, so solving is the easy part of working the equations. Once you have written your fraction, the numerator is the dividend and the denominator is the divisor.

Before you can divide the equation, you can convert the fraction so you have a whole number for the denominator. To do this you simply move the decimal point place in both the numerator and the denominator the same number of places needed to make the whole number denominator. If you move the decimal point 2 places, it is the same as multiplying the numerator and the denominator by 100, as there are 2 zeros in 100. If you move the decimal point 3 places, it is the same as multiplying both the numerator and the denominator by 1000, as there are 3 zeros.

Now you are ready to complete the division problem. The last and most important thing you need to do when dividing decimals is place the decimal in the proper place in the quotient. If the numerator in the fractional equation has a decimal, simply align the decimal of the *quotient* with the decimal of the numerator.

EXAMPLE 1 ▶ Divide $0.8 \div 0.02$

1. Write the problem as a fraction: $\frac{0.8}{0.02}$
2. Move the decimal point two places to the right in both the numerator and the denominator. The denominator is now a whole number.

$$\frac{0.8}{0.02} = \frac{8}{0.2} = \frac{80}{2}$$

(This step is equivalent to multiplying $\frac{0.8}{0.02} \times \frac{100}{100}$)
3. Complete the division.

$$2\overline{)80} \quad \begin{array}{c} 40 \\ \underline{80} \end{array} \quad \text{so} \quad 0.8 \div 0.02 = 40$$

EXAMPLE 2 ▶ Divide $0.066 \div 0.11$

1. Write the problem as a fraction $\frac{0.066}{0.11}$
2. Move the decimal point two places to the right so that the denominator (divisor) is a whole number.

$$\frac{0.066}{0.11} = \frac{.0 \rightarrow 6 \rightarrow 6}{0.1 \rightarrow 1 \rightarrow} = \frac{6.6}{11}$$

(This step is equivalent to multiplying $\frac{0.066}{0.11} \times \frac{100}{100}$)
3. Complete the division.

$$11\overline{)6.6} \quad \begin{array}{c} 0.6 \\ \underline{6.6} \end{array} \quad \text{so} \quad 0.066 \div .011 = 0.6$$

Align the decimal point of the quotient with the decimal point of the numerator (dividend).

Super Tech . . .

Open the CD-ROM that accompanies your textbook and select Chapter 1, Exercise 1-19. Review the animation and example problems, and then complete the practice problems.

✳ Tech Check

Accuracy Counts

If the physician's drug order reads "Take $2\frac{1}{2}$ tablets with breakfast and $1\frac{1}{4}$ tablets with dinner," how many tablets will the patient take each day?

Follow through All Steps of the Problem

$$2 + 1 + \frac{1}{2} + \frac{1}{4} = 3 + \frac{2+1}{4} = 3\frac{3}{4} = 3.75$$

You answered this same problem in fractions in your last Tech Check, and the fractional form was $3\frac{3}{4}$, which is equal to your decimal of 3.75.

✅ Review and Practice 1-15 Dividing Decimals

Divide the following numbers. When necessary, round to the nearest thousandth.

1. $3.2 \div 1.6$
2. $48.6 \div 1.8$
3. $25.4 \div 0.2$
4. $0.004 \div 0.002$
5. $1.25 \div 0.5$
6. $0.32 \div 0.8$

✅ Chapter 1 Review

Test Your Knowledge

Multiple Choice

Select the best answer and write the letter on the line.

_____ 1. The 10 Arabic numbers are referred to as:
   A. Numbers
   B. Values
   C Digits
   D. Decimals

_____ 2. What is the value of the Roman numeral V?
   A. 10
   B. 5
   C. 1
   D. 50

_____ 3. In a fraction, what does the numerator represent?
   A. The whole
   B. A percent
   C. Parts of the whole
   D. None of the above

_____ 4. In the decimal 8475.26 what value place is the 7 in?
   A. Ones
   B. Tens
   C. Hundreds
   D. Thousands

_____ 5. In the decimal 8475.26 what value place is the 2 in?
   A. Ones
   B. Tenths
   C. Hundredths
   D. Thousandths

Practice Your Knowledge

Convert the following mixed numbers to fractions.

1. $2\frac{3}{8}$

2. $1\frac{2}{7}$

3. $9\frac{9}{10}$

4. $12\frac{11}{12}$

Reduce the following fractions to their lowest terms.

5. $\frac{12}{36}$

6. $\frac{39}{48}$

7. $\frac{45}{9}$

8. $\frac{58}{8}$

Find the least common denominator. Then write an equivalent fraction for each.

9. $\frac{3}{10}$ and $\frac{4}{5}$

10. $\frac{5}{6}$ and $\frac{4}{9}$

11. $\frac{3}{8}$, $\frac{3}{4}$, and $\frac{1}{6}$

12. $\frac{7}{10}$, $\frac{1}{4}$, and $\frac{2}{3}$

Place >, <, or = between the following pairs of fractions to make a true statement.

13. $\frac{3}{10}$ ___ $\frac{3}{16}$

14. $\frac{3}{2}$ ___ $\frac{8}{5}$

15. $1\frac{2}{3}$ ___ $1\frac{16}{24}$

16. $\frac{4}{25}$ ___ $\frac{16}{75}$

Perform the following calculations. Give the answer in the proper form.

17. $\frac{9}{4} + \frac{2}{3}$

18. $\frac{3}{5} + 1\frac{2}{5}$

19. $\frac{2}{10} + \frac{1}{100} + \frac{4}{50}$

20. $3 - \frac{2}{7}$

21. $\frac{11}{9} - \frac{1}{3}$

22. $\frac{4}{5} - \frac{3}{4}$

23. $\frac{5}{6} \times \frac{2}{3}$

24. $\frac{7}{9} \times \frac{3}{14}$

25. $\frac{3}{8} \times 11$

26. $\frac{12}{13} \div \frac{3}{52}$

27. $\frac{1}{7} \div \frac{3}{4}$

28. $2\frac{5}{8} \div \frac{1}{6}$

Place >, <, or = between the following pairs of decimals to make a true statement.

29. 5.7 _____ 5.09

30. 0.04 _____ 0.004

31. 6.3 _____ 6.300

Round to the nearest hundredth.

32. 0.229 _____

33. 7.091 _____

34. 46.001 _____

35. 9.885 _____

Round to the nearest tenth.

36. 4.34 _____

37. 3.65 _____

38. 6.991 _____

39. 0.073 _____

Round to the nearest whole number.

40. 8.96 _____

41. 20.6 _____

42. 0.931 _____

43. 12.449 _____

Convert the following fractions to decimals.

44. $\dfrac{7}{14}$ _____

45. $\dfrac{5}{8}$ _____

46. $2\dfrac{3}{5}$ _____

47. $\dfrac{32}{4}$ _____

Convert the following decimals to fractions. Reduce the answers to lowest terms.

48. 0.82 _____

49. 0.65 _____

50. 3.5 _____

51. 1.001 _____

Perform the following calculations.

52. 7.23 + 12.38

53. 4.59 + 0.2

54. 0.031 + 0.99

55. 7.49 − 0.38

56. 4.28 − 3.39

57. 0.852 − 0.61

58. 14.01 − 0.7888

59. 2.3 × 4.9

60. 0.33 × 0.002

61. 5 × 0.999

62. 38.85 ÷ 2.1

63. 4.875 ÷ 3.25

64. 2.2 ÷ 0.11

Apply your Knowledge

Controlling the Numbers

You are the pharmacy technician working in the pharmacy. You need to determine how much medication should be dispensed by the Pharmacist to the patient. The physician's drug order on the prescription reads: "Take $\frac{1}{2}$ tablet in the morning and take $\frac{1}{4}$ tablet at bedtime for eight days." The medication has 100 milligrams in each tablet.

Answer the following questions:

1. How many tablets need to be dispensed for eight days?

   _____

2. How many tablets will the patient take each day?

   _____

3. How many milligrams will the patient take each day?

   _____

Internet Activity

Visit one of the following sites or a website of your own choice for more practice of completing fraction and decimal problems. You might search for "Dosage Calculations Practice Problems," "Math and Dosage Practice Problems," or "Fractions and Decimals Practice."

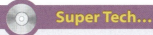

Super Tech...

Open the CD-ROM that accompanies your textbook and a final review of Chapter 1. For a final evaluation, take the chapter test and email or print your results for your instructor. A score of 95 percent or above indicates mastery of the chapter concepts.

2

Working with Percents, Ratios, and Proportions

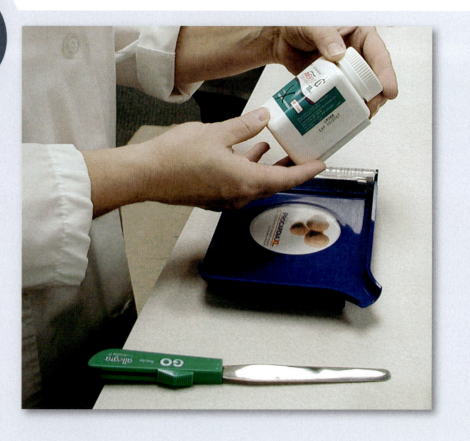

Key Terms

Cross-multiplying
Dosage strength
Fraction proportion
Means and extremes
Percent
Proportion
Ratio
Ratio proportion
Ratio strength
Solute
Solution
Solvent (diluent)
Strengths of mixtures

Learning Outcomes

When you have successfully completed Chapter 2, you will have mastered skills to be able to:

▶ Calculate equivalent measurements, using percents, ratios, decimals, and fractions.

▶ Indicate solution strengths by using percents and ratios.

▶ Explain the concept of proportion.

▶ Calculate missing values in proportions by using ratios (means and extremes) and fractions (cross-multiplying).

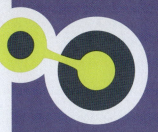

Introduction

As a pharmacy technician, you may be responsible for preparing solutions and solids in varying amounts. To do this, you must be 100 percent accurate when working with percents, ratios, and proportions. This chapter focuses on the first step in many dosage calculations, which is the process of finding the missing value in a ratio or fraction proportion problem. When you have worked all of Chapter 2, you will be able to solve the mystery of the missing value. Ready to compare the numbers? Let's get started!

Critical Thinking in the Pharmacy
Comparing the Numbers

You are the pharmacy technician working in the pharmacy. You need to determine how much medication should be dispensed by the pharmacist to the patient. The physician's drug order on the prescription reads: "Take $\frac{1}{2}$ tablet in the morning and take 1 tablet at bedtime for 6 days." The medication has 100 milligrams in each tablet.

After you have completed Chapter 2, you will be able to determine how many tablets need to be dispensed, how many milligrams the patient will take each day, and how to write a proper ratio of tablets to milligrams.

PTCB Correlations

When you have completed this chapter you will have the mathematical building block of knowledge needed to assist you in performing dosage calculations.

▶ Knowledge of pharmacy calculations (for example, algebra, ratio and proportions, metric conversions, IV drip rates, IV admixture calculations) (Statement I-50).

Percents

Percent: Means per 100 or divided by 100.

Percents, like decimals and fractions, provide a way to express the relationship of parts to a whole. Indicated by the symbol %, **percent** literally means "per 100" or "divided by 100" The whole is always 100 units. Table 2-1 shows the same number expressed as a decimal, a fraction, and a percent.

Table 2-1   Comparing Decimals, Fractions, and Percents

Words	Decimal	Fraction	Percent
Eight hundredths	0.08	8/100	8%
Twenty-three hundredths	0.23	23/100	23%
Seven-tenths	0.7	7/10	70%
One	1.0	1/1	100%
One and five-tenths or one and one-half	1.5	$1\frac{5}{10}$ or $1\frac{1}{2}$	150%

Working with Percents

As a pharmacy technician, you may be responsible for preparing solutions and solids in varying amounts. To do this, you must have a solid understanding of percents, ratios, and proportions.

Converting between percents and decimals requires dividing and multiplying by 100.

Converting a percent to a decimal is basically dividing a number by 100. If the percent is a fraction or a mixed number, first convert it to a decimal. Then divide by 100, moving the decimal point two places to the left. Always write a zero before the decimal point when writing your answer. For example: 0.12

To convert a percent to a decimal, remove the percent symbol. Then divide the remaining number by 100.

Memory tip Count the number of zeros to determine the number of spaces to move, there are two zeros in 100, so you move two spaces.

EXAMPLE 1 ▶   Convert 56% to decimal form.

$$56\% = 56.0 \div 100 = 0.56$$

The decimal place moved two places to the left so that the 6 is in the hundredths place. (You move the decimal point two places to the left, as there are 2 zeros in 100).

Insert the zero before the decimal point in you written answer.

EXAMPLE 2 ▶   When you move the decimal point to the left, you may need to insert zeros. Convert 0.3 percent to a decimal.

$$0.3\% = 0.3 \div 100 = 0.003$$

The decimal place moved two places to the left so that the 3 is in the thousandths place.

EXAMPLE 3 ▶ Convert $\frac{3}{4}\%$ to decimal form.

First convert $\frac{3}{4}$ to a decimal.

$$\frac{3}{4} = 4\overline{)3.00}^{\,0.75} = 0.75$$

$$\frac{3}{4}\% = 0.75\% = 0.75 \div 100 = 0.0075$$

Insert the zero before the decimal point in you written answer.

The decimal place moved two places to the left so that the 5 is in the hundred-thousandths place.

┌───┐
  ◉   **Super Tech . . .**

Open the CD-ROM that accompanies your textbook and select Chapter 2, Exercise 2-1. Review the animation and example problems, and then complete the practice problems.
└───┘

Converting a decimal to a percent is basically multiplying a number by 100. Multiplying a number by 100 percent does not change its value since 100% equals 1.

To convert a decimal into a percent, multiply the decimal by 100 and add the % sign.

EXAMPLE 1 ▶ Express 1.42 as a percent.

$$1.42 \times 100\% = 142\%$$

The decimal place moved two places to the right. (You move the decimal point two places to the right, as there are 2 zeros in 100).

EXAMPLE 2 ▶ Express 0.02 as a percent.

$$0.02 \times 100\% = 2.00\% = 2\%$$

The decimal place moved two places to the right so that the 2 is in the ones place.

EXAMPLE 3 ▶ When you move the decimal point to the right, you may need to insert zeros. Express 0.8 as a percent.

$$0.8 \times 100\% = 80.0\% = 80\%$$

The decimal place moved two places to the right so that the 8 is in the tens place.

EXAMPLE 4 ▶ Express $\frac{1}{2}$ as a percent.

First convert $\frac{1}{2}$ to a decimal.

$$\frac{1}{2} = 1 \div 2 = 0.5$$

Now convert the decimal to a percent.

$$\frac{1}{2} = 0.5 = 0.5 \times 100\% = 50\%$$

The decimal place moved two places to the right so that the 5 is in the tens place.

Remember that when you divide a number by 100, you move the decimal point two places to the left. When you multiply a number by 100, you move the decimal point two places to the right.

Super Tech . . .

Open the CD-ROM that accompanies your textbook and select Chapter 2, Exercise 2-2. Review the animation and example problems, and then complete the practice problems.

Because percent means "per 100" or "divided by 100," you can easily convert percents to fractions.

To convert a fraction to a percent, first convert the fraction to a decimal. Round the decimal to the nearest hundredth. Then follow the rule for converting a decimal to a percent.

EXAMPLE 1 ▶ Express $\frac{1}{2}$ as a percent.

First convert $\frac{1}{2}$ to a decimal.

$$\frac{1}{2} = 1 \div 2 = 0.5$$

Now convert the decimal to a percent.

$$\frac{1}{2} = 0.5 = 0.5 \times 100\% = 50\%$$

You can write this as $0.5 = 0.50 = 0. \to 5 \to 0.\% = 50\%$.

EXAMPLE 2 ▶ Express $1\frac{3}{4}$ as a percent.

Change $1\frac{3}{4}$ to the fraction $\frac{7}{4}$.

$$1\frac{3}{4} = \frac{7}{4} = 1.75 = 1.75 \times 100\% = 175\%$$

You can write this as $1\frac{3}{4} = 1. \to 7 \to 5.\% = 175\%$.

An alternative method for converting a fraction to a percent is to multiply the fraction by 100 percent.

EXAMPLE 1 ▶ Convert $\frac{1}{2}$ to a percent.

$$\frac{1}{2} \times 100\%$$

$$\frac{1}{2} \times \frac{100\%}{1} = \frac{100}{2} = 50\%$$

EXAMPLE 2 ▶ Convert $1\frac{3}{4}$ to a percent.

Change $1\frac{3}{4}$ to the fraction $\frac{7}{4}$.

$$\frac{7}{4} \times \frac{100\%}{1} = \frac{700}{4} = 175\%$$

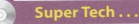

Super Tech . . .

Open the CD-ROM that accompanies your textbook and select Chapter 2, Exercise 2-3. Review the animation and example problems, and then complete the practice problems.

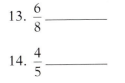

Review and Practice 2-1 Percents

Convert the following percents to decimals.

1. 14% _____
2. 30% _____
3. 2% _____
4. 9% _____
5. 103% _____
6. 300% _____

Convert the following decimals to percents.

7. 4.04 _____
8. 2.3 _____
9. 0.7 _____
10. 0.33 _____
11. 0.06 _____
12. 0.013 _____

Convert the following fractions to percents. Round to the nearest percent.

13. $\frac{6}{8}$ _____
14. $\frac{4}{5}$ _____
15. $\frac{1}{6}$ _____
16. $\frac{5}{9}$ _____
17. $1\frac{1}{10}$ _____
18. $2\frac{1}{4}$ _____

Ratios

Ratio: Expression of the relationship of a part to the whole.

Pharmacy technicians will work with **ratios** and need to understand how ratios express the relationship of a part to the whole. They may relate a quantity of liquid drug to a quantity of solution, or can also be used to calculate dosages of dry medication such as tablets. When ratios describe dry medications, the whole unit is often 1, as in 1 tablet. If there are 25 milligrams (mg) of drug to one tablet, the ratio would be written as 25:1. This concept of ratio is important when you calculate a dosage.

Ratios can also be written as fractions but are usually written in the form *A:B*. The colon tells you to compare *A* to *B*, and *A:B* is read "*A* to *B*."

EXAMPLE A 1:100 drug solution ("one to one hundred") describes a solution that has 1 part drug to every 100 parts of solution.

The ratio 1:100 is equivalent to the fraction $\frac{1}{100}$, the decimal 0.01, and the percent 1%.

Working with Ratios

You may use only whole numbers when you write a ratio.

Correct ratios include 8:1, 2:5, and 1:100
Incorrect ratios include 2.5:10, 1:4.5, and $\frac{1}{2}$:100
Ratios should almost always be expressed in lowest terms. Just as $\frac{4}{100}$ reduces to $\frac{1}{25}$ the ratio 4:100 should be written 1:25

Similarly, you would reduce 2:10 to 1:5 and 10:12 to 5:6

You will reduce a ratio as you would a fraction. Find the largest whole number that divides evenly into both values A and B.

EXAMPLE ▶ Reduce 2:12 to its lowest terms.

Both values 2 and 12 are divisible by 2

$$2 \div 2 = 1 \qquad 12 \div 2 = 6$$

2:12 reduced is written 1:6

Super Tech . . .

Open the CD-ROM that accompanies your textbook and select Chapter 2, Exercise 2-4. Review the animation and example problems, and then complete the practice problems.

Because a ratio relates two quantities, value A and value B, ratios can be written as fractions.

Within this textbook, for simplicity, when two numbers are expressed as $A:B$, this is a ratio. When two numbers are expressed as $\frac{A}{B}$ this is a fraction.

When you convert between ratios and fractions, you do not have to perform any calculations. You simply rearrange the presentation of the numbers.

To convert a ratio to a fraction, write value A (the first number) as the numerator and value B (the second number) as the denominator, so that $A:B = \frac{A}{B}$. Convert a mixed number to a ratio by first writing the mixed number as an improper fraction.

EXAMPLE ▶ Convert the following ratios to fractions.

a. $1:2 = \frac{1}{2}$

b. $4:5 = \frac{4}{5}$

c. $1:100 = \frac{1}{100}$

Super Tech . . .

Open the CD-ROM that accompanies your textbook and select Chapter 2, Exercise 2-5. Review the animation and example problems, and then complete the practice problems.

To convert a fraction to a ratio, write the numerator as the first value A and the denominator as the second value B.

Convert a mixed number to a ratio by first writing the mixed number as a fraction.

EXAMPLE ▶ Convert the following to ratios.

a. $\frac{7}{12} = 7:12$

b. $\frac{3}{10} = 3:10$

c. $2\frac{1}{2} = \frac{5}{2} = 5:2$

Super Tech . . .

Open the CD-ROM that accompanies your textbook and select Chapter 2, Exercise 2-6. Review the animation and example problems, and then complete the practice problems.

Let's take it one step further now and convert a ratio to a fraction and then to a decimal.

EXAMPLE ▶ Convert $1:10$ to a decimal.

Write the decimal as a fraction.

$$1:10 = \frac{1}{10}$$

Convert the fraction to a decimal.

$$\frac{1}{10} = 1 \div 10 = 0.1 \qquad \text{So } 1:10 = \frac{1}{10} = 0.1$$

Now, reverse the process and convert a decimal to a ratio.
Write the decimal as a fraction.

$$0.1 = \frac{1}{10}$$

Rewrite the number as a ratio.

$$\frac{1}{10} = 1:10 \qquad \text{So } 0.1 = \frac{1}{10} = 1:10$$

Super Tech . . .

Open the CD-ROM that accompanies your textbook and select Chapter 2, Exercise 2-7. Review the animation and example problems, and then complete the practice problems.

Remember that you can write a percent as a fraction with the denominator of 100. This step helps you to convert a ratio to a percent and a percent to a ratio.

To convert a ratio to a percent, first convert the ratio to a decimal, write the decimal as a percent by multiplying the decimal by 100, and add the percent symbol.

EXAMPLE ▶ Convert $1:50$ to a percent.

1. Convert the ratio to a decimal.

$$1:50 = \frac{1}{50} = 0.02$$

2. Multiply 0.02 by 100 and add the percent symbol.

$$0.02 \times 100\% = 2\%$$

To convert a percent to a ratio, first write the percent as a fraction, reduce the fraction to lowest terms, then write the fraction as a ratio by writing the numerator as value A and the denominator as value B, in the form $A:B$.

EXAMPLE ▶ Convert 25 percent to a ratio.

1. Write the percent as a fraction.

$$25\% = \frac{25}{100}$$

2. Reduce the fraction.

$$\frac{25}{100} = \frac{1}{4}$$

3. Restate the fraction as a ratio. Write the numerator as value A and the denominator as value B.

$$\frac{1}{4} = 1:4 \qquad \text{So, } 25\% = \frac{1}{4} = 1:4$$

Super Tech . . .

Open the CD-ROM that accompanies your textbook and select Chapter 2, Exercise 2-8. Review the animation and example problems, and then complete the practice problems.

✓ Review and Practice 2-2 Ratios

Convert the following ratios to fractions or mixed numbers.

1. $3:4$ _____   3. $5:3$ _____   5. $1:20$ _____

2. $4:9$ _____   4. $10:1$ _____   6. $1:250$ _____

Convert the following fractions to ratios.

7. $\frac{2}{3}$ _____   8. $\frac{6}{7}$ _____   9. $\frac{5}{4}$ _____   10. $\frac{7}{3}$ _____

Convert the following ratios to decimals. Round to the nearest hundredth, if necessary.

11. $1:4$ _____   12. $1:8$ _____   13. $3:4$ _____   14. $2:5$ _____

Convert the following ratios to percents. If necessary, round to the nearest percent.

15. 1:4 _____   16. 1:25 _____   17. 2:9 _____   18. 7:17 _____

Convert the following percents to ratios.

19. 14% _____   20. 65% _____   21. 400% _____   22. 175% _____

Ratio Strengths

Ratio strength: The amount of drug in a solution or the amount of drug in a solid dosage form such as a tablet or capsule; dosage strength.

Dosage strength: The amount of drug per dosage unit.

Ratio strengths can be used to express the amount of drug in a solution or the amount of drug in a solid dosage form such as a tablet or capsule. This relationship represents the **dosage strength** of the medication, which is the amount of drug per dosage unit. The first number of the ratio represents the amount of drug, while the second number represents the amount of solution or the number of tablets or capsules. For example, a 1 mg:5 mL dosage strength represents 1 mg of drug in every 5 mL of solution. A 250 mg:1 tablet dosage strength means that each tablet contains 250 mg of drug.

EXAMPLE 1 ▶ Write the ratio strength to describe 50 mL of solution containing 3 g of a drug.

The first number in the ratio strength always represents the amount of drug, which is 3 g.
The second number represents the amount of solution, 50 mL.
The ratio is 3 g:50 mL.

EXAMPLE 2 ▶ Write the ratio strength to describe 25 mg of a drug dissolved in 150 mL of solution.

The amount of the drug is 25 mg, while the amount of solution is 150 mL.
The ratio is 25 mg:150 mL.

Recall from the previous section that ratios should always be reduced to lowest terms. Since both numbers in the ratio can be divided by 25, the ratio needs to be reduced. The ratio should be written 1 mg:6 mL.

EXAMPLE 3 ▶ Write the ratio strength to describe 3 tablets containing 75 mg of a drug.

Remember that the amount of drug always goes first in the ratio. The amount of the drug is 75 mg. The ratio is 75 mg:3 tablets, which is then reduced to 25 mg:1 tablet.
Look at this example as the following 2 fractions:

$$\frac{75 \text{ mg}}{3 \text{ tablets}} = \frac{25 \text{ mg}}{1 \text{ tablet}}$$

If you knew that 25 mg:1 tablet and the doctor ordered 75 mg, could you determine how many tablets to give?
The equation would be set up like this:

$$\frac{25 \text{ mg}}{1 \text{ tablet}} = \frac{75 \text{ mg}}{? \text{ tablet}}$$

You will master this type of equation later in this chapter.

> ⚠️ **Caution!**
>
> Do not forget the units of measurement.

Including units in the dosage strength will help you to avoid some common errors. Consider the case in which we have two solutions of a drug. One of the solutions contains 1 **g** of drug in 50 **mL;** the other contains 1 **mg** of drug in 50 **mL.** While both of these solutions have ratio strengths of 1 : 50, they are obviously different from each other. To distinguish between them, the first solution could be written as 1 **g** : 50 **mL** while the second is written 1 **mg** : 50 **mL.**

> ✳ **Tech Check**
>
> *Reversing Terms in a Ratio Strength*
>
> A pharmacy technician is preparing 1000 mL of a 1 g : 10 mL solution of dextrose. He mixes 10,000 g of dextrose in 1000 mL of solution. The technician has mistakenly reversed the terms and prepared a 10 g : 1 mL solution.

> ✤ **Think Before You Act**
>
> The technician should have used 100 g of dextrose in 1000 mL.
>   Note that 100 g : 1000 mL = 1 g : 10 mL.
>   Thinking critically about the task, the technician should have realized that, in a 1 g : 10 mL solution, the number of grams should be smaller than the number of milliliters. The fact that 10,000 is larger than 1000 should have alerted the technician to the error.

✓ Review and Practice 2-3 Ratio Strengths

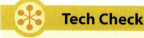

Write a ratio to describe the dosage strength in each of the following. Reduce the ratio to its lowest terms.

1. 100 mL of solution contains 5 g of drug. _____

2. 500 mL of solution contain 25 g of dextrose. _____

3. Each capsule contains 5 mg of drug. _____

4. 40 mg of drug is in every tablet. _____

5. 20 mg of drug is in 100 mL of solution. _____

6. 150 mg of drug is in 1500 mL of solution. _____

7. 250 mL of solution contains 50 g of drug. _____

8. 500 mg of drug in each capsule. _____

9. 500 mg of drug in 1000 mL of solution. _____

10. Two tablets contain 500 mg of drug. _____

Proportions

Proportion: A mathematical statement that two ratios are equal.

A **proportion** is a mathematical statement that two ratios are equal. Because ratios are often written as fractions, a proportion is also a statement that two fractions are equal. If you share a pizza with a friend and each of you gets half, it doses not matter if you cut it into 2, 4, 6, or 8 slices; no matter how you cut it, you still have half of a pizza. This could be expressed as $\frac{1}{2} = \frac{2}{4}$ or $\frac{3}{6} = \frac{4}{6}$ for example. These are proportions.

Writing Proportions

*When you write proportions, you **do not** reduce the ratios to their lowest terms.*

The ratio $2:3$ is read "two to three." To write a proportion, a double colon is used between two ratios. The double colon means *as*. The proportion $2:3::4:6$ reads "two is to three as four is to six." This **ratio proportion** states that mathematically the two ratios are equal; 2 to 3 is the same as the relationship of 4 to 6.

Ratio proportion: Mathematical statement that indicates two ratios are equal.

You can also write proportions by replacing the double colon with an equal sign.

Thus, $2:3::4:6$ is the same as $2:3 = 4:6$.

You can also write a proportion with fractions.

For example, $2:3::4:6$ can be written $\frac{2}{3} = \frac{4}{6}$.

Fraction proportion: Mathematical statement that indicates two fractions are equal.

This format is also referred to as a **fraction proportion,** which is a mathematical statement that indicates two fractions are equal.

> **Super Tech . . .**
>
> Open the CD-ROM that accompanies your textbook and select Chapter 2, Exercise 2-9. Review the animation and example problems, and then complete the practice problems.

To write a ratio proportion as a fraction proportion, simply change the double colon to an equal sign and then convert both ratios to fractions.

EXAMPLE ▶ Write $3:4::9:12$ as a fraction proportion.

1. Change the double colon to an equal sign.
$$3:4::9:12 \rightarrow 3:4 = 9:12$$

2. Convert both ratios to fractions.
$$3:4 = \frac{3}{4} \quad \text{and} \quad 9:12 = \frac{9}{12} \quad \text{So } 3:4 = 9:12 \rightarrow \frac{3}{4} = \frac{9}{12}$$

To write a fraction proportion as a ratio proportion, simply convert both fractions to ratios and then change the equal sign to a double colon.

EXAMPLE ▶ Write $\frac{3}{6} = \frac{1}{2}$ as a ratio proportion.

1. Convert each fraction to a ratio.

$$\frac{3}{6} = 3:6 \quad \text{and} \quad \frac{1}{2} = 1:2 \quad \text{So } 3:6 = 1:2$$

2. Change the equal sign to a double colon.

$$3:6 = 1:2 \rightarrow 3:6::1:2$$

Super Tech ...

Open the CD-ROM that accompanies your textbook and select Chapter 2, Exercise 2-10. Review the animation and example problems, and then complete the practice problems.

Tech Check

Accuracy Counts

A physician's drug order reads: "Take $\frac{1}{2}$ tablet with breakfast and $\frac{1}{2}$ tablet with dinner." There are 100 mg of medicine in each tablet. How many milligrams to tablets will the patient take each day?

Follow through all steps of the problem

Daily dose is $\frac{1}{2} + \frac{1}{2} = \frac{2}{2} = 1$ tablet per day.
Each tablet has 100 mg of medication, so your ratio is 100 mg:1 tablet.

✓ Review and Practice 2-4 Proportions

Write the following ratio proportions as fraction proportions.

1. $4:5::8:10$ _____   3. $1:10::100:1000$ _____

2. $5:12::10:24$ _____   4. $2:3::20:30$ _____

Write the following fraction proportions as ratio proportions.

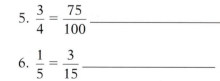

5. $\frac{3}{4} = \frac{75}{100}$ _____

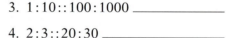

7. $\frac{8}{4} = \frac{2}{1}$ _____

6. $\frac{1}{5} = \frac{3}{15}$ _____

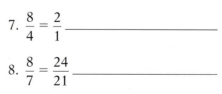

8. $\frac{8}{7} = \frac{24}{21}$ _____

Cross-Multiplying

Now you will learn to cross-multiply to find the missing value in a fraction proportion. To find the missing value in a fraction proportions cross-multiply between numerators and denominator of the fractions. Write an equation setting the products equal to each other then solve the equation to find the missing value.

EXAMPLE ▶ Find the missing value in $\frac{3}{5} = \frac{6}{?}$.

1. Cross-multiply.

$$\frac{3}{5} = \frac{6}{?} \rightarrow 3 \times ? = 5 \times 6$$

$$5 \times 6 = 30 \qquad \text{So } 3 \times ? = 30$$

2. Solve the equation. Here, divide both sides by 3

$$\frac{3 \times ?}{3} = \frac{30}{3}$$

Here $30 \div 3 = 10$ So $? = 10$

3. Restate the proportion, inserting the missing value.

$$\frac{3}{5} = \frac{6}{10}$$

4. Check your work by cross-multiplying. (Note that the fractions are equivalent since 6/10 can be obtained by multiplying both the numerator and the denominator of 3/5 by 2).

$$3 \times 10 = 5 \times 6$$

$$30 = 30$$

The proportion is true.
The missing value is 10.

Super Tech . . .

Open the CD-ROM that accompanies your textbook and select Chapter 2, Exercise 2-11. Review the animation and example problems, and then complete the practice problems.

Canceling Units

If the units of the numerator of the two fractions are the same, they can be dropped or canceled before you set up a proportion. Likewise, if the units from the denominator of the two fractions are the same, they can be canceled.

EXAMPLE 1 ▶ If 100 mL of solution contains 20 mg of drug, how many milligrams of the drug will be in 500 mL of the solution?

Start by setting up the fractions.

$$\frac{20 \text{ mg}}{100 \text{ mL}} \qquad \text{and} \qquad \frac{?}{500 \text{ mL}}$$

Compare the units used in the two fractions to see if any can be canceled. In this case, the units for the denominators of both fractions are milliliters. These can be canceled when you set up the proportion.

$$\frac{20 \text{ mg}}{100} = \frac{?}{500}$$

Now solve for ?, the missing value.

1. $100 \times ? = 20 \text{ mg} \times 500$

2. $\dfrac{100 \times ?}{100} = \dfrac{20 \text{ mg} \times 500}{100}$

3. $? = 100 \text{ mg}$

The second solution will contain 100 mg of drug in 500 mL of solution.

EXAMPLE 2 ▶   15 grams of drug is dissolved in 300 mL of solution. If you need 45 g of the drug, how many milliliters of the solution are needed?

Set up the fractions.

$$\dfrac{15 \text{ g}}{300 \text{ mL}} \quad \text{and} \quad \dfrac{45 \text{ g}}{?}$$

Cancel units and set up the proportion.

$$\dfrac{15}{300 \text{ mL}} = \dfrac{45}{?}$$

Solve for the missing value.

1. $300 \text{ mL} \times 45 = 15 \times ?$

2. $\dfrac{300 \text{ mL} \times 45}{15} = \dfrac{15 \times ?}{15}$

3. $900 \text{ mL} = ?$

You will need 900 mL of the solution to have 45 g of drug.

Canceling units in fraction proportions

You have a solution containing 200 mg of drug in 5 mL, and you are asked to determine how many milliliters of a solution contain 500 mg of drug. You can solve the problem by using the following two fractions. We can cancel units in fraction proportions. Now, however, we need to compare the units used in the top and bottom of the two fractions in the proportion.

$$\dfrac{200 \text{ mg}}{5 \text{ mL}} \quad \text{and} \quad \dfrac{500 \text{ mg}}{?}$$

In this case, the units for the numerators of the fraction are milligrams. Canceling the units leaves us with the following proportion.

$$\dfrac{200}{5 \text{ mL}} = \dfrac{500}{?}$$

The missing value can now be found by cross-multiplying and solving the equation as before.

1. $200 \times ? = 5 \text{ mL} \times 500$

2. $\dfrac{200 \times ?}{200} = \dfrac{5 \text{ mL} \times 500}{200}$

3. $200 \times ? = 200? \div 200 = ?$ and $5 \text{ mL} \times 500 = 2500 \text{ mL} \div 200 = 12.5 \text{ mL}$

4. $? = 12.5$

Super Tech . . .

Open the CD-ROM that accompanies your textbook and select Chapter 2, Exercise 2-12. Review the animation and example problems, and then complete the practice problems.

 Tech Check

Setting Up the Correct Proportion

A physician's order calls for a patient to receive 250 mg of amoxicillin oral suspension 3 times a day. Amoxicillin oral suspension is a dry medication that is mixed with water before being given to the patient. Each 5 mL of suspension contains 125 mg of drug. The pharmacy technician needs to calculate how many milliliters he will need to add for each dose. The technician sets up the proportion as 5 mL/125 mg = 250 mg/?.

Think Before You Act

The pharmacy technician realizes while solving the equation that he will not be able to cancel any units, and that his answer will contain both milligrams and milliliters. After looking at the proportion once again, he discovers that he has set up the proportion incorrectly, and that the first fraction is written upside down. The technician rewrites the proportion as 125 mg/mL = 250 mg/?. The pharmacy technician solves the equation correctly and determines that each dose is 10 mL.

Critical thinking is especially important when you use a calculator. Had the technician ignored the units and simply punched in the numbers, he would have come up with the wrong dose. Always include the units when you perform drug calculations.

✓ Review and Practice 2-5 Cross-Multiplying

Determine if the following proportions are true.

1. $\dfrac{7}{16} = \dfrac{28}{48}$

2. $\dfrac{6}{9} = \dfrac{24}{36}$

3. $\dfrac{100}{250} = \dfrac{150}{375}$

4. $\dfrac{50}{125} = \dfrac{125}{300}$

Cross-multiply to find the missing value.

5. $\dfrac{3}{15} = \dfrac{?}{5}$? = _____

6. $\dfrac{2}{?} = \dfrac{8}{100}$? = _____

7. $\dfrac{?}{20} = \dfrac{120}{100}$? = _____

8. $\dfrac{50}{75} = \dfrac{100}{?}$? = _____

Means and Extremes

Pharmacy technicians often work with proportions to calculate dosages. You must learn to set up the proportion correctly. If you set up the proportion incorrectly, you could give the wrong amount of medication, with serious consequences for the patient. Later in this book you will learn to read physicians' orders and drug labels, which are the sources for the information that goes into the proportion. But first you have to master the skill of setting up ratio proportions correctly and finding missing values.

When you set up a ratio proportion in the form $A:B::C:D$, the inner values B and C are the **means** and the outer values A and D are the **extremes.** If you have trouble remembering which is which, think, "Means are in the middle. Extremes are on the ends." In any true ratio proportion, the product of the means always equals the product of the extremes. See Figure 2.1.

Means and Extremes: For the equation A:B::C:D, B and C are the means (middle) and A and D are the extremes (ends).

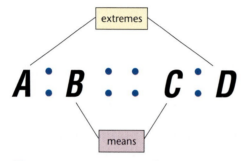

Figure 2-1 Means and Extremes

To determine if a ratio proportion is true, multiple the means and then multiple the extremes. If the products of both the means and extremes are equal then the proportion is true.

EXAMPLE 1 ▶ Determine if $1:2::3:6$ is a true proportion.

1. Multiply the means: $2 \times 3 = 6$

2. Multiply the extremes: $1 \times 6 = 6$

3. Compare the products of the means and the extremes.

$$6 = 6$$

The statement $1:2::3:6$ is a true proportion.

EXAMPLE 2 ▶ Determine if $100:20::5:4$ is a true proportion.

1. Multiply the means: $20 \times 5 = 100$

2. Multiply the extremes: $100 \times 4 = 400$

3. Compare the products of the means the extremes.

$$400 \neq 100$$

The proportion $10:20::5:4$ is not a true proportion.

When you know only three of four values of a proportion, you need to find the missing value. You will learn to find the missing value in both a ratio proportion and in a fractional proportion. Both methods lead to the same answer. Which method you select to use is a matter of personal preference.

You will use the means and extremes to find a missing value in a proportion. Remember that in a true proportion the product of the means must equal the product of the extremes. To find the missing value in a ratio proportion, write an equation setting the means equal to the extremes then solve the equation for the missing value.

In the proportion $2:4::?:12$ the ? represents the missing value. To find the value of ?, write your multiplication equations for the means and extremes using an equals sign, setting the means equal to the extremes. You can multiply the extremes in this equation to help find the missing value in the means.

$$4 \times ? = 2 \times 12 = 24$$

The product of the extremes is 24, and to have a true proportion you know that the product of means must equal 24.

$$4 \times ? = 2 \times 12$$
$$2 \times 12 = 24 \qquad \text{So } 4 \times ? = 24$$

Here you simply divide both sides by the know number in the means equation, or 4.

$$\frac{4 \times ?}{4} = \frac{24}{4}$$

Here $24 \div 4 = 6$ So $? = 6$
Now check that the proportion is true:

$$2:4::6:12$$
$$4 \times 6 = 24 \quad \text{and} \quad 2 \times 12 = 24 \quad \text{So } 4 \times 6 = 2 \times 12$$

The proportion is true.
Remember, taking the time to check your work will help you avoid errors.

EXAMPLE ▶ Find the missing value in $25:5::50:?$.

1. Write an equation setting the product of the means equal to the product of the extremes.

$$5 \times 50 = 25 \times ?$$
$$5 \times 50 = 250 \qquad \text{So } 25 \times ? = 250$$

2. Solve the equation. Divide both sides by 25.

$$\frac{250}{25} = \frac{25 \times ?}{25}$$

Here 250 ÷ 25 = 10   So ? = 10

3. Restate the proportion, inserting the missing value:

$$25:5::50:10$$

4. Check your work.

$$5 \times 50 = 25 \times 10$$
$$250 = 250$$

The proportion is true.

Super Tech . . .

Open the CD-ROM that accompanies your textbook and select Chapter 2, Exercise 2-14. Review the animation and example problems, and then complete the practice problems.

Cross-Multiplying

Cross-multiplying: Multiplying the numerator of the first fraction by the denominator of the second fraction and the denominator of the second fraction by the numerator of the first fraction.

Earlier in this chapter, you learned that a proportion can be written with ratios or with fractions. Writing a proportion as A:B::C:D is the same as writing it as $\frac{A}{B} = \frac{C}{D}$. Remember to determine whether a proportion is true, you compare the products of the means (*B* and *C*) with the product of the extremes (*A* and *D*). When a proportion is written with fractions, you will use the method of **cross-multiplying** to determine if it is true by multiplying the numerator of the first fraction by the denominator of the second fraction and the denominator of the second fraction by the numerator of the first fraction. See Figure 2-2. The numerator of the first fraction, *A*, and the denominator of the second fraction, *D*, are the extremes of the ratio proportion. The denominator of the first fraction, *B*, and the numerator of the second fraction, *C*, are the means. Just as with ratio proportions, simply multiply the means and extremes to determine if the fraction proportion is true.

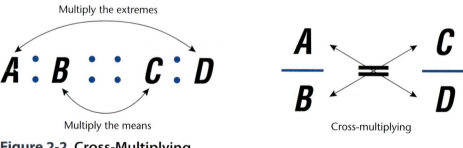

Figure 2-2 Cross-Multiplying

To determine if a fraction proportion is true, cross-multiply. Multiply the numerator of the first fraction with the denominator of the second fraction. Next, multiply the denominator of the first fraction with the numerator of the second fraction, and then compare the products. The products must be equal.

EXAMPLE 1 ▶   Determine if $\frac{2}{5} = \frac{10}{25}$ is a true proportion.

1. Cross-multiply.

$$\frac{2}{5} = \frac{10}{25} \rightarrow 2 \times 25 = 5 \times 10$$

2. Compare the products on both sides of the equal sign.

$$2 \times 25 = 5 \times 10$$
$$50 = 50$$

The proportion $\frac{2}{5} = \frac{10}{25}$ is true.

EXAMPLE 2 ▶   Determine if $\frac{5}{8} = \frac{40}{72}$ is a true proportion.

1. Cross-multiply.

$$\frac{5}{8} = \frac{40}{72} \rightarrow 5 \times 72 = 8 \times 40$$

2. Compare the products on both sides of the equal sign.

$$5 \times 72 = 8 \times 40$$
$$360 \neq 320$$

The proportion $\frac{5}{8} = \frac{8}{40}$ is not true.

Super Tech . . .

Open the CD-ROM that accompanies your textbook and select Chapter 2, Exercise 2-15. Review the animation and example problems, and then complete the practice problems.

✓ Review and Practice 2-6 Means and Extremes

Determine whether the following proportions are true.

1. $6:12::12:24$ _____

2. $3:8::9:32$ _____

3. $5:75::15:250$ _____

4. $8:100::20:250$ _____

Use the means and extremes to find the missing values.

5. $10:?::5:8$? = _____

6. $10:4::20:?$? = _____

7. $4:25::16:?$? = _____

8. $?:15::100:75$? = _____

Strength of Mixtures

Strengths of mixtures: Are used to indicate the concentration of ingredients in mixtures such as solutions, lotions, creams, and ointments.

When you are in the pharmacy you will work with medications that have a percent strength. **Strengths of mixtures** are commonly used to indicate the concentration of ingredients in mixtures such as solutions, lotions, creams, and ointments. While mixtures may contain many different components, it is the amount of the medication or medications in the mixture that is important when you are calculating doses.

Mixtures can be divided into two different categories: fluid and solid or semisolid.

Fluid mixtures are those that flow. One example is a solution. Other fluid mixtures include suspensions and lotions.

These terms are important to understanding solutions: solute, solvent or diluent, and solution.

Solute: Chemicals dissolved in a solvent, making a solution; drug or substance being dissolved in a solution.

Solvent or diluent: Liquid used to dissolve other chemicals, making a solution.

Solution: The combined mixture of solvent or diluent.

- The **solute** is the chemicals dissolved in a solvent, making a solution; drug or substance being dissolved in a solution.
- The **solvent (diluent)** is the liquid used to dissolve other chemicals, making a solution.
- The **solution** is the combined mixture of solvent or diluent.

Let's break it down, when you dissolve 1 teaspoon (tsp) of sugar into 8 oz of tap water. The sugar is the solute. The tap water is the solvent or diluent. The sugar water is the solution. Solid or semisolid mixtures are creams and ointments.

For fluid mixtures prepared with a dry medication, the **percent strength** represents the number of grams of the medication contained in **100 mL** of the solution. In a solution with a 3 percent strength, there are 3 grams of medication in each 100 mL of the solution.

This can be written as the fraction $\frac{3\text{ g}}{100\text{ mL}}$.

For fluid mixtures prepared with a liquid medication, the percent strength represents the number of milliliters of medication contained in **100 mL** of the mixture. In a mixture with a 5 percent strength, there are 5 mL of medications in each 100 mL of the mixture.

This can be written as the fraction $\frac{5\text{ mL}}{100\text{ mL}}$.

To determine the amount of hydrocortisone powder in 300 mL of 2 percent hydrocortisone lotion, we know that each percent represents 1 gram (g) of hydrocortisone per 100 mL of lotion. Therefore 2 percent hydrocortisone lotion contains 2 g of hydrocortisone power in every 100 mL of the mixture. We need to find how many grams of hydrocortisone powder are in 300 mL of a 2 percent hydrocortisone mixture.

EXAMPLE ▶ $\dfrac{2\text{ g}}{100\text{ mL}} \times \dfrac{?}{300\text{ mL}}$

Cross-multiply.

$$100 \times ? = 100\ ?$$
$$2\text{ g} \times 300 = 600\text{ g}$$
$$100? = 600\text{ g}$$
$$? = 6\text{ g}$$

There are 6 g of 2 percent hydrocortisone powder in a 300 mL mixture.

EXAMPLE 1 ▶ Determine the amount of ethanol in 500 mL of a 30 percent ethanol solution. (Ethanol is a liquid.) The percent strength (30 percent) tells us that every 100 mL of the solution contains 30 mL of ethanol.

$$\frac{30 \text{ mL}}{100 \text{ mL}} \times \frac{?}{500 \text{ mL}}$$

Cross-multiply.

$$100 \times ? = 100?$$
$$30 \text{ mL} \times 500 = 15{,}000 \text{ mL}$$
$$100? = 15{,}000 \text{ mL}$$
$$? = 150 \text{ mL}$$

Since percent means "per 100," the percent strength of a solution is always calculated on the amount of a drug per 100 mL. Solutions with higher percent strengths contain more of the drug in each 100 mL and, therefore, are stronger solutions. For example, a 10 percent solution has twice as much drug (10 g per 100 mL) as a 5 percent solution (5 g per 100 mL). See Table 2-2 to compare solution strengths.

Table 2-2   Comparing Solution Strengths

Amount of Solution	Solution Strength	Dry Drug	Liquid Drug
50 mL	1%	0.5 g	0.5 mL
100 mL	1%	1 g	1 mL
200 mL	1%	2 g	2 mL
50 mL	2%	1 g	1 mL
100 mL	2%	2 g	2 mL
200 mL	2%	4 g	4 mL
100 mL	5%	5 g	5 mL
50 mL	10%	5 g	5 mL
100 mL	10%	10 g	10 mL
200 mL	10%	20 g	20 mL

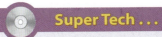

Super Tech . . .

Open the CD-ROM that accompanies your textbook and select Chapter 2, Exercise 2-16. Review the animation and example problems, and then complete the practice problems.

Review and Practice 2-7 Strength of Mixtures

Note: 100 mL = 100 cc. The abbreviation *cc* represents cubic centimeters and *mL* represents milliliters. Measurements and abbreviations such as mL and cc will be discussed in Chapter 3.

1. How many grams of drug are in 100 mL of a 5 percent solution?

2. How many grams of drug are in 100 mL of a 6 percent solution?

3. How many grams of drug are in 100 mL of a 10 percent solution?

4. How many grams of dextrose will a patient receive from 20 mL of a 5 percent solution?

5. The drug label states that 50 mL of pure drug is contained in 100 mL of solution. What is the strength of the solution in percent?

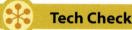 **Tech Check**

Confusing Multiplying Fractions with Cross-Multiplying

A pharmacy technician is preparing a 5 percent solution of dextrose in batches of 500 cubic centimeters or milliliters (mL). She sets up the calculation as follows: $\frac{5\,g}{100\,mL} = \frac{?}{500\,mL}$.

Distracted by a call, she returns to the calculation and computes:

$$5 \times ? = 100 \times 500 = 50,000$$

This calculation leads to:

$$? = 10,000$$

Think Before You Act

The technician realizes that mixing 10,000 g for a solution with 500 mL is not reasonable. Looking at her work, she realizes she has treated the problem as if she were multiplying fractions rather than solving a proportion problem. She has mistakenly multiplied the two numerators and set their product equal to the product of the two denominators.

To calculate correctly, the technician should cross-multiply 100 × ? and 5 × 500. In turn, 100 × ? = 2500 and ? = 25

The technician will need 25 g, *not* 10,000 g, of dextrose.

The technician did not double-check her answer by making sure that the answer gave a true proportion. If she had, she would have found that 5 g/100 mL is not equal to 10,000 g/500 mL. Fortunately, the answer that she calculated was not reasonable, and she was able to detect the error. Sometimes, however, even a wrong answer can be reasonable. *Always double-check your answer when performing dosage calculations.*

✓ Chapter 2 Review

Test Your Knowledge

Multiple Choice

Select the best answer and write the letter on the line.

_____ 1. What is a combined mixture?
   A. The solution
   B. The solute
   C The diluent
   D. The solvent

_____ 2. What is the liquid with which the solute is combined?
   A. The solvent
   B. The solute
   C. The diluent
   D. Both A and C

_____ 3. What is the substance being dissolved in a combined mixture?
   A. The solvent
   B. The solute
   C. The diluent
   D. The solution

Practice Your Knowledge

In each row of the table below, use the information to calculate the equivalent values. For instance, in row 1, convert the ratio 2 : 3 to a fraction, a decimal, and a percent. Where necessary, round decimals to the nearest hundredth. Round the percents to the nearest whole percent. Do not reduce ratios and fractions.

	Fraction	Decimal	Ratio	Percent
1.			2:3	
2.	$\frac{5}{4}$			
3.				28%
4.		0.03		
5.	$\frac{40}{8}$			
6.			4:12	
7.	$\frac{9}{27}$			
8.		1.4		
9.				0.5%
10.			3:50	
11.				25%
12.		6		
13.	$\frac{1}{9}$			
14.				150%
15.			6:97	
16.		12.8		

Find the missing value.

17. $1:10::4:?$

18. $3:27::?:9$

19. $?:6::8:12$

20. $5:?::10:50$

21. $\dfrac{4}{8} = \dfrac{24}{?}$

22. $\dfrac{?}{14} = \dfrac{5}{70}$

23. $\dfrac{3}{?} = \dfrac{30}{20}$

24. $\dfrac{1}{25} = \dfrac{?}{125}$

25. If 1 tablet contains 25 mg of drug, how many milligrams of drug are in 3 tablets?

26. If 100 mL of drug is in 600 mL of solution, how many milliliters of drug are in 1800 mL of solution?

27. A solution is 5 percent dextrose. How many grams (g) of dextrose are in 500 cc of solution?

28. A solution contains 1 g of drug for every 50 mL of solution. How much solution would you need to give a patient to administer 3 g of drug?

29. 10 mL of a liquid medication contains 250 mg of drug. How many milliliters contain 50 mg of drug?

30. If 30 g of drug is in 100 mL of solution, what is the ratio strength of the solution?

Apply your Knowledge

Comparing the Numbers

You are the pharmacy technician working in the pharmacy. You need to determine how much medication should be dispensed by the pharmacist to the patient. The physician's drug order on the prescription reads: "Take $\frac{1}{2}$ tablet in the morning and take 1 tablet at bedtime for 6 days." The medication has 100 milligrams in each tablet.

Answer the following questions:

1. How many tablets need to be dispensed?

   _____

2. How many milligrams will the patient take each day?

   _____

3. How many tablets will the patient take each day?

   _____

4. Convert the fraction of daily tablets to a decimal.

   _____

5. Write the daily ratio of mg to tablets.

   _____

Internet Activity

To obtain a better understanding of solutions, lotions, creams, suspensions, and ointments, search for these terms on the Internet. Find their definitions and at least three example medications of each type. You can start with an online dictionary such as found on www.refdesk.com and then search websites such as www.fda.gov or www.rxlist.com for example medications.

Super Tech...

Open the CD-ROM that accompanies your textbook and do a final review of Chapter 2. For a final evaluation, take the chapter test and e-mail or print your results for your instructor. A score of 95 percent or above indicates mastery of the chapter concepts.

3

Systems of Measurement and Weight

Key Terms

Centi (c)
Dram (ʒ)
Grain (gr)
Gram (g)
International unit (IU)
Kilo (k)
Liter (L)
Meter (m)
Micro (mc)
Milli (m)
Milliequivalents (mEq)
Minim (♏)
Ounce (ʒ)
Unit (there is no symbol used for unit)

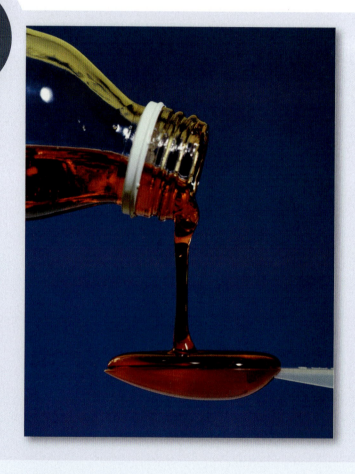

Learning Outcomes

When you have successfully completed Chapter 3, you will have mastered skills to be able to:

▸ Summarize metric notation.

▸ Calculate equivalent measurements within the metric system.

▸ Identify the most frequently used equivalent measurements among metric, household, and apothecaries' measurements.

▸ Convert measurements between the metric, household, and apothecary systems of measurement.

▸ List the fundamental units of the metric system for length, weight, and volume.

▸ Recognize the symbols for dram, ounce, grain, and drop.

▸ Calculate temperature and time conversions.

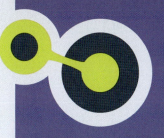

Introduction

Understanding and converting systems of weights and measures are required skills of a pharmacy technician. Most medications taken by patients are measured in grams or milligrams. These are basic units of the metric system. As a pharmacy technician it is imperative that you master the concepts of the systems of measurements and weights. You need to be able to "measure up to the mark," so to speak, as you will use units of measurement and weight in all dosage calculations.

Critical Thinking in the Pharmacy
Measuring up to the Mark

You are the pharmacy technician working in the pharmacy. A patient suffering from pink-eye (conjunctivitis) and a cold is given two prescriptions. One prescription reads: "Take 15 mL of cough suppressant every 8 h for 10 days." The other, for eye drops, reads: "Use 2 drops in each eye twice a day for 5 days." The patient will be using a household measuring device to measure the dose of cough suppressant. How many milliliters of each medication need to be dispensed?

After you have completed Chapter 3 you will be able to determine how many milliliters need to be dispensed, how many teaspoons and/or tablespoons the patient will take each day, and convert between systems of measurement.

PTCB Correlations

When you have completed this chapter you will have the mathematical building block of knowledge needed to assist you in performing dosage calculations.

▶ Knowledge of pharmacy calculations (for example, algebra, ratio and proportions, metric conversions, IV drip rates, IV admixture calculations (Statement I-50).

▶ Knowledge of measurement systems (for example metric and avoirdupois) (Statement I-51).

Metric System

Meter: The basic unit of length in the metric system.

The metric system is the most widely used system of measurement in the world today. The system, which was defined in 1792, gets its name from the **meter,** the basic unit of length in the metric system.

Units of measurement in the metric system are sometimes referred to as SI units, an abbreviation for International System of Units. This system was established in 1960 to make units of measurement for the metric system standard throughout the world.

Table 3-1 lists the basic metric units for weight and volume.

Table 3-1   Basic Units of Metric Measurement

Type of Measure	Basic Unit	Abbreviation
Weight (or mass)	gram	g
Volume	liter	L

Gram- : The basic unit of measurement for weight in the metric system.

Liter: The basic unit for measurement of volume in the metric system.

Gram (g) the basic unit of measurement for weight in the metric system, is abbreviated with a lowercase letter, but **liter (L),** the basic unit for measurement of volume in the metric system, is abbreviated with an uppercase L. Using the uppercase L minimizes the chance of confusing the lowercase letter L (l) with the digit 1. As a pharmacy technician you will use weight and volume frequently when you calculate dosages.

Most dosages and drug strengths are expressed using the metric system. (see Figure 3.1)

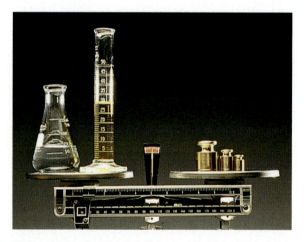

Figure 3-1 Most dosages and drug strengths are measured in weight or volume.

Understanding Metric Notation

The metric system is based on multiples of 10 just like the decimal system and the dollar. The greater confidence you have working with decimals, the more comfortable you will be working with metric units. To review decimals, see Chapter 1.

If you think of everything in terms of money it may help you understand the system better. For example, a half milliliter is written as 0.5 mL, and a

Kilo- : The metric prefix that indicates the basic unit multiplied by 1000.

Milli- : The metric prefix that indicates one-thousandth of the basic unit.

Centi- : The metric prefix that indicates one-hundredth of the basic unit.

Micro- : The metric prefix that indicates one-millionth of the basic unit.

half dollar is written as 0.50. So you could think about half a milliliter as 50 cents.

As stated earlier, the basic unit of measurement for weight in the metric system is gram (g). A prefix before the basic unit indicates relative size. For example, **kilo- (k)** is the metric prefix that indicates that the basic unit is multiplied by 1000. A kilogram is 1000 grams, and a kiloliter is 1000 liters. When you divide 1 gram into 1000 equal parts, each part is 1 milligram. The metric prefix **milli- (m)** indicates one-thousandth of the basic unit. A milliliter is one-thousandth of a liter, and a milligram is one-thousandth of a gram. **Centi- (c)** is the metric prefix that indicates one-hundredth of the basic unit and **micro- (mc)** is the metric prefix that indicates one-millionth of the basic unit. Table 3-2 lists several common prefixes, their abbreviations, and their value relative to the basic unit. As a pharmacy technician, you will use metric prefixes in dosage calculations such as kilo-, milli-, centi- and micro-.

Table 3-2 Combining Prefixes and Units

Prefix	Weight (Mass) (gram)	Volume (liter)
kilo- ($\times$1000)	kilogram kg	kiloliter kL
centi ($\div$100)	centigram cg	centiliter cL
milli- ($\div$1000)	milligram mg	milliliter mL
micro- ($\div$1,000,000)	microgram mcg	microliter mcL

Writing Units of Metric Measurements

To write units of metric measurements follow these simple rules:

- Use Arabic numbers with decimals to represent any fractions. To represent $1\frac{1}{4}$ g, you would write 1.25 g.
- If the quantity is less than 1, include a 0 before the decimal point. Delete any other zeros that are not necessary. Three quarters $\left(\frac{3}{4}\right)$ of a dollar is 75 cents. You would write this as $0.75.
- Always write the unit of measurement after the quantity with a space between them. Thirty milligrams is written as 30 mg.
- Use uppercase L to represent liter and use lowercase letters for all other metric abbreviations. Write mg and write mL, *not* ml. While ml is also technically correct, writing mL will help you avoid errors in dosage calculations.

Now, using the above rules, let's determine the correct metric notation for six and two-eighths milliliters. First, $6\frac{2}{8}$ must be converted to decimals. Always reduce to lowest terms; $\frac{2}{8}$ can be reduced to $\frac{1}{4}$ and $\frac{1}{4}$ converts to the decimal 0.25 by dividing 1 by 4.

$$6\frac{2}{8} = 6.25$$

Next, write the unit of measurement after the quantity, leaving a space between them and using the abbreviation mL for milliliters. The correct metric notation for six and two-eighths milliliters is 6.25 mL.

Determine the correct metric notation to write one-half milligram.

$$\frac{1}{2} = 0.5$$

Place a zero in front of the decimal point, and delete any unnecessary zeros. 0.5

Place the unit of measurement after the quantity with a space between them.

The correct metric notation for one-half milligram is 0.5 mg.

Super Tech . . .

Open the CD-ROM that accompanies your textbook and select Chapter 3, Exercise 3-1. Review the animation and example problems, and then complete the practice problems. Continue to the next section of the book once you have mastered the information presented.

Review and Practice 3-1 Metric System

In Exercises 1–10, select the correct metric notation.

1. Two and one-half kilograms

   a. 2.5 Kg
   b. 2.05 kg
   c. $2\frac{1}{2}$ kg
   d. 2.5 kg

2. Seven-tenths of a milliliter

   a. $\frac{7}{10}$ mL
   b. .7 mL
   c. ml 0.7
   d. 0.7 mL

3. Four-hundredths of a gram

   a. 400 G
   b. 0.4 g
   c. 0.04 g
   d. .04 g

4. Thirty-one milliliters

   a. 31ml
   b. 0.031 mL
   c. 31.0 ml
   d. 31 mL

5. Eight liters

   a. 8.0 l
   b. 8 L
   c. 8.0 L
   d. 0.8 l

6. One hundred twenty-five micrograms

   a. 125 mg
   b. 0.125 mcg
   c. 125 mcg
   d. 125mg

7. Seventy-eight grams

   a. 78 gm
   b. 78.0 gm
   c. 0.78 g
   d. 78 g

8. Two hundred fifty microliters

   a. mcL 250   b. 250 mcL   c. 25.0 mcL   d. 250 mL

9. Nine and one-quarter milligrams

   a. $9\frac{1}{4}$ mg   b. 9.25 mg   c. 9.75 mg   d. 9.25 mgm

10. Four-tenths of a liter

    a. 0.4 L   b. $\frac{4}{10}$ L   c. 0.40 L   d. 0.40 l

In Exercises 11–20, write the indicated amounts.

11. Four and one-half milliliters _____

12. Sixty-two hundredths of a gram _____

13. Three-quarters of a milliliter _____

14. Seven-tenths of a gram _____

15. Twelve liters _____

16. Nine-twelfths of a kilogram _____

17. One hundred fifty-seven kilograms _____

18. Seven and three-quarters liters _____

19. Ninety-three micrograms _____

20. Eight-hundredths of a milligram _____

Converting within the Metric System

When you calculate dosages, you will work most often with four metric units of weight and three metric units of volume. The four units of weight are kilogram (kg), gram (g), milligram (mg), and microgram (mcg). Two of the units of volume are liter (L) and milliliter (mL). The third is cubic centimeter (cc), which is equivalent to milliliter (mL).

Although the abbreviation cc for cubic centimeter may be seen in practice, it should not be used as it can be mistaken for units (U). Instead use the abbreviation mL for milliliter.

In Chapter 1 you learned that when you multiply a decimal number by 100, you get a larger number and the decimal point moves two places to the right. When you divide a decimal number by 100, you get a smaller number and the decimal point moves two places to the left.

Converting one metric unit of measurement to another is similar to multiplying and dividing decimal numbers. For example, if you travel 1 kilometer, you travel 1000 meters. When you convert from the larger unit of measurement (kilometer) to the smaller unit of measurement (meter), the number of units increases. When you multiply, the decimal point moves to the right.

If you convert from meters to kilometers, the quantity of units decreases. If you travel 1000 meters, you travel 1 kilometer. When you convert from a smaller unit of measurement (meter) to a larger unit of measurement

Memory tip *Count the number of zeros to determine how many spaces your decimal point will move when converting from or to the basic unit of measure.*

(kilometer), the number of units decreases. When you divide, the decimal point moves to the left.

The four units of weight, or mass, are related to each other by a factor of 1000. A kilogram is 1000 times larger than a gram. A gram is 1000 times larger than a milligram, which is 1000 times larger than a microgram. The same relationship is true for liters and milliliters; a liter is 1000 times larger than a milliliter. Table 3-3 lists four of the most commonly used equivalent measurements. Because they are so important to dosage calculations, you should memorize them.

Table 3-3   Equivalent Metric Measurements

1 kg = 1000 g	1 mg = 1000 mcg
1 g = 1000 mg	1 L = 1000 mL

To convert a quantity from one unit of metric measurement to another:

To convert from a larger ***unit of measurement*** to a smaller ***unit of measurement,*** divide, which moves your decimal point to the left because it has a lesser value.

To convert from a smaller ***unit of measurement*** to a larger ***unit of measurement,*** multiply, which moves your decimal point to the right because it has a greater value.

Figure 3-2 will help you determine both the direction and the number of places to move the decimal point when you convert between units of metric measurement. For example, as shown in figure 3-2, milliliter is three places to the right of the basic unit of a liter.

Prefix	kilo-	hecto-	deca-	Base Unit	deci-	centi-	milli-	decimilli-	centimilli-	micro-
Value	1000	100	10	1	$\frac{1}{10}$	$\frac{1}{100}$	$\frac{1}{1000}$	$\frac{1}{10,000}$	$\frac{1}{100,000}$	$\frac{1}{1,000,000}$
Abbreviation	kg			gram			mg			mcg
	kL			liter			mL			mcL
Value relation to Base Unit	1000	100	10	1	0.1	0.01	0.001	0.0001	0.00001	0.000001

Figure 3-2 Metric System Place Values—To convert a quantity from liters (larger) to milliliters (smaller), multiply by 1000 (which moves the decimal point three places to the right). Similarly, to convert a quantity from grams (smaller) to kilograms (larger), divide by 1000 (which moves the decimal point three places to the left).

EXAMPLE 1 ▶ Convert 4 L to milliliters (mL).

A milliliter (mL) is smaller than a liter (L); a quantity will have more milliliters than liters. Using Figure 3-2, you can see that there are 1000 milliliters in each liter. The number of units increases by a factor of 1000 and decimal point for 4 liters moved three places to the right to indicate the number of milliliters.

$$4 \text{ L} \times 1000 = 4.0 \text{ L} \times 1000 = 4000 \text{ mL}$$

EXAMPLE 2 ❯   Convert 4.5 mcg to milligrams (mg).

You are converting from a smaller unit to a larger one. Divide 4.5 by 1000, moving the decimal point three places to the left.

$$4.5 \text{ mcg} \div 1000 = 0004.5 \text{ mcg} \div 1000 = 0.0045 \text{ mg}$$

EXAMPLE 3 ❯   Convert 62 kg to grams (g).

You are converting from a larger unit to a smaller one. Multiply 62 by 1000 moving the decimal point three places to the right.

$$62 \text{ kg} \times 1000 = 62.000 \text{ kg} \times 1000 = 62,000 \text{ g}$$

Super Tech . . .

Open the CD-ROM that accompanies your textbook and select Chapter 3, Exercise 3-2. Review the animation and example problems, and then complete the practice problems. Continue to the next section of the book once you have mastered the information presented.

⚠ Caution!

Remember: The larger the unit, the smaller the quantity. The smaller the unit, the larger the quantity.

You may be tempted to multiply when you convert from a smaller unit to a larger unit, thinking that you are increasing in size. If you find yourself confused, think about conversions you have made all your life.

For example, a dollar bill is a larger unit of money than a quarter, which is a larger unit of money than a penny. When you write their relationship, look at how the quantity changes:

$$1 \text{ dollar bill} = 4 \text{ quarters} = 100 \text{ pennies}$$

When you convert from the larger unit of measure to the smaller one, the quantity increases. Writing the money relationship as:

$$100 \text{ pennies} = 4 \text{ quarters} = 1 \text{ dollar bill}$$

This shows you that as the unit of measurement increases in size, the quantity actually decreases. You see the same relationship with units of time and in the metric system:

$$1 \text{ hour} = 60 \text{ minutes} = 3600 \text{ seconds}$$
$$1 \text{ g} = 1000 \text{ mg} = 1,000,000 \text{ mcg}$$

Tech Check

Placing the Decimal Point Correctly

You are the pharmacy technician working in the pharmacy. The physician orders 0.05 mg of medication for a child. You quickly calculate that 0.05 mg = 500 mcg, and you give the medication to the pharmacist for verification. Fortunately, the pharmacist catches the error before the medication is sold. The child should be given 50 mcg, not 500 mcg of medication.

Think Before You Act

When you convert quantities from one unit of measure to another, pay close attention to the decimal point. In going from milligrams (mg) to micrograms (mcg), the quantity should be multiplied by 1000; the decimal should move three places to the right.

$$0.05 \text{ mg} \times 1000 = 0.050 \text{ mg} \times 1000 = 50 \text{ mcg}$$

Be even more careful when the patient is a child. Dosages that are perfectly safe for adults may be life-threatening for children.

✓ Review and Practice 3-2 Converting within the Metric System

In Exercises 1–20, complete the conversions.

1. 7 g = _____ mg

2. 1200 mg = _____ g

3. 23 g = _____ kg

4. 8 kg = _____ g

5. 8.01 L = _____ mL

6. 100 mL = _____ L

7. 3.6 L = _____ mL

8. 5233 mg = _____ g

9. 500 mL = _____ L

10. 3.25 kg = _____ g

11. 0.25 mg = _____ mcg

12. 462 mg = _____ mcg

13. 250 mcg = _____ mg

14. 75 mcg = _____ mg

15. 0.06 g = _____ mcg

16. 0.5 g = _____ mcg

17. 8000 mcg = _____ g

18. 20,000 mcg = _____ g

Other Systems of Measurement

Milliequivalent: A unit of measure based on the chemical combining power of the substance; one-thousandth of an equivalent of a chemical.

Pharmacy technicians must be able to work with all systems of measurement used in medication orders. The most commonly used is the metric system of measurement. There are two other systems of measurement still used, the apothecary and household systems. There are also two other measures, **milliequivalent,** which is a unit of measure based on the chemical combining power of the substance, defined as one-thousandth of an equivalent of a chemical, and units that are used for certain medications, such as insulin.

Apothecary System

The apothecary system is an old system of measurement. Used first by apothecaries (early pharmacists), it traveled across Europe from Greece and Rome to France and England. Eventually, it crossed the Atlantic to colonial America. The household system familiar to most Americans evolved from the apothecary system. Although this system is not widely used today, you must still be familiar with it. Certain medications, especially older ones such as aspirin and morphine, are still measured in apothecary units.

Units of measure

Grain: The basic unit of weight in the apothecary system.

The basic unit of weight in the apothecary system is the **grain (gr).**

Originally, the grain was defined as the weight of a single grain of wheat, hence its name.

Minim: Common unit of volume in the apothecary system.

Three units of volume in the apothecary system are the **minim (m),** the **dram (ʒ),** and the **ounce (ʒ).** The apothecary ounce has become part of the common system of measures used in the United States. There are 8 ounces (oz) to 1 cup (c) in our commonly used household system of measures. The minim is seldom used these days, although many syringes continue to have marks that indicate minims. The dram symbol is most frequently used as an abbreviation for a teaspoonful, which has nearly the same volume.

Dram: Common unit of volume in the apothecary system.

Ounce: Common unit of volume in the apothecary system.

Apothecary notation

The system of apothecary notation has special rules that combine fractions, Roman and Arabic numerals, symbols, and abbreviations. Even the order in which information is written differs from the order you are used to. Recall that Roman numerals may be written with a bar above them.

Rules to remember when you are writing a value in the apothecary system:

1. If a value is less than 1, write it as a fraction. However, if the value is one-half, write it as the abbreviation "ss."
2. Write values with lowercase Roman numerals.
3. Use the abbreviation "gr" to represent grain. Use the symbols **m, ʒ, ʒ,** and to represent minim, dram, and ounce, respectively.
4. Write the abbreviation, symbol, or unit before the quantity.

EXAMPLE 1 ▶ Write *four grains,* using apothecary notation.

Use lowercase Roman numerals to represent four as iv. Abbreviate grains as gr, and place it before the quantity: gr iv or gr $\overline{\text{iv}}$.

EXAMPLE 2 ▶ Write *twelve ounces,* using apothecary notation.

Use the Roman numeral xii. Use the symbol for ounces and place it before the quantity: ʒ xii.

EXAMPLE 3 ▶ Write *two* and *one-half grains,* using apothecary notation.

Use lowercase Roman numerals to represent two as ii. Abbreviate one-half as ss, writing two and one-half as iiss. The abbreviation for grain is written before the quantity: gr iiss.

> ⚠️ **Caution!**
>
> Do not confuse grains and grams.

A grain is a measure in the apothecary system and a gram is a measure in the metric system. Often grains (gr) and grams (g) are confused because they have names and abbreviations that are similar. If you are not sure whether an order refers to grains or grams, check with the physician or pharmacist. For *most* conversions, 1 grain equals 60 milligrams (mg), which means:

$$1 \text{ gr} = 60 \text{ mg} = 0.06 \text{ g}$$

1 grain is significantly smaller than 1 gram. Medications that are measured in grains do not all use the same conversion. The conversion varies from 60 mg to 66.7 mg per grain. The most common conversion is that 1 grain = 60 mg. You will need to use information from the drug label or a drug reference to help you determine which equivalent measure to use for a given drug.

However, their labels list the metric units as well.

> ⚠️ **Caution!**
>
> Do not confuse the symbols for drams (℥) and ounces (℥).

The symbols for drams and ounces appear similar. When they are typed, the symbol for dram looks similar to the numeral 3; the symbol for ounce has an extra line at the top. When they are handwritten, the symbol for dram can look like the written letter *z*. Again, the symbol for ounce has an extra line at the top. As always, if you are in doubt about which symbol is used, check with the physician or pharmacist.

> 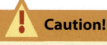 **Super Tech . . .**
>
> Open the CD-ROM that accompanies your textbook and select Chapter 3, Exercise 3-3. Review the animation and example problems, and then complete the practice problems. Continue to the next section of the book once you have mastered the information presented.

Household System

The household system of measurement is still commonly used today. Patients who take medication at home are more likely to use everyday household measures than metric ones. Many over-the-counter medications provide instructions for patients based on household measures. For instance, a patient will be told to take two teaspoons of a cough syrup, which is equivalent to 10 mL.

Units of measure

Basic units of volume in the household system, from smallest to largest, include the drop, teaspoon, tablespoon, ounce, cup, pint, quart, and gallon. Of these, the four smallest measures are most commonly used for medications.

When working with medications and dosage calculations, the word *ounce* generally implies volume; it represents a fluid ounce of a liquid medication.

Household notation

Like the metric system, household notation places the quantity in Arabic numbers before the abbreviation for the unit. Table 3-4 summarizes the standard abbreviations. To write *six drops*, using household notation, write the quantity with the Arabic number before the abbreviation for the unit of measurement: 6 gtt. To write *twelve ounces*, using household notation, write the quantity with the Arabic number before the abbreviation for the unit of measurement: 12 oz.

Table 3-4   Abbreviations for Household Measures

Unit of Measurement	Abbreviation
Drop	gtt
Teaspoon	tsp, t, or ℨ*
Tablespoon	tbsp, tbs or T
Ounce	oz or ℨ*
Cup	cup or c
Pint	pt
Quart	qt
Gallon	gal

* When you refer to the apothecary symbols for teaspoon and ounce, Roman numerals are used.

Apothecary and Household Equivalents

Most all units of measurement found in both the apothecary and the household systems are equal; for example, an apothecary ounce equals a household ounce. Unlike the metric system, neither the apothecary system nor the household system is based on multiples of 10. You must become familiar with their equivalent measures (see Table 3-5). In practice, the size of a drop depends on the dropper and the liquid. A drop by itself is not a reliably accurate form of measurement.

Table 3-5   Apothecary, Metric, and Household Equivalent Measures

Household	Apothecary Equivalent	Metric Equivalent
Drop	1 drop = 1 minim	15 to 20 drops* = 1 mL
Teaspoon	1 teaspoon = 60 drops	1 teaspoon = 5 mL
Tablespoon	1 tablespoon = 3 teaspoons	1 tablespoon = 15 mL
Ounce	1 ounce = 2 tablespoons = 8 drams	1 ounce = 30 mL
Cup	1 cup = 8 ounces	1 cup = 240 mL

* In practice, the size of a drop depends on the dropper and the liquid.

EXAMPLE 1 ▶ How many teaspoons of solution are contained in 1 ounce (oz) of solution?

From Table 3-6, you can see that 1 ounce contains 2 tablespoons. In turn, each tablespoon contains 3 teaspoons. Therefore, one ounce of solution contains six teaspoons of solution.

EXAMPLE 2 ▶ How many tablespoons are in $\frac{1}{2}$ cup of solution?

Convert 1 cup to ounces, then ounces to tablespoons. From Table 2-6, you know that 1 cup = 8 oz and that 1 oz = 2 tbsp:

$$\frac{1}{2}\text{ cup} = \frac{1}{2} \times \text{cup} = \frac{1}{2} \times 8\text{ oz} = 4\text{ oz} = 4 \times 1\text{ oz} = 4 \times 2\text{ tbsp} = 8\text{ tbsp}$$

One-half cup of solution contains eight tablespoons of solution.

Milliequivalents and Units

Some drugs are measured in milliequivalents (mEq). A unit of measure based on the chemical combining power of the substance, one milliequivalent is defined as an equivalent weight of a chemical. Electrolytes, such as sodium and potassium, are often measured in milliequivalents. Sodium bicarbonate and potassium chloride are examples of drugs that are prescribed in milliequivalents. You do not need to learn to convert from milliequivalent to another system of measurement.

Unit: The amount of a medication required to produce a certain effect.

International unit: The amount of medication needed to produce a certain effect, standardized by international agreement.

Medications such as insulin, heparin, and penicillin are measured in *USP units*. (See Chapter 4 to learn more about USP.) A **unit** is the amount of a medication required to produce a certain effect. The size of a unit varies for each drug. Some medications, such as vitamins, are measured in standardized units called **international units (IU).**

These IUs represent the amount of medication needed to produce a certain effect, but they are standardized by international agreement. As with milliequivalents, you do not need to convert from units to other measures. Medications that are ordered in units will also be labeled in units.

✳ Tech Check

Understanding Abbreviations

A medication order on a prescription reads 450 mL. How many ounces should the pharmacy technician have the pharmacist dispense?

✳ Think Before You Act

The pharmacy technician needs to convert from milliliters to ounces, so he needs to know off the top of his head that there are 30 mL in an ounce, then divide the number of milliliters by 30 to solve the equation. The pharmacy technician needs 15 ounces of the medication.

✓ Review and Practice 3-3 Other Systems of Measurement

In Exercises 1–10, write the symbols or abbreviations.

1. Minim _____

2. Dram _____

3. Grain _____

4. Ounce _____

5. Drop _____

6. Teaspoon _____

7. Tablespoon _____

8. Pint _____

9. Milliequivalent _____

10. Unit _____

In Exercises 11–25, write the amounts, using either apothecary or household notation, as appropriate. (Some may require you to write the amount using both notations.)

11. Seven grains _____

12. Five drams _____

13. Three ounces _____

14. Eight ounces _____

15. Fourteen grains _____

16. Seventeen grains _____

17. One-half teaspoon _____

18. One-half tablespoon _____

19. One-half grain _____

20. One-half ounce _____

Converting among Metric, Apothecary, and Household Systems

When you calculate dosages, you must often convert among the metric, apothecary, and household systems of measurement. To do this, you will need to know how the measure of a quantity in one system compares with its measure in another system. For example, you learned the relationships between milliliter and liter and between teaspoon and tablespoon. To convert between systems, you may also need to know the relationship between milliliter and teaspoon. When you convert between systems, you lose a certain amount of exactness, especially when you round numbers. This may result in two measures often being approximately the same, but not exactly the same.

Equivalent Volume Measurements

Table 3-6 summarizes several important volume relationships.

A standard equivalent measure is that 1 tsp = 5 mL.

$$1 \text{ tsp} = 5 \text{ mL}$$

You can now determine most relationships between household or apothecary systems and metric systems. For instance, because 1 tbsp = 3 tsp,

$$1 \text{ tbsp} = 3 \text{ tsp} = 3 \times 1 \text{ tsp} = 3 \times 5 \text{ mL} = 15 \text{ mL}$$

We now know that 1 tbsp = 15 mL, and because 1 oz = 2 tbsp,

$$1 \text{ oz} = 2 \text{ tbsp} = 2 \times 1 \text{ tbsp} = 2 \times 15 \text{ mL} = 30 \text{ mL}$$

and

$$1 \text{ oz} = 30 \text{ mL}$$

Table 3-7 shows that 1 oz = 8 dr.
We now know that 1 oz = 8 dr = 2 tbsp = 30 mL.

Table 3-6   Approximate Equivalent Measures for Volume

Metric	Household	Apothecary
5 mL	1 tsp	1 dram*
15 mL	1 tbsp	3 drams*
30 mL	2 tbsp = 1 oz	1 oz = 8 drams*
240 mL	8 oz = 1c	8 oz
480 mL	2c = 1 pt	16 oz
960 mL	2 pt = 1 qt	32 oz

* The dram (dr) is used today to represent 1 tsp or 5 mL. Actually the dram has an exact volume of 3.7 mL.

Equivalent Weight Measurements

Earlier you learned that 1 grain is equivalent to 60 milligrams:

$$\text{gr i} = 60 \text{ mg}$$

The relationship between grains and milligrams or grams is actually more complex. The conversion varies from 60 mg to 66.7 mg per grain. You will need to use information from the drug label or a drug reference to help you determine which equivalent measure to use for a given drug.

In cases where you use 60 mg as the equivalent measure, one way to remember the relationship between grains and milligrams is to think of a clock (see Figure 3-3). If each "minute" is one milligram, then an entire hour is one grain. This image of the clock may help you when you need to find the equivalent of $\frac{1}{2}$ grain (gr ss) or $\frac{1}{4}$ grain $\left(\text{gr } \frac{1}{4}\right)$. Each half of an "hour" or grain is 30 "minutes" or milligrams. Similarly, each quarter of an "hour" or grain is 15 "minutes" or milligrams.

Table 3-7 summarizes important weight equivalent measures, including the relationship between kilograms and pounds (lb).

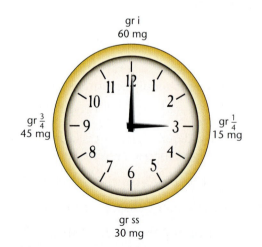

Figure 3-3 Use a clock and a round image to help you remember the comparison between 60 mg and 1 gr.

Table 3-7   Approximate Equivalent Measures for Weight Metric Apothecary

Metric	Apothecary
60 mg or 65 mg	gr i (1 grain)
45 mg	gr $\frac{3}{4}$
30 mg	gr ss ($\frac{1}{2}$ grain)
15 mg	gr $\frac{1}{4}$
1 mg	gr $\frac{1}{60}$
1g (1000 mg)	gr xv (15 grains)
0.5 g	gr viiss ($7\frac{1}{2}$ grains)
1 kg	2.2 lb

Conversion Factors

A conversion factor is a fraction made of two quantities that are equal to each other but are expressed in different units. For example, Table 3-8 tells us that 1 kg and 2.2 lb are equal to each other. Forming a fraction from these two quantities gives us a conversion factor. Two different conversion factors can be formed from these quantities, 1 kg/2.2 lb and 2.2 lb/1 kg. The first conversion factor, 1 kg/2.2 lb, is used to convert from pounds to kilograms, and the second conversion factor, 2.2 lb/1 kg, is used to convert from kilograms to pounds. As a pharmacy technician you will need to be able to do these conversions to perform dosage calculations, most commonly for pediatric patients. For example, a drug order may read: "Give 5 mg per kg of patient's weight." When you are writing conversion factors. the two quantities in the conversion factor must be equal to each other.

EXAMPLE ▶   Write a conversion factor for converting from milliliters to ounces.

According to Table 3-7, 30 mL is equivalent to 1 oz. Since we wish to convert to ounces, write the quantity with ounces as the numerator of the conversion factor. The conversion factor is 1 oz/30 mL. (*Note:* Other conversion factors from Table 3-7 include 8 oz/240 mL, 16 oz/480 mL, and 32 oz/960 mL. Each of these factors can be reduced to 1 oz/30 mL, but using the reduced conversion factor will make the conversion easier to solve.)

Super Tech . . .

Open the CD-ROM that accompanies your textbook and select Chapter 3, Exercise 3-4. Review the animation and example problems, and then complete the practice problems. Continue to the next section of the book once you have mastered the information presented.

Using Conversion Factors

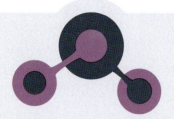

The Fraction Proportion Method

Cross-multiplying can be used to convert from one unit to another if you know a conversion factor. Recall from Chapter 2 that you can solve proportions for an unknown value by cross-multiplying. One of the fractions in your proportion is the conversion factor itself. The other fraction contains the unknown value in the numerator and the value that you wish to convert in the denominator.

When you are converting by the fraction proportion method, write a conversion factor with the units needed in the numerator and the units you are converting from in the denominator. Then write a fraction with the unknown, or ?, in the numerator and the number that you need to convert in the denominator. Set the two fractions up as a proportion, cancel units of measurement, cross-multiply, then solve for the unknown value.

EXAMPLE 1 ▶   Convert 66 lb to kilograms.

1. Table 3-8 tells us that 1 kg is equal to 2.2 lb. Since we are converting to kilograms, kilograms must appear in the numerator of our conversion factor. Our conversion factor is 1 kg/2.2 lb.
2. The other fraction for our proportion has the unknown (?) for a numerator and 66 lb as the denominator.
3. Setting the two fractions into a proportion gives us the following equation:

$$\frac{?}{66 \text{ lb}} = \frac{1 \text{ kg}}{2.2 \text{ lb}}$$

4. Cancel units of measurement.

$$\frac{?}{66} = \frac{1 \text{ kg}}{2.2}$$

5. Solve for the unknown by cross-multiplying.

$$2.2 \times ? = 1 \text{ kg} \times 66$$
$$\frac{2.2 \times ?}{2.2} = \frac{1 \text{ kg} \times 66}{2.2}$$

$$? = 30 \text{ (So the solution is 66 lb equals 30 kg.)}$$

EXAMPLE 2 ▶   A patient needs to take 10 mL of a medication, but is going to be measuring the medication with a teaspoon. How many teaspoons should he use?

1. Table 3-7 tells us that 5 mL is equal to 1 tsp. Since we are converting to teaspoons, our conversion factor is $\frac{1 \text{ tsp}}{5 \text{ mL}}$.
2. The other fraction for our proportion is $\frac{?}{10 \text{ mL}}$.
3. Setting the two fractions into a proportion gives us the following equation:

$$\frac{?}{10 \text{ mL}} = \frac{1 \text{ tsp}}{5 \text{ mL}}$$

4. Cancel units of measurement.

$$\frac{?}{10} = \frac{1 \text{ tsp}}{5}$$

5. Solve for the unknown.

$$5 \times ? = 1 \text{ tsp} \times 10$$
$$\frac{5 \times ?}{5} = \frac{1 \text{ tsp} \times 10}{5}$$
$$? = 2 \text{ tsp}$$

Super Tech . . .

Open the CD-ROM that accompanies your textbook and select Chapter 3, Exercise 3-5. Review the animation and example problems, and then complete the practice problems. Continue to the next section of the book once you have mastered the information presented.

Using Conversion Factors

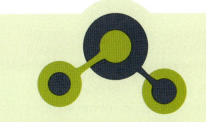

The Ratio Proportion Method

By writing a conversion factor as a ratio, you can use means and extremes to convert a quantity from one unit of measure to another. Recall from Chapter 2 that you can use means and extremes to find a missing value in ratio proportion.

When you are converting by the ratio proportion method, Write the conversion factor as a ratio $A:B$ so that A has the units needed in the answer. Write a second ratio $C:D$ so that C is the missing value and D is the number that is being converted. Write the proportion in the form $A:B::C:D$. Cancel units of measurement and solve the proportion by multiplying the means and extremes.

EXAMPLE 1 ▶ Convert 66 lb to kilograms.

1. Since we are converting to kilograms, our conversion ratio will have kilograms as the first part. Since 1 kg = 2.2 lb, our first ratio is 1 kg:2.2 lb.
2. The second ratio is ?:66 lb.
3. Our proportion is 1 kg:2.2 lb::?:66 lb.
4. Cancel like units.

$$1 \text{ kg}:2.2 \text{ lb}::?:66 \text{ lb}$$
$$1 \text{ kg}:2.2::?:66$$

5. Solve for the missing value.

$$2.2 \times ? = 1 \text{ kg} \times 66$$

$$\frac{2.2 \times ?}{2.2} = \frac{1 \text{ kg} \times 66}{2.2}$$

$$? = 30 \text{ (So the solution is 66 lb equals 30 kg.)}$$

EXAMPLE 2 ▸ A patient needs to take 10 mL of a medication, but is going to be measuring the medication with a teaspoon. How many teaspoons should he use?

1. We are converting to teaspoons, so they must appear in the first part of the conversion ratio. Our conversion ratio is 1 tsp : 5 mL.
2. The second ratio is ? : 10 mL.
3. Our proportion is 1 tsp : 5 mL :: ? : 10 mL
4. Cancel units.

$$1 \text{ tsp} : 5 :: ? : 10$$

5. Solve for the missing value.

$$5 \times ? = 1 \text{ tsp} \times 10$$

$$\frac{5 \times ?}{5} = \frac{1 \text{ tsp} \times 10}{5}$$

$$? = 2 \text{ tsp}$$

 Super Tech . . .

Open the CD-ROM that accompanies your textbook and select Chapter 3, Exercise 3-6. Review the animation and example problems, and then complete the practice problems. Continue to the next section of the book once you have mastered the information presented.

Tech Check

Selecting the Correct Conversion Factor

The pharmacist is reviewing instructions on the medication label for a patient on how much liquid medication to take. The physician has ordered 30 mL of milk of magnesia, and the patient will be using teaspoons to measure her medication. Using a conversion chart, the technician confuses 1 tbsp with 1 tsp, and he reads 1 tsp = 15 mL. Using the incorrect information, he calculates the dose and types the patient instruction label: "Take 2 tsp of milk of magnesia." The pharmacist realizes that this amount is only one-third of the amount that the physician ordered; the patient would not get the relief desired.

Think Before You Act

Even though the pharmacy technician set up the proportion correctly, he used the wrong conversion factor. Certain equivalent measures, such as 1 tsp = 5 mL, are so commonly used that you should memorize them. When you are using a conversion chart, always double-check that you select the correct unit of measure and be sure that you read across the same line.

Had the technician used the correct conversion, he would have calculated as follows:

$$\frac{?}{30 \text{ mL}} = \frac{1 \text{ tsp}}{5 \text{ mL}}$$

$$? \times 5 = 1 \text{ tsp} \times 30$$

$$? = 6 \text{ tsp}$$

The patient would be told to take 6 tsp of medication, not 2 tsp.

✓ Review and Practice 3-4 Converting among Metric, Apothecary, and Household Systems

In Exercises 1–10, convert the measures from one system of measurement to another. When necessary, round to the nearest tenth.

1. 4 dr = _____ tsp

2. 125 mL = _____ tsp

3. 120 mL = _____ tsp

4. 240 mL = _____ oz

5. 15 mg = gr _____

6. gr 15 = _____ mg

7. 10 mg = gr _____

8. 2.5 g = gr _____

9. 42 kg = _____ lb

10. 44 lb = _____ kg

11. If an order calls for the patient to receive 2 tsp of cough syrup, how many milliliters of syrup should the patient receive?

12. A patient weighs 65 kg. How many pounds does she weigh?

13. A patient weighs 187 lb. How many kilograms does he weigh?

14. A physician orders 8 dr of liquid medication. How many tablespoons should the patient take?

15. A patient drinks 4 c of liquid during the morning. How many milliliters did the patient drink?

Temperature

Both the Fahrenheit (F) and Celsius (C) temperature scales are used in health care settings. The Celsius temperature scale is also known as the centigrade (C) temperature scale. If you examine the two thermometers in Figure 3-4, you will notice that the Fahrenheit scale sets the temperature at which water freezes at 32 degrees, or 32°F. It also measures the temperature at which water boils as 212°F. On the Celsius scale, water freezes at 0°C and boils at 100°C. In Fahrenheit, average body temperature is 98.6°F. In Celsius, average body temperature is 37°C.

As a pharmacy technician, you may need to convert between these two temperature scales. The following formula can be used for converting between the two systems:

$$5°F - 160 = 9°C$$

In these formulas, F represents the temperature in degrees Fahrenheit and C represents the temperature in degrees Celsius.

You may also use these formulas to convert between temperature scales. From Fahrenheit to Celsius use:

$$\frac{°F - 32}{1.8} = °C$$

From Celsius to Fahrenheit use:

$$(1.8 \times °C) + 32 = °F$$

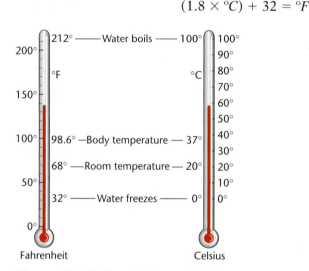

Figure 3-4 Fahrenheit and Celsius scales.

To convert between temperature systems, use any of the following formulas to convert a temperature between Fahrenheit to Celsius.

EXAMPLE 1 ▶   Convert 98.6°F to degrees Celsius.

Substituting 98.6° for °F in the first formula gives us:
(Multiply before subtracting.)

$$(5 \times 98.6°) - 160 = 9°C$$
$$493 - 160 = 9°C$$
$$333 = 9°C$$

Since $\frac{9}{9}$ equals 1, divide both sides by 9 to solve for C.

$$\frac{333}{9} = \frac{9°C}{9}$$

$$37 = C$$

Thus 98.6°F = 37°C; both measures represent normal body temperature.

EXAMPLE 2 ❯ Convert 100°C to degrees Fahrenheit.

Substituting 100 for C in the first formula gives us:

$$5F - 160 = 9 \times 100$$
$$5F - 160 = 900$$

Add 160 to both sides.

$$5F - 160 + 160 = 900 + 160$$
$$5F - 160 + 160 = 5F$$
$$900 + 160 = 1060$$
$$5F = 1060$$

Since $\frac{5}{5}$ equals 1, divide both sides by 5 to solve for F.

$$\frac{5F}{5} = \frac{1060}{5}$$

$$F = 212$$

So, 100°C = 212°F; both measures represent the boiling point of water.

EXAMPLE 3 ❯ Convert 37°C to degrees Fahrenheit.

Substituting 37 for °C in the third formula gives:

$$(1.8 \times 37) + 32 = 66.6 + 32 = 98.6$$

Thus 37°C = 98.6°F.

💿 Super Tech . . .

Open the CD-ROM that accompanies your textbook and select Chapter 3, Exercise 3-7. Review the animation and example problems, and then complete the practice problems. Continue to the next section of the book once you have mastered the information presented.

✔ Review and Practice 3-5 Temperature

In Exercises 1–10, convert the temperatures. Round to the nearest tenth, when necessary.

1. 34°C = _____ F

2. 41°C = _____ F

3. 95°F = _____ C

4. 102°F = _____ C

5. 45.3°F = _____ C

6. 212°F = _____ C

7. 25°C = _____ F

8. 100°C = _____ F

9. 59°F = _____ C

10. 67°C = _____ F

Time

Many health care facilities use a clock with 24 hours (h), known as military or international time. A traditional 12-h clock is a source of errors in administering medication. On the 12-h clock, each time occurs twice a day. For instance, the hour 10:00 is recorded as both 10:00 a.m. and 10:00 p.m. The abbreviation "a.m." means *ante meridian* or before noon; "p.m." means *post meridian* or after noon. If these abbreviations are not clearly marked, the patient could receive medication at the wrong time.

The 24-h clock (international time) bypasses this opportunity for error. Each time occurs only once per day. In international time, 10:00 a.m. is written as 1000, whereas 10:00 p.m. is written as 2200. (See Figure 3-5.)

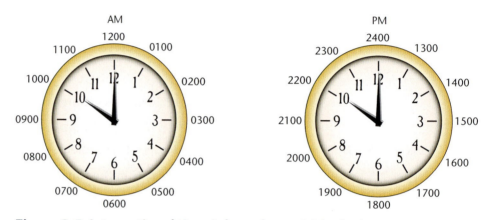

Figure 3-5 International time is based on a 24-h clock.

When you write the time using a 12-h clock, you separate the hour from the minutes by a colon. You then add a.m. or p.m. to indicate before or after noon. When you write the time using a 24-h clock, you use a four-digit number with no colon. The first two digits represent the hour; the last two digits, the minutes.

When you are using a 24-h clock for international time:

1. Write 00 as the first two digits to represent the first hour after midnight.
2. Write 01, 02, 03, . . . , 09 as the first two digits to represent the hours 1:00 a.m. through 9:00 a.m.
3. Add 12 to the first two digits to represent the hours 1:00 p.m. through 11:00 p.m., so that 13, 14, 15, . . . , 23 represent these hours.
4. Write midnight as either 2400 (international) or 0000 (military time).

EXAMPLE 1 ❯ Convert 9:00 a.m. to international time.

Remove the colon and the abbreviation a.m. Write the hour 9 with two digits, starting with zero.

$$9{:}00 \text{ a.m.} = 0900$$

EXAMPLE 2 ❯ Convert 12:19 a.m. to international time.

Remove the colon and the abbreviation a.m. Because this time occurs in the first hour after midnight, use 00 for the hour.

$$12{:}19 \text{ a.m.} = 0019$$

EXAMPLE 3 ▶ Convert 4:28 p.m. to international time.

Remove the colon and the abbreviation p.m. Because this time is after noon, add 12 to the hour.

$$4:28 \text{ p.m.} = 1628$$

EXAMPLE 4 ▶ Convert 1139 to traditional time.

Insert a colon to separate the hour from the minutes. Because this time occurs before noon, add a.m. after the time.

$$1139 = 11:39 \text{ a.m.}$$

EXAMPLE 5 ▶ Convert 1515 to traditional time.

Insert a colon to separate the hour from the minutes. Subtract 12 from the hour, and add the abbreviation p.m.

$$1515 = 3:15 \text{ p.m.}$$

Super Tech . . .

Open the CD-ROM that accompanies your textbook and select Chapter 3, Exercise 3-8. Review the animation and example problems, and then complete the practice problems. Continue to the next section of the book once you have mastered the information presented.

To state the time using military time:

1. Say *zero* if the first digit is a zero.
2. Say *zero* if the first two digits are both zero.
3. If the minutes are represented by 00, then say *hundred* before you say the word "hours."

EXAMPLE 1 ▶ State the time 0900.

Say *zero nine* for the hours and *hundred* for the minutes. Thus, 0900 is stated as *zero nine hundred hours*.

EXAMPLE 2 ▶ State the time 1139.

Say *eleven* for the hours and *thirty-nine* for the minutes. Thus, 1139 is stated as *eleven thirty-nine hours*.

EXAMPLE 3 ▶ State the time 0023.

Say *zero* for the hours and *twenty-three* for the minutes. Thus, 0023 is stated *zero twenty-three hours*.

Super Tech . . .

Open the CD-ROM that accompanies your textbook and select Chapter 3, Exercise 3-9. Review the animation and example problems, and then complete the practice problems. Continue to the next section of the book once you have mastered the information presented.

✓ Review and Practice 3-6 Time

In Exercises 1–10, convert the times to international time.

1. 2:35 a.m.

2. 7:57 a.m.

3. 12:08 a.m.

4. 12:55 a.m.

5. 1:49 p.m.

6. 3:14 p.m.

7. 11:54 p.m.

8. 10:19 p.m.

9. 6:59 p.m.

10. 4:26 a.m.

In Exercises 11–20, convert the times to traditional time.

11. 0011

12. 0036

13. 0325

14. 0849

15. 1313

16. 1527

17. 2145

18. 2359

19. 2037

20. 1818

✓ Chapter 3 Review

Test Your Knowledge

Multiple Choice

Select the best answer and write the letter on the line.

_____ 1. A standard household teaspoon is equivalent to how many milliliters?
   A. 15 mL
   B. 10 mL
   C. 5 mL
   D. 12 mL

_____ 2. A standard household tablespoon is equivalent to how many milliliters?
   A. 10 mL
   B. 15 mL
   C. 1 mL
   D. 50 mL

_____ 3. How many drops are in a mL?
   A. 10 to 15
   B. 15 to 20
   C. 25 to 30
   D. 30 to 35

_____ 4. 2200 hours is what time in traditional time?
   A. 9:00 a.m.
   B. 10:00 a.m.
   C. 9:00 p.m.
   D. 10:00 p.m.

_____ 5. 98.6° Fahrenheit is normal body temperature, what is the normal body temperature in Celsius?
   A. 37° C
   B. 41° C
   C. 38.6° C
   D. 32° C

Practice Your Knowledge

In Exercises 1–8, write the indicated amounts, using numerals and abbreviations.

1. Twenty-five and one-half kilograms _____

2. Forty-five hundredths of a centimeter _____

3. Forty micrograms _____

4. Three-quarters of a liter _____

5. Nine-tenths of a milligram _____

6. One and one-half grains _____

7. Three hundred seventy-five thousandths of a gram _____

8. Twelve milliliters _____

In Exercises 9–30, calculate the conversions.

9. 0.06 g = _____ mg

10. 125 mcg = _____ mg

11. 0.004 km = _____ m

12. 0.75 mg = _____ g

13. 965 mL = _____ L

14. 0.008 L = _____ mL

15. 0.32 kg = _____ g

16. 0.05 mg = _____ mcg

17. 988 m = _____ km

18. 1725 mg = _____ g

19. 368 mg = _____ g

20. 247 g = _____ kg

21. 8 g = gr _____

22. gr iiss = _____ mg

23. 90 mL = _____ tbsp

24. 5 tsp = _____ mL

25. 8 dr = _____ mL

26. 1200 mL = _____ oz

27. 540 mg = gr _____

28. $\frac{3}{4}$ gr = _____ mg

29. 178.2 lb = _____ kg

30. 47 kg = _____ lb

31. An order is placed for gr v of medication. If the medication is supplied in milligrams, how many milligrams should be given? (For this example, assume gr i = 65 mg.)

32. If a patient weighs 44 lb, how many kilograms does she weigh?

33. A physician orders $\frac{1}{2}$ oz of medication for a patient. How many milliliters of medication should the patient be given?

34. The maximum dose of a medication is 3 tbsp. What is the maximum number of milliliters that the patient should be given?

35. A physician tells a patient to drink 2400 mL of fluid per day. How many quarts of liquid should this patient drink?

36. Several months ago, a patient weighed 95 kg. When he comes in for his next appointment, he tells you he has lost 11 lb. If he is correct, how many kilograms should he weigh?

Convert the following temperatures to Celsius. Round to the nearest tenth, when necessary.

37. 97.6°F _____

38. 72°F _____

39. 57.4°F _____

40. 82.8°F _____

Convert the following temperatures to Fahrenheit. Round to the nearest tenth, when necessary.

41. 24°C _____

42. 43.8°C _____

43. 15.6°C _____

44. 8.8°C _____

Convert the following times to international time.

45. 3:21 a.m. _____

46. 4:42 p.m. _____

47. 10:47 p.m. _____

48. 11:20 a.m. _____

Convert the following times to traditional time.

49. 0029 _____

50. 1417 _____

51. 2053 _____

52. 0912 _____

Apply Your Knowledge

Measuring up to the Mark

You are the pharmacy technician working in the pharmacy.
A patient suffering from pink-eye (conjunctivitis) and a cold is given two prescriptions. One prescription reads: "Take 15 mL of cough suppressant every 8 h for 10 days." The other, for eye drops, reads: "Use 2 drops in each eye twice a day for 5 days." The patient will be using a household measuring device to measure the dose of cough suppressant. How many milliliters of each medication need to be dispensed?

Answer the following questions:

1. Which household device should the patient use to take the cough medication?

   _____

2. How much cough medication should the patient take, given the device you recommend?

   _____

3. How many milliliters of cough medication will the patient take each day?

   _____

4. What is the ratio of milliliters to teaspoons of cough medication for one dose?

   _____

5. How many milliliters of cough medication need to be dispensed?

   _____

6. How many milliliters of eye drops need to be dispensed?

   _____

Internet Activity

Find a reliable metric conversion chart on the Internet and use it to convert the following.

1. Your weight in pounds to your weight in kilograms.

2. A temperature of 98.2°F to degrees Celsius.

3. A 500-mg dose of medication to grams.

4. A 2-tbsp dose of medication to ounces.

Super Tech . . .

Open the CD-ROM that accompanies your textbook and do a final review of Chapter 3. For a final evaluation, take the chapter test and e-mail or print your results for your instructor. A score of 95 percent or above indicates mastery of the chapter concepts.

4

Drug Orders

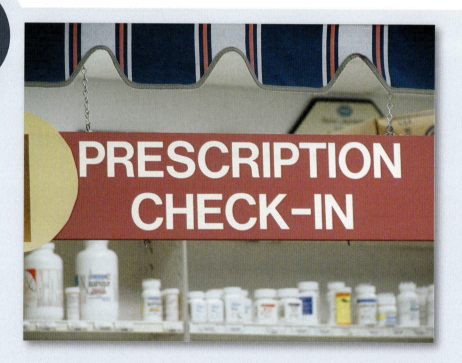

Learning Outcomes

When you have successfully completed Chapter 4, you will have mastered skills to be able to:

▶ Summarize the Rights of Medication Administration.

▶ Interpret a written drug order.

▶ Identify the information on a medication order needed to dispense medications.

▶ Locate the information needed to administer medication on medication administration records or medication cards.

▶ Recognize incomplete drug orders.

▶ Identify and verify DEA numbers.

▶ Recognize classifications of controlled substances.

▶ Recognize prescription errors and forged or altered prescriptions.

▶ Interpret and use pharmaceutical and medical abbreviations and terminology.

▶ Use various medication reference materials.

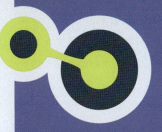

Introduction

One of the most important responsibilities of a pharmacy technician is performing accurate dosage calculations. There is more to assisting the pharmacist in dispensing medications than just doing the math. You need to learn how to read all over again. You must be 100 percent accurate in interpreting medication orders. In this chapter you will gain new skills to be able to read what is written in a medication order. You will also develop and/or sharpen your attention to detail skills.

Critical Thinking in the Pharmacy
Reading What Is Written

You are the pharmacy technician working in a retail pharmacy. An elderly patient gives you a prescription and tells you that his wife died yesterday, and his doctor thinks he should get this medication. The patient asks you to fill the prescription and asks if the pharmacist could tell him how to take it.

The prescription reads: Xanax® 0.5 mg, quantity 120, sig: I tab po tid with meals, refills: 1.

After you have completed Chapter 4 you will be able to read what is written in this prescription.

The Rights of Medication Administration

When you interpret a medication order, you can be held responsible if an error occurs, regardless of its source. You must be able to interpret and confirm all physicians' medication orders with 100 percent accuracy. To assist you, the medical field has created guidelines, called the Rights of Medication Administration (see Table 4-1). As a pharmacy technician you may only be responsible for some of the rights in your daily duties, but you must be aware of all the rights.

Table 4-1   The Rights of Medication Administration

1. Right patient	6. Right reason
2. Right drug	7. Right to know
3. Right dose	8. Right to refuse
4. Right route	9. Right technique
5. Right time	10. Right documentation

Right patient

Before any medication is given to a patient, check that the name on the medication order is exactly the same as the name of the patient. Verify the full name. Two patients with the same last name may have the same first initials, or even the same first names. Ask the patient to state his or her full name. If the patient is unable to do so, ask the parent or caregiver to state the patient's full name. Compare the name to the medication order. In out-patient settings, you may be required to ask for the patient's date of birth, phone number, home address, and photographic identification, such as a driver's license. In an inpatient setting, check the room and bed number and the patient's identification number.

Right drug

To be certain that a patient receives the *right drug*, always check the medication three times: when you take it off the shelf, when you prepare it, and when you replace it on the shelf. Check the medication three times even if the dose is prepackaged, labeled, and ready to be administered.

Only prepare drugs you have pulled yourself and that are clearly and completely labeled. Check that the drug order has not expired and that the medication is still in date.

If a patient questions a medication, recheck the original order. Be sure you have the correct drug. Patients are often familiar with their medications. Listening to them may prevent an error. A patient *always* has the right to refuse medication. If this happens, follow your facility's guidelines for recording the patient's refusal and notifying the physician.

Right dose

The patient must take the *right dose* of medication. In later chapters, you will learn to convert from the *dosage ordered* by the physician to the *desired dose*—the amount of drug that a patient should receive at any one time. You will also learn to calculate dosages, factoring in the strength of the medication and the equipment you are using.

Right route

You must ensure the patient's medications are taken by the *right route*. A drug intended for one route is often not safe if administered via another route. For example, drugs labeled *for topical use only* should be applied to the affected area and not ingested.

Some medications are produced in different versions for different routes. The drug label will indicate the intended route. For example, Compazine® is available as a suppository, a tablet, and an injection. Always check that the route listed on the drug label matches the route ordered by the physician.

Right time

Medications must be taken at the *right time*. The right time may refer to an absolute time, such as 6:00 p.m., or to a relative time, such as "before breakfast."

Some medications, such as insulin, antibiotics, and cardiac drugs, must be given at specific times because of how they interact with food or the patient's body. Other medications may be spaced over waking hours without changing their effectiveness. The drug order must identify special timing considerations to be followed.

Right reason

The health care professional who administers the medication should know the reason the drug is given. This should be the right reason. Depending upon health care profession, it may be your responsibility to ensure that a medication is given for the right reason. You may need to check the patient's medication and/or with the prescribing physician to be certain the medication ordered is correct for the patient.

Right to know

All patients have the right to be educated about the medications they are receiving. This should include the reason, the effect and the side effects of medications. This basic "right to know" is an essential right of all patients. When a medication is administered in a health care facility, this information must be provided to the patient by a health care professional.

Right to refuse

Every patient has the *right to refuse* a medication. If a patient does refuse a medication, this information should be documented in the patient's medical record.

Right technique

Be familiar with the *right technique* needed to administer a medication. For example, both buccal and sublingual medications are applied to the mucous membranes of the mouth. A buccal medication is placed between the cheek and the gum, whereas a sublingual medication is placed under the tongue. If you are not familiar with the correct technique to use, check resources such as **Facts and Comparisons, Remington: *The Science and Practice of Pharmacy,*** and the ***Physicians' Desk Reference* (PDR)** or other drug reference material for more information.

Right documentation

Be sure that the *right documentation* is completed. For example, inpatient facilities administer medication to the patient. The health professional who administered the medication must, *immediately after* the patient takes the medication, sign the **medication administration record (MAR)** (or

Facts and Comparisons: A comprehensive drug information reference available in print, online, or on a PDA; updated on a monthly basis.

Remington: *The Science and Practice of Pharmacy:* Comprehensive reference book with 10 sections providing essential information on the practice of pharmacy; published every five years.

Physicians' Desk Reference (PDR): A compilation of information from package inserts of medications; reprinted every year.

Medication administration record (MAR): A record that contains a list of medications ordered for a patient and space to document the administration of those medications.

similar form), which is a record that contains a list of medications ordered for a patient and space to document the administration of those medications. Until a procedure is documented, it is not complete. As a pharmacy technician in an inpatient facility you may need to review this documentation when preparing medications for the patients.

❋ Tech Check

The Importance of the Right Dose

A physician's order reads Compazine® supp i pr q4h PRN/nausea. The pharmacy technician interprets this order as "Administer 1 Compazine® suppository rectally every four hours as necessary for nausea."

The pharmacy technician assumes that the patient is an adult and dispenses 25-mg suppositories, the normal adult dose. In turn the nurse, who does not notice that the dose is not specified in the order, administers the 25-mg suppository to the patient, a 6-year-old boy.

The usual dose of Compazine® for children is a 2.5-mg suppository. The pediatrician who wrote the order did not include the dose, assuming the staff would know this information. The child receives 10 times the normal dose of Compazine®. He has a seizure and develops fever, respiratory distress, severe low blood pressure, and a rapid heartbeat because of drug toxicity. He is admitted to the intensive care unit for treatment.

⊕ Think Before You Act

The pediatrician made the initial error by not specifying the dose. This error does not relieve the pharmacist, pharmacy technician, and nurse of their responsibilities. All of them should have recognized that one of the rights—the right dose—was missed in this order. They should have called the physician to clarify the desired dose.

◉ Super Tech . . .

Open the CD-ROM that accompanies your textbook and select Chapter 4, Exercise 4-1. Review the animation and example problems, and then complete the practice problems. Continue to the next section of the book once you have mastered the information presented.

✓ Review and Practice 4-1 The Rights of Drug Administration

Match the rights of drug administration with an example of that right.

a. Right patient   c. Right dose   e. Right time   g. Right documentation

b. Right drug   d. Right route   f. Right technique

_____ 1. The medication bottle said *for rectal use*.

_____ 2. The medication was to be given under the tongue.

_____ 3. James E. Jones received medication for James E. Jones.

_____ 4. The nurse charted a medication on the medication record before the patient had taken the medication.

_____ 5. The physician ordered Uracel®, and the patient received uracil.

_____ 6. The dose to be administered was 1 tsp, and the patient received 5 mL.

_____ 7. The medication was ordered at bedtime, and the patient took it at 9 p.m.

Abbreviations

As a pharmacy technician you will need to know many different pharmaceutical and medical abbreviations in order to be able to interpret medical orders. Medical abbreviations approved for use vary among different facilities. The Joint Commission on Accreditation of Healthcare Organizations (JCAHO), a regulating agency for health care facilities, has established a list of abbreviations, as well as "Do not use" and "Undesirable" abbreviations (see Tables 4-2, 4-3, and 4-4). These lists were developed after research indicated that use of the listed abbreviations increased the number of medication errors. Be certain to check abbreviations carefully when you read drug orders. You may notice some slight difference in the way they are written. Some may be written in either uppercase or lowercase letters, with or without punctuation marks and some may also be spelled slightly different. Examples would be susp, or susp., sol, or soln. and dil, or dil.

Some physicians use lowercase Roman numerals, such as ii, to indicate numbers. You may see these numerals with a line over them, such as $\overline{ii}$. Physicians often use this format for apothecary measurements such as grains. They may also put a line over general and frequency abbreviations, such as _a, ac, c, p,_ and _s,_ when the abbreviations are lowercase.

Now that you are prepared for the variations, let's learn the most widely used abbreviations.

Table 4-2   Abbreviations Commonly Used in Drug Orders

General Abbreviations			
Abbreviation	**Meaning**	**Abbreviation**	**Meaning**
aq	water	**NPO, n.p.o.**	nothing by mouth
aq dist	distilled water	**$\overline{p}$, p**	after
a, $\overline{a}$	before, ante	**q, q., $\overline{q}$**	every
aa, $\overline{aa}$	of each	**qs**	quantity sufficient
BP	blood pressure	**R**	take
c, $\overline{c}$	with	**$\overline{s}$**	without
d.c., D/C*	discontinue	**sig. s**	write on label
disp	dispense	**ss, $\overline{ss}$**	one-half
et	and	**sys**	Systolic
iss, $\overline{iss}$	one and one-half	**tbs, T**	tablespoon
NKA	no known allergies	**tsp, t**	teaspoon
NKDA	no known drug allergies	**ut dict, ud**	as directed

(continued)

Table 4-2   *(continued)*

Form of Medication			
Abbreviation	**Meaning**	**Abbreviation**	**Meaning**
cap, caps	capsule	**MDI**	metered-dose inhaler
comp	compound	**sol, soln.**	solution
dil.	dilute	**SR**	slow-release
EC	enteric-coated	**supp.**	suppository
elix.	elixir	**susp.**	suspension
ext.	extract	**syr, syp.**	syrup
fld., fl	fluid	**syr**	syringe
gt, gtt	drop, drops	**tab**	tablet
H	hypodermic	**tr, tinct, tinc.**	tincture
LA	long-acting	**ung, oint**	ointment
liq	liquid		

Route (Where to Administer)			
Abbreviation	**Meaning**	**Abbreviation**	**Meaning**
ad, A.D., AD*	right ear	**od, O.D., OD**	right eye
as, A.S., AS*	left ear	**os, O.S., OS**	left eye
au, A.U., AU*	both ears	**ou, O.U., OU**	both eyes

Route (How to Administer)			
Abbreviation	**Meaning**	**Abbreviation**	**Meaning**
GT	gastrostomy tube	**NG, NGT, ng**	nasogastric tube
IVPB	intravenous piggyback	**NJ**	nasojejunal tube
IVSS	intravenous soluset	**per**	per, by, through
ID	intradermal	**po, p.o., PO, P.O.**	by mouth; orally
IM, I.M.	intramuscular	**R, P.R., p.r.**	rectally
IV, I.V.	intravenous	**sc,* SC,* s.c.,* sq,* SQ,* sub-q, Sub-q**	subcutaneous, beneath the skin
IVP	intravenous push	**SL, sl**	sublingually, under the tongue
KVO, TKO	keep vein open	**top, TOP**	topical, applied to skin surface

(continued)

Table 4-2   *(concluded)*

Frequency			
Abbreviation	**Meaning**	**Abbreviation**	**Meaning**
a.c., ac, AC, a̅c̅	before meals	**qam, q.a.m.**	every morning
ad. lib, ad lib	as desired, freely	**qpm, o.n., q.n.**	every night
b.i.d., bid, BID	twice a day	**q.d.,* qd***	daily
b.i.w.	twice a week	**q.h., qh**	every hour
h, hr	hour	**q. ___ hrs, q ___ h**	every ___ hours
h.s.,* hs,* HS*	hour of sleep, at bedtime	**qhs, q.h.s.**	every night, at bedtime
LOS	length of stay	**q.i.d., qid, QID**	4 times a day
min	minute	**q.o.d.,* qod***	every other day
non rep	do not repeat	**rep**	repeat
n, noc, noct	night	**SOS, s.o.s.**	once if necessary, as necessary
od	every day	**stat**	immediately
p.c., pc, PC, p̅c̅	after meals	**t.i.d., tid, TID**	3 times a day
p.r.n., prn, PRN	when necessary, when required, as needed	**t.i.w.***	3 times a week

* Indicates a "Do not use" or "undesirable" abbreviation according to JCAHO.

Table 4-3 "Do Not Use" Abbreviations, Potential Problems, and Preferred Terms

Abbreviation	**Potential Problem**	**Preferred Term**
U (for unit)	Mistaken as zero, four, or cc.	Write *unit*
IU (for international unit)	Mistaken as IV (intravenous) or 10.	Write *international unit*
Q.D., Q.O.D. (Latin abbreviations for once daily and every other day)	Mistaken for each other. The period after the Q can be mistaken for an I and the O can be mistaken for I.	Write *daily* and *every other day*
Trailing zero (3.0 mg) [Note: Prohibited only for medication-related notations] Lack of leading zero (.3 mg)	Decimal point is missed.	Never write a zero by itself after a decimal point (3 mg), and always use a zero before a decimal point (0.3 mg).
MS MSO$_4$ MgSO$_4$	Confused for one another. Can mean morphine sulfate or magnesium sulfate.	Write *morphine sulfate* or *magnesium sulfate*

Table 4-4   Undesirable Abbreviations

Abbreviation	Potential Problem	Preferred Term
μg (for microgram)	Mistaken for mg (milligrams), resulting in 1000-fold dosing overdose.	Write *mcg*
H.S. (for half-strength, or Latin abbreviation for bedtime)	Mistaken for either half-strength or hour of sleep (at bedtime). q.H.S. mistaken for every hour. All can result in a dosing error.	Write out *half-strength* or *at bedtime*
T.I.W. (for 3 times a week)	Mistaken for 3 times a day or twice weekly, resulting in an overdose.	Write *3 times weekly* or *three times weekly*
S.C. or S.Q. (for subcutaneous)	Mistaken as SL for sublingual, or "5 every."	Write *Sub-Q, subQ,* or *subcutaneously*
D/C (for discharge)	Interpreted as discontinue whatever medications follow (typically discharge medications).	Write *discharge*
c.c. (for cubic centimeter)	Mistaken for U (units) when poorly written.	Write *mL* for milliliters.
A.S., A.D., A.U. (Latin abbreviation for left, right, and both ears)	Mistaken for OS, OD, and OU.	Write *left ear, right ear,* or *both ears*

Tech Check

Understanding Abbreviations

A medication order on a prescription reads 2 gtts in A.D. BID. What instructions are to be typed on the patient's medication label?

Think Before You Act

The pharmacy technician needs to interpret the medical order, so he needs to know off the top of his head that gtts means drops, BID means twice a day, and A.D. is right ear. The pharmacy technician needs to type "Instill two drops in the right ear twice a day."

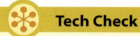

Review and Practice 4-2 Abbreviations

Refer to Table 4-2 and write the correct abbreviation for each of the following:

1. immediately _____

2. twice a day _____

3. hour of sleep, at bedtime _____

4. after meals _____

5. when necessary, when required, as needed _____

6. every morning _____

7. daily _____

8. 4 times a day _____

9. 3 times a day _____

10. before meals _____

11. right ear _____

12. both ears _____

13. left ear _____

14. right eye _____

15. both eyes _____

16. left eye _____

17. discontinue _____

18. dispense _____

19. one and one-half _____

20. no known drug allergies _____

21. nothing by mouth _____

22. after _____

23. every _____

24. without _____

25. write on label _____

26. as directed _____

27. teaspoon _____

28. tablespoon _____

29. capsule _____

30. compound _____

31. dilute _____

32. enteric-coated _____

33. elixir _____

34. extract _____

35. fluid _____

36. drop, drops _____

37. hypodermic _____

38. long-acting _____

39. liquid _____

40. metered-dose inhaler _____

41. solution _____

42. slow-release _____

43. suppository _____

44. suspension _____

45. syrup _____

46. syringe _____

47. tablet _____

48. tincture _____

49. ointment _____

50. by mouth; orally _____

51. rectally _____

52. subcutaneous, beneath the skin _____

53. sublingually, under the tongue _____

54. topical, applied to the skin surface _____

55. intramuscular _____

Interpreting Physicians' Orders and Prescriptions

Always verify that a drug order contains all information needed to carry it out safely and accurately. If an order is unclear, talk with the physician before you carry it out.

Drug orders should include the following:

1. The full name of the patient.
2. The full name of the drug.
3. The dose, the route, the time and frequency.
4. The signature of the prescribing physician.
5. The date of the order.
6. A prn order must include the reason for administering the medication.

Outpatient Settings

Prescriptions: A written or computerized form for medication orders; used in outpatient settings.

For outpatient settings, physicians' orders are given as **prescriptions,** a written or computerized form for medication orders used in outpatient settings. They are filled at a pharmacy or through the mail. Prescriptions include all the elements of a physician's order, as well as the physician's name and prescriber number, the quantity to be dispensed, the number of refills permitted, and instructions for the label of the container. These instructions are preceded by the abbreviation **sig,** which means write on label/directions/instructions.

Figure 4-1 shows that a prescription should include the following:

1. The physician's name.
2. The physician's prescriber number.
3. The full name of the patient.
4. The full name of the drug.
5. The quantity to be dispensed.
6. Sig: The dose, the route, the time, and the frequency.
7. The number of refills.
8. The signature of the prescribing physician.
9. The date of the order.
10. A prn order must include the reason for administering the medication.

I. Heal, MD

Best Medical Clinic

123-456-7890

Name Sonny Daze   Date May 12, 2012

Address _____

Rx: Doxycycline 100 mg

QUANTITY: # 20

SIG: i cap po BID pc

Refills: 0 (zero)

AH1234567   *I. Heal. MD*

Prescriber ID #

Figure 4-1 Sample of an outpatient prescription.

The patient is Sonny Daze. The drug is Doxycycline. The dose is 100 mg. From the sig line, the instructions on the label should read, "Take one capsule twice a day after meals" or one capsule (i cap), twice a day (BID), by mouth (po), after meals (pc). Dosage form, number, route, frequency, and timing are all shown. The quantity (quan) of capsules is 20. The prescription cannot be refilled. The physician's name, prescriber number, and signature are present. This order contains all the required elements.

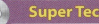

Super Tech . . .

Open the CD-ROM that accompanies your textbook and select Chapter 4, Exercise 4-2. Review the animation and example problems, and then complete the practice problems. Continue to the next section of the book once you have mastered the information presented.

✔ Review and Practice 4-3 Interpreting Physicians' Orders and Prescriptions

In Exercises 1–5, refer to prescription A.

1. What components, if any, are missing from prescription A?

2. How many Lopressor® tablets should the pharmacy technician dispense?

3. How often should the patient take Lopressor®?

4. What strength tablets should be dispensed?

5. If the patient gets all the refills permitted, how long will the medication covered by this prescription last?

In Exercises 6–10, refer to prescription B.

6. What components, if any, are missing from prescription B?

7. How much Amoxil® should the pharmacy technician dispense?

8. How much Amoxil® should the patient take at one time?

9. How many times can this prescription be refilled?

10. How often should the patient take Amoxil®?

I. Heal, MD

Best Medical Clinic

123-456-7890

Name Anna Versary   Date April 19, 2012

Address _____

Rx: Lopressor 50 mg

QUANTITY: # 90

SIG: i tab po tid

Refills: 5

AH1234567   *I. Heal. MD*

Prescriber ID #

Prescription A

I. Heal, MD

Best Medical Clinic

123-456-7890

Name Mark Theeway   Date June 21, 2012

Address _____

Rx: Amoxil-oral susp

QUANTITY: 100 mL

SIG: i tsp po q8h

Refills: 0 (zero)

AH1234567   *I. Heal. MD*

Prescriber ID #

Prescription B

In Exercises 11–15, refer to prescription C.

11. How many components, if any, are missing from prescription C?

12. How many Norvasc® tablets should the pharmacy technician dispense?

13. How much Norvasc® should the patient take at a time?

14. How many times can this prescription be refilled?

15. If the patient gets all the refills permitted, how long will the medication covered by the prescription last?

I. Heal, MD

Best Medical Clinic

123-456-7890

Name Melody   Date May 3, 2012

Address _____

Rx: Norvasc

QUANTITY: # 30

SIG: i po

Refills: 2

AH1234567   *I. Heal. MD*

Prescriber ID #

Prescription C

Super Tech . . .

Open the CD-ROM that accompanies your textbook and select Chapter 4, Exercise 4-3. Review the animation and example problems, and then complete the practice problems. Continue to the next section of the book once you have mastered the information presented.

Controlled Substances

Controlled substance: A drug that has the potential for addiction, abuse, or chemical dependency.

A **controlled substance** is a drug that has the potential for addiction, abuse, or chemical dependency, also referred to as a narcotic. There are five categories of controlled substances listed by schedule (see Table 4-5).

There are specific federal and state requirements for controlled substances. Some states may have more restrictions than federal law requires. Be sure to research your state laws for distribution of controlled substances. All labels on controlled substances are marked with a C and the schedule number. (See Figure 4-2)

Table 4-5 Controlled Substance Schedules

Schedule I

Drugs have a high level for potential abuse and are unacceptable for medical use in the United States.

These drugs are not to be prescribed.

Example: Heroin

Schedule II

Drugs have a high level for potential abuse and dependency. Drug orders must be on a written or typed hard copy order and have DEA number and prescriber signature. Referred to as narcotics. Quantities are limited and NO REFILLS are allowed.

Examples: opium, morphine, oxycodone

Schedule III

Drugs have less potential for abuse than schedule I and II drugs, but still have a moderate potential for dependency. Drug orders may be ordered by phone or in writing and may have five refills in a six-month period.

Examples: anabolic steroids, hydrocodone/codeine

Schedule IV

Drugs have a low level for potential abuse, and limited potential for dependency. Drug orders may be ordered by phone or in writing and may have five refills in a six-month period.

Examples: alprazolam (Xanax®), diazepam (Valium®), zolpidem (Restoril®)

Schedule V

Drugs have a low level for potential abuse, and limited potential for dependency.

Drug orders may be ordered by phone or in writing and may have five refills in a six-month period.

Examples: diphenoxylate (Lomotil®), pregabalin (Lyrica®)

Note: Schedules III, IV, and V may be ordered by phone or in writing and may have five refills in a six-month period.

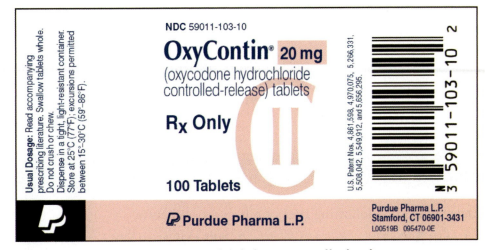

Figure 4-2 OxyContin® is a Schedule II controlled substance (narcotic).

DEA Numbers

The Drug Enforcement Administration (DEA) of the Justice Department passed the Controlled Substances Act in 1970. It regulates the distribution of controlled substances. Federal law mandates that any prescriber that writes a medication order for a controlled substance must be registered with the DEA and is given a DEA number that must be listed on the controlled substance orders. A DEA number always consists of two letters followed by seven numbers. The second letter is the initial of the prescriber's last name. An example of a DEA number is AH1234567. Medicare and Medicaid are requesting that providers use a 10-digit National Provider Identification (NPI) number for prescriptions. This number is used to meet Health Insurance Portability and Accountability Act (HIPAA) requirements on electronic transmissions for billing and protects provider information.

Formula to verify DEA numbers

To ensure that a DEA number is authentic, the following formula is used for verification: Using the example DEA number of AH1234567, add the first, third, and fifth digits together; next add the second, fourth, and sixth digits together and multiply the sum by 2; then add the two answers together. The last digit in your answer of the formula must be the same as the last digit of the DEA number for it to be authentic.

Step 1. Add the first, third, and fifth numbers.

$$1 + 3 + 5 = 9$$

Step 2. Add second, fourth, and sixth numbers and multiply by 2.

$$2 + 4 + 6 = 12$$
$$12 \times 2 = 24$$

Step 3. Add the two answers together.

$$9 + 24 = 33$$

If the answer in step 3 of the formula ends in the same number as the last number of the DEA numbers, it could be an authentic number. In working the formula we see that the example DEA is not an authentic number; if it were, it would have ended with the number 3.

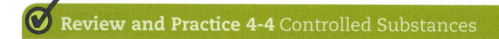

✓ Review and Practice 4-4 Controlled Substances

Determine if the following DEA numbers are authentic.

1. AB1725247
2. CD9314864

3. EF5432671
4. GH6718948

5. IJ1352468

Super Tech . . .

Open the CD-ROM that accompanies your textbook and select Chapter 4, Exercise 4-4. Review the animation and example problems, and then complete the practice problems. Continue to the next section of the book once you have mastered the information presented.

Detecting Errors and Forged or Altered Prescriptions

Because of the potential for addiction to and abuse of controlled substances, it is important to know how to detect errors and forged or altered prescriptions. As a pharmacy technician you need to know federal and state restrictions for all schedules of controlled substances. It is imperative that you verify the date, DEA number, and prescriber's signature on all controlled substance drug orders. On Schedule II drug orders, verify the allowable quantity limits and that there are NO refills written. Inspect the hard copy for paper type and the order for consistent handwriting style. If a prescription looks altered or forged in any way, follow your facility's protocol.

Inpatient Settings

For inpatient settings, drug orders are usually written on **physicians' order forms,** with space for multiple orders. Orders may also be entered into a computer. The patient's name and the physician's signature appear once on the form. Under *Medication Orders,* the physician writes the components of each medication requested in the following sequence: name of drug, dose, route, frequency, and additional instructions.

The form in Figure 4-3 shows several medication orders.

Verbal Orders

Usually, orders must be written or personally signed by a physician. However, if a physician is not able to write an order that must be carried out quickly, verbal orders may be permitted. State laws govern which personnel may accept such orders and how soon the physician must countersign them.

If you are legally permitted to accept a telephone order, write it carefully and legibly *as* you receive it, *not after* the call. In some cases, you may write the order on the physician's order form, identifying it as a verbal order. Always read the order back to the physician. Verify that you have transcribed it correctly. If you are not certain of the spelling of the drug name, ask the physician to spell it. Many drugs have names that are pronounced or spelled similarly.

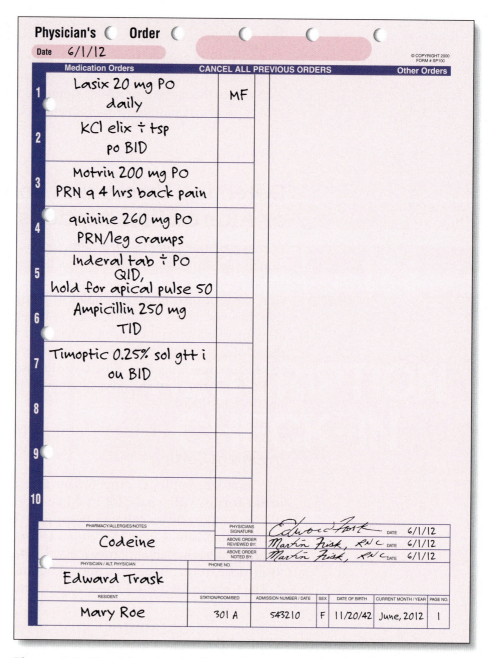

Figure 4-3 Physicians' order form. Can you determine the incomplete order?

If you must prepare a medication from a verbal order, take special precautions. Double-check that you have prepared the medication accurately.

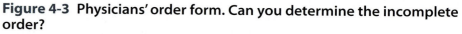

⚠️ **Caution!**

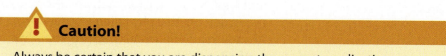

Always be certain that you are dispensing the correct medication.

Many drugs have names that are very similar. Read the order carefully and, when in doubt, contact the prescribing physician. The following list gives just a few examples of how similar the names of different drugs can look and sound. It is especially easy to confuse them when they are written rather than printed or typed.

Acular®—ocular
Benadryl®—Bentyl®
Cafergot®—Carafate®
Darvon®—Diovan®
digitoxin—digoxin
Eurax®—Urex®
iodine—Lodine®
Nicobid®—NitroBid®
Pavabid®—Pavased®
phenaphen—Phenergan®
quinidine—quinine
Uracel®—uracil

Medication Reference Materials

As a pharmacy technician, when you prepare medications, you need to know their effects. Hundreds of drugs exist. New ones are produced and approved all the time. You cannot memorize all the information you might need to know. Therefore, you need to be familiar with drug information sources.

Package inserts provided by the manufacturers with each medication are important reference tools. They describe intended effects, possible side effects, typical doses, dosage forms available, conditions under which the drug should not be used, and special precautions to be taken while using the drug. Information from package inserts is also printed in the *Physicians' Desk Reference* (PDR). Other versions feature nonprescription medications and herbal medications. The PDR has information about most currently available prescription drugs. A new volume is produced each year. Many physicians' offices, pharmacies, and health care facilities have the PDR available for employee use.

Many other guides are available for health care professionals, including the *United States Pharmacopeia/National Formulary*, found in most pharmacies. Most are updated every year or two. Other books have titles suggesting they are for nurses, but they are useful to all health care workers. Their information is similar to that of the PDR, but they often have simpler language. *Drug Facts and Comparisons* is a commonly used reference in pharmacies and includes resources for pharmacists and health care professionals, comparative data, drug interaction guides, and patient counseling resources. *Drug Facts and Comparisons* can be accessed on the internet at www.factsandcomparisons.com.

The *Orange Book—Approved Drug Products with Therapeutic Equivalence Evaluations* identifies drug products approved on the basis of safety and effectiveness by the Food and Drug Administration under the Federal Food, Drug, and Cosmetic Act. The *Orange Book* can be accessed on the internet at www.orangebook.com.

Internet users can access information about the 200 most commonly prescribed drugs at www.rxlist.com/top200.htm. This site provides information about the most frequently prescribed drugs based on a list published in *American Druggist*. For each drug listed, the site lists appropriate doses of the drug for specific indications, available dosages and dosage forms, descriptions of the pills or liquids, and the drug's effects. Another Internet site, www.druginfonet.com, lists drug information, allows searches by brand or generic names, and provides many other useful features.

Also available are software programs designed to run on a handheld computer, known as a *personal digital assistant*, or PDA. One such program is called Epocrates. Used mostly by physicians, this program is updated regularly and is a handy resource for any health care professional needing the latest medication information. Epocrates can also be accessed on the internet at www.epocrates.com.

✓ Review and Practice 4-5 Detecting Errors and Forged or Altered Prescriptions

Match the medication reference material with its description.

a. PDR

b. Package insert

c. Rxlist.com

d. Epocrates

e. The *Orange Book*

f. *Drug Facts and Comparisons*

_____ 1. Provides information about one medication.

_____ 2. Includes a list of the top 200 drugs used.

_____ 3. Software used on a PDA to reference medications.

_____ 4. Compilation of package inserts, updated yearly.

_____ 5. Commonly used reference in pharmacies, includes resources for pharmacists.

_____ 6. Identifies drug products approved on the basis of safety and effectiveness.

✓ Chapter 4 Review

Test Your Knowledge

Multiple Choice

Select the best answer and write the letter on the line.

_____ 1. What is the potential for addiction or abuse of Schedule I controlled substances?
A. Low
B. High
C. Moderate
D. None

_____ 2. What is the potential for addiction or abuse of Schedule II controlled substances?
A. Low
B. High
C. Moderate
D. None

_____ 3. What is the potential for addiction or abuse of Schedule III controlled substances?
   A. Low
   B. High
   C. Moderate
   D. None

_____ 4. What is the potential for addiction or abuse of Schedule IV controlled substances?
   A. Low
   B. High
   C. Moderate
   D. None

_____ 5. What is the potential for addiction or abuse of Schedule V controlled substances?
   A. Low
   B. High
   C. Moderate
   D. None

Practice Your Knowledge

Fill in the meanings of the abbreviations in the table below.

General Abbreviations			
Abbreviation	**Meaning**	**Abbreviation**	**Meaning**
aq		NPO, n.p.o.	
aq dist		$\overline{p}$, p	
a, $\overline{a}$		q, q., $\overline{q}$	
aa, $\overline{aa}$		qs	
BP		R	
c, $\overline{c}$		$\overline{s}$	
d.c., D/C*		sig. s	
disp		ss, $\overline{ss}$	
et		sys	
iss, $\overline{iss}$		tbs, T	
NKA		tsp, t	
NKDA		ut dict, ud	
Form of Medication			
Abbreviation	**Meaning**	**Abbreviation**	**Meaning**
cap, caps		MDI	
comp		sol, soln.	
dil, dil.		SR	

(continued)

Form of Medication

Abbreviation	Meaning	Abbreviation	Meaning
EC		supp, supp.	
elix, elix.		susp, susp.	
ext, ext.		syr, syp.	
fld., fl		syr	
gtt, gtts		tab	
H		tr, tinct, tinc.	
LA		ung, oint	
liq			

Route (Where to Administer)

Abbreviation	Meaning	Abbreviation	Meaning
ad, A.D., AD*		od, O.D., OD	
as, A.S., AS*		os, O.S., OS	
au, A.U., AU*		ou, O.U., OU	

Route (How to Administer)

Abbreviation	Meaning	Abbreviation	Meaning
GT		NG, NGT, ng	
IVPB		NJ	
IVSS		per	
ID		po, p.o., PO, P.O.	
IM, I.M.		R, P.R., p.r.	
IV, I.V.		sc,* SC,* s.c.,* sq,* SQ,* sub-q, Sub-q	
IVP		SL, sl	
KVO, TKO		top, TOP	

Frequency

Abbreviation	Meaning	Abbreviation	Meaning
a.c., ac, AC, $\overline{ac}$		qam, q.a.m.	
ad. lib, ad lib		qpm, o.n., q.n.	
b.i.d., bid, BID		q.d.,* qd*	
b.i.w.		q.h., qh	
h, hr		q. _____ hrs, q _____ h	
h.s.,* hs,* HS*		qhs, q.h.s.	

(continued)

Frequency			
Abbreviation	**Meaning**	**Abbreviation**	**Meaning**
LOS		q.i.d., qid, QID	
min		q.o.d.,* qod*	
non rep		rep	
n, noc, noct		SOS, s.o.s.	
od		stat	
p.c., pc, PC, p̄c̄		t.i.d., tid, TID	
p.r.n., prn, PRN		t.i.w.*	

In Exercises 1–3, refer to prescription 1.

I. Heal, MD

Best Medical Clinic

123-456-7890

Name Melody Song   Date May 3, 2012

Address _____

Rx: Timoptic 0.5%

QUANTITY: 5 mL

SIG: ii gtts od qid

Refills: 2

AH1234567   *I. Heal. MD*

Prescriber ID #

Prescription 1

1. What instructions should be printed for the patient?

2. How many times can this prescription be refilled?

3. By what route should this medication be administered?

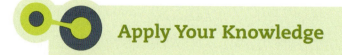

Apply Your Knowledge

Reading What Is Written

You are the pharmacy technician working in a retail pharmacy. An elderly patient gives you a prescription and tells you that his wife died yesterday, and his doctor thinks he should get this medication. The patient asks you to fill the prescription and asks if the pharmacist could tell him how to take it.

The physician gave the patient the following prescription:

I. Heal, MD

Best Medical Clinic

123-456-7890

Name <u>Manny Sadd</u>   Date <u>May 3, 2012</u>

Address _____

Rx: Xanax 0.5 mg

QUANTITY: # 120

SIG: i tab po tid with meals

Refills: 1

<u>AH1234567</u>   *I. Heal, MD*

Prescriber ID #

Answer the following questions:

1. You are filling the prescription. How many tablets will be dispensed to the patient?

   _____

2. How many refills are on the prescription?

   _____

3. What directions will be typed on the label?

   _____

4. What will the pharmacist tell the patient about how to take the medication?

   _____

Internet Activity

You receive a physician's order for cephalexin 500 mg q6h. In the past, you have given only 250-mg doses. You want to verify that 500 mg is safe. Use the Top 200 Prescribed Drugs list from the Internet to check the safety of this dose.

Assignment: Type www.rxlist.com in the address bar of your Internet search program. Find cephalexin, then read "Dosage and Administration."

Determine whether the ordered dose is safe.

Super Tech . . .

Open the CD-ROM that accompanies your textbook and a final review of Chapter 4. For a final evaluation, take the chapter test and email or print your results for your instructor. A score of 95 percent or above indicates mastery of the chapter concepts.

5

Drug Labels and Package Inserts

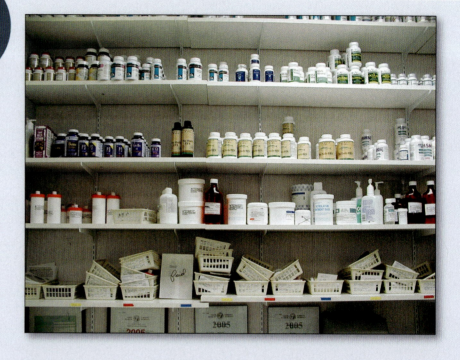

Learning Outcomes

When you have successfully completed Chapter 5, you will have mastered skills to be able to:

▶ Identify on a drug label the drug name, form, dosage strength, route, warnings, and manufacturing and storage information.

▶ Locate directions on drug labels and package inserts for reconstituting and diluting medications.

▶ Recognize different types of tablets and capsules.

▶ Distinguish administration routes for medications.

▶ Locate additional information in a package insert.

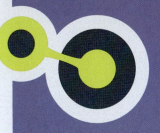

Introduction

Now that you have learned basic math and drug orders, it is time to learn a little bit about drugs. The information you need to perform dosage calculations must be read carefully. This information can be found on the drug label and on the **package insert,** which is a paper insert that provides complete and authoritative information about a medication. Make sure you know exactly what is found on a drug label, and do not forget to read the fine print. Very essential information is located there.

Critical Thinking in the Pharmacy
Which Is Right?

You are the pharmacy technician working in a retail pharmacy. The pharmacist receives a faxed drug order for erythromycin for a 3-year-old patient. The prescribed dose is available in tablet and liquid forms. The drug order does not list which form to dispense.

After you have completed Chapter 5 you will be able to identify different drug forms and their routes of administration.

PTCB Correlations

When you have completed this chapter you will have the mathematical building block of knowledge needed to assist you in performing dosage calculations.

▶ Knowledge of generic and brand names of pharmaceuticals (Statement I-5).

▶ Knowledge of proper storage conditions (Statement I-31).

▶ Knowledge of NDC number components (Statement I-34).

▶ Knowledge of the purpose for lot numbers and expiration dates (Statement I-35).

Package insert: Paper insert that provides complete and authoritative information about a medication.

Drug Labels and Package Inserts

To prepare drugs, you must understand information that appears on drug labels, including the drug name, form, dosage strength, total amount in the container, route of administration, warnings, storage requirements, manufacturing information and references.

Locating Information on Drug Labels

United States Pharmacopeia (USP) and National Formulary (NF)

United States Pharmacopeia (USP): The official public standards-setting authority for all prescription and over-the-counter medicines, dietary supplements, and other health care products manufactured and sold in the United States.

The *United States Pharmacopeia (USP)* is the official public standards-setting authority for all prescription and over-the-counter medicines, dietary supplements, and other health care products manufactured and sold in the United States. USP sets standards for the quality of these products and works with health care providers to help them reach the standards. USP's standards are also recognized and used in more than 130 countries. These standards have been helping to ensure good pharmaceutical care for people throughout the world for more than 185 years.

USP is an independent, science-based public health organization. As a self-sustaining nonprofit organization, USP is funded through revenues from the sale of products and services that help to ensure good pharmaceutical care. USP's contributions to public health are enriched by the participation and oversight of volunteers representing pharmacy, medicine, and other health care professions as well as academia, government, the pharmaceutical industry, health plans, and consumer organizations.

National Formulary (NF): A book of public phramacopeial standards.

The *United States Pharmacopeia—National Formulary* (USP–NF) is a book of public pharmacopeial standards. It contains standards for medicines, dosage forms, drug substances, excipients, medical devices, and dietary supplements.

Drug Names, Trade and Generic

Generic name: A drug's official name.

Every drug has an official name—its **generic name.** By law, this name must appear on the drug's label. It is also recorded with a national listing of drugs: the *United States Pharmacopeia* (USP) and the *National Formulary* (NF). If USP appears on the label, it indicates that this drug's name is recorded with the *United States Pharmacopeia.*

Trade name: The name of the drug owned by a specific company also referred to as *brand name* or *proprietary name.*

Some drug labels list only a generic name. Many also include the **trade name,** which is the name of the drug owned by a specific company, also referred to as *brand name* or *proprietary name,* used to market the drug. A trade name is the property of a specific drug company. The registered mark® indicates the name has been legally registered with the U.S. Patent and Trademark Office, Figure 5-1. Several companies may manufacture a drug but market it under different trade names. Generally speaking, trade names begin with a capital letter and generic names begin with a lowercase letter.

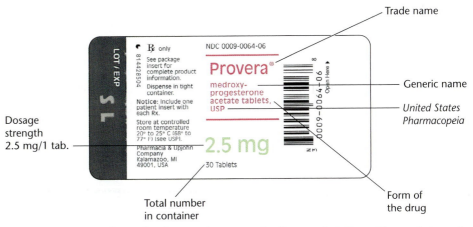

Figure 5-1 An® beside the trade name indicates it is legally registered with the U.S. Patent and Trademark Office.

Physicians can write drug orders using either generic or trade names (see Figures 5-2 and 5-3). Some companies produce drugs under their generic names and market them at a lower cost than that of the trade name equivalents. For example, ibuprofen is sold under its generic name, as well as trade names, such as Advil® and Motrin®. As a pharmacy technician you must know both the generic and trade names of drugs.

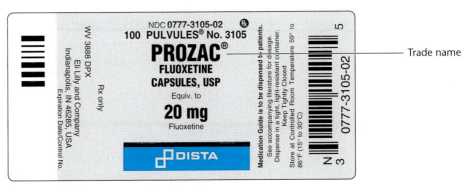

Figure 5-2 Prozac® is the trade name.

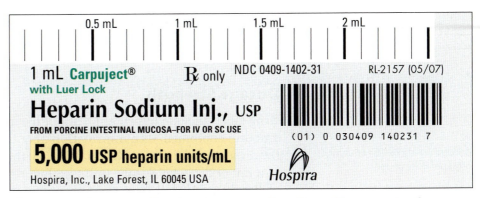

Figure 5-3 Some medications are generic only and have no trade name.

Tech Check

Recognizing Generic and Trade Names of Drugs

The patient profile indicates that the patient is allergic to Vicodin®, a narcotic painkiller. The medication order from the physician is written for Lortab®. What do you tell the pharmacist?

Think Before You Act

You need to alert the pharmacist that the patient is allergic to Vicodin®. The generic drugs in Vicodin®—hydrocodone bitartrate and acetaminophen— are also found in the trade name drugs Anexsia®, Lortab®, and Zydone®. If you administer one of these drugs as an alternative to Vicodin®, the patient may have a similar allergic reaction. Resources such as the PDR *(Physicians' Desk Reference)* provide information about a drug's ingredients.

Super Tech . . .

Open the CD-ROM that accompanies your textbook and select Chapter 5, Exercise 5-1. Review the animation and example problems, and then complete the practice problems. Continue to the next section of the book once you have mastered the information presented.

Drug Form

Manufacturers may offer the same drug in different forms (see Figure 5-4). For example, penicillin is available as a tablet, a capsule, a liquid for oral administration, and an injection. Every label indicates the drug's form. Solid oral medications come in the form of tablets, capsules, gelcaps, and caplets. Liquid forms include oral, injections, inhalants, drops, sprays, and mists. Other forms of medication include ointments, creams, gels, lotions, patches, suppositories, and shampoos.

Dosage Strength

Dosage strength: The amount of drug per dosage unit.

Drug labels include information about the amount of the drug present. This amount, combined with information about the form of the drug, identifies the drug's **dosage strength.** On the label, the dosage strength is stated as the amount of drug per dosage unit (see Figure 5.5). In most cases, the amount of the drug is listed in grams (g), milligrams (mg), micrograms (mcg), or grains (gr). In certain cases, such as insulin, the amount is listed in units.

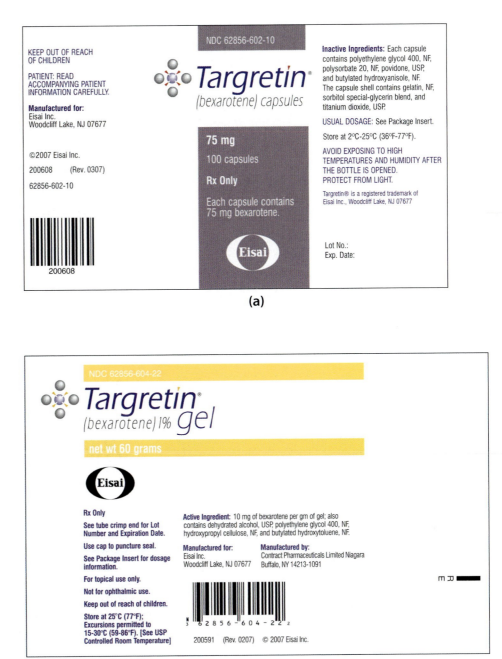

Figure 5-4 Targretin® is a medication offered in different forms: (a) capsules; (b) gel.

Certain liquid drugs, such as hydrogen peroxide and glycerin, may list the amount in milliliters (mL).

For solid medications, the dosage strength is the amount of drug present per tablet, capsule, or other forms.

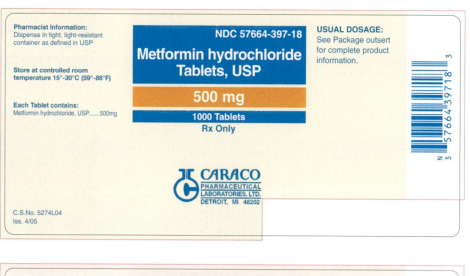

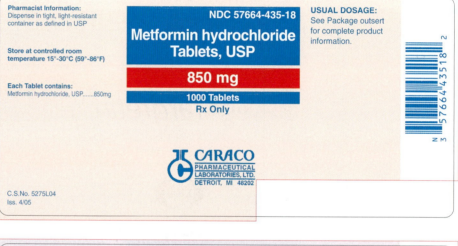

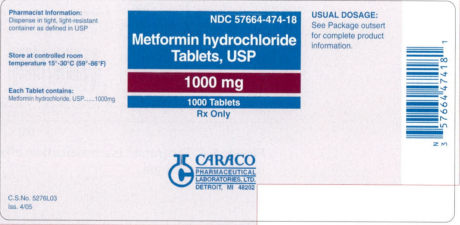

Figure 5-5 Metformin is a medication offered in different dosage strengths.

For liquid medications, the dosage strength is the amount of the drug present in a certain quantity of solution. Recall from Chapter 2 that a solute (the drug) is mixed with a solvent or diluent (such as saline) to create a solution. You need to know both the amount of the drug and the amount of the total solution in which it is contained. The amount of solution that is considered a dosage unit varies. Pharmaceutical companies manufacture medications with dosage strengths corresponding to commonly prescribed doses. This practice reduces the risk of medical error by reducing the number of dosage calculations.

Total Number or Volume in Container

Many medications are packaged separately in *unit doses*. These packages may contain a single dosage unit, for example, a single tablet or a vial with 2 mL of solution for injection. If the container holds more than one dosage unit, the total number or volume must be listed on the label. Nonprescription medications are often packaged in multiple-dose containers. Be careful not to confuse the total amount of drug in the container with the dosage strength (see Figure 5-6). Additional information can be found in the package insert. In Figure 5-7, the container of Famotidine provides a unit dose of 20 mg/2mL. The term *single dose* is on the label. The label's directions indicate that the drug is to be administered intravenously and any unused portion is to be discarded. The container is used once.

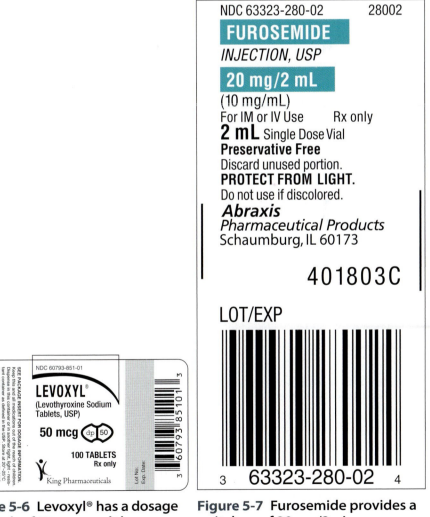

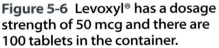

Figure 5-6 Levoxyl® has a dosage strength of 50 mcg and there are 100 tablets in the container.

Figure 5-7 Furosemide provides a unit dose of 20 mg/2mL.

Reconstituting Drugs

Reconstitute: Process of adding liquid to a powder medication.

Some drugs, such as antibiotics for pediatric use, are packaged in powder form. You **reconstitute** the drug (add liquid to the powder) shortly before administering it. Reconstituted medications remain potent for only a short time. The label indicates the time period within which they can be safely administered (see Figure 5-8). Other drugs must be diluted before they are administered. They, too, must be used within a limited time. Directions for reconstituting or diluting a drug appear on the label.

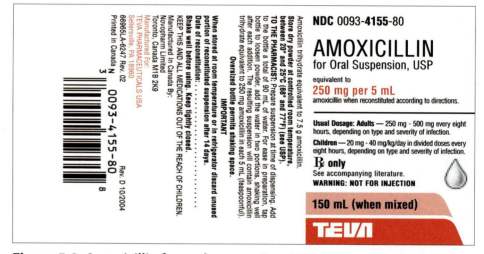

Figure 5-8 Amoxicillin for oral suspension, USP 250 mg per 5 mL.

Super Tech . . .

Open the CD-ROM that accompanies your textbook and select Chapter 5, Exercise 5-2. Review the animation and example problems, and then complete the practice problems. Continue to the next section of the book once you have mastered the information presented.

Route of Administration

Route: Method by which a medication is to be delivered to a patient.

The **route of administration** is the method by which a medication is to be delivered to a patient.

Directions for the route of administration may be specified on the label. This information may not be included for oral medications. However, if a tablet or a capsule is not to be swallowed, additional information will be provided. For example, the label for Nitrostat® (see Figure 5-9) shows it is administered sublingually (under the tongue). Chewable tablets will be labeled as such. Topical medications will also be labeled as such (see Figure 5-10).

Sublingual

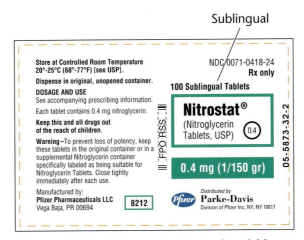

Figure 5-9 Sublingual tablets should be placed only under the tongue.

Topical

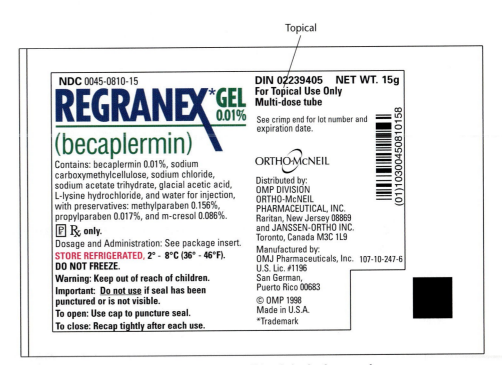

Figure 5-10 Topical medications will be labeled as such.

Intradermally (ID): Medication administered between the layers of the skin by injection.

Intravenously (IV): Medication administered delivered directly into the bloodstream through a vein.

Intramuscularly (IM): Medication administered into a muscle by injection.

Subcutaneously (Sub-Q): Medication administered under the skin by injection.

Liquid medications may be given orally or injected (see Figures 5-11 and 5-12). Labels will indicate whether an injection is given **intradermally (ID)** (administered between the layers of the skin by injection), **intravenously (IV)** (delivered directly into the bloodstream through a vein), **intramuscularly (IM)** (administered into a muscle by injection), or **subcutaneously (Sub-Q)** (administered under the skin by injection). Labels will indicate other routes as well. For example, Aerobid®-M for oral inhalation only (see Figure 5-13).

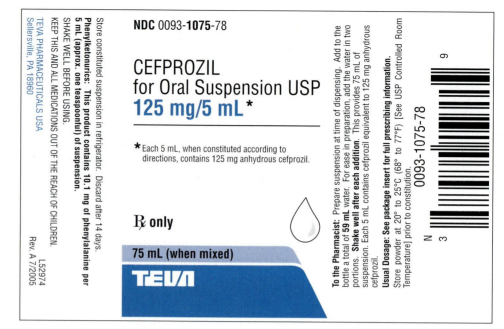

Figure 5-11 For oral suspension.

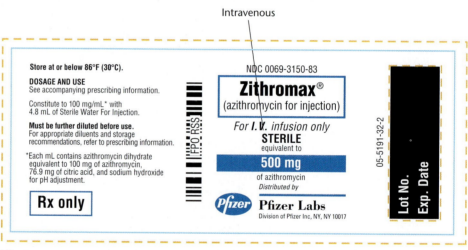

Figure 5-12 For Intravenous (IV) administration only.

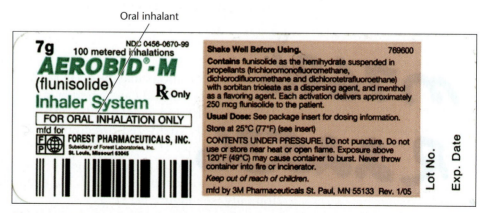

Figure 5-13 For oral inhalation only.

Tech Check

Read Labels Carefully

A pharmacy technician is filling an order for Synthroid® 0.05 mg p.o. q.d. Synthroid® is available in tablets of 11 different strengths, each in a different color. The technician has access to tablets in 0.025-mg (orange), 0.05-mg (white), 0.125-mg (brown), and 0.15-mg (blue) doses.

Looking quickly at the labels, the technician sees a Synthroid® label with "5" on it. Without realizing it is for 0.15 mg, he removes a tablet. When he fills it, the pharmacist tells him that the usual pill is white, not blue. The technician checks the order and replaces the incorrect tablets with the correct tablets.

Think Before You Act

In this example, the pharmacy technician made an initial mistake. He did not carefully compare the drug order with the drug label. He did, however, listen to the pharmacist and rechecked his work. The technician should have read the label three times before dispensing the drug. This rule is especially important when you dispense a drug that is available in different dosage strengths or is designed for different routes of administration.

Fortunately, the pharmacist gave the technician an opportunity to correct the error. If the pharmacist had not caught the error the patient may have been dispensed 3 times the amount of the drug that was ordered.

Warnings and Interactions

Warnings on labels help health care workers administer drugs safely. They include statements such as "It is recommended that drug dispersing should not exceed weekly supply. Dispensing should be contingent upon the results of a WBC count." Controlled substances such as Lortab® warn: "May be habit-forming." Other labels indicate that the contents are poisonous. Labels may carry warnings for specific groups of patients. Some labels state that the product is not safe for pregnant women or for children (see Figure 5-14). Other labels describe harmful effects resulting from combinations with other products.

Every facility follows guidelines for disposing of drugs that are not used. The guidelines for medications that carry warnings are especially strict. For example, in some cases, you destroy (e.g., flush) narcotics with a coworker as witness, then provide appropriate documentation.

Storage Information

Some drugs must be stored under specific conditions to maintain their potency and effectiveness. Storage information will appear on the drug's label. The label may have information about storage temperature, exposure to light, or the length of time the drug will remain potent after the container has been opened. Storage at the wrong temperature or exposure to light can trigger a chemical reaction that makes the drug unusable. (See Figure 5-15 for storage information.)

Warning label

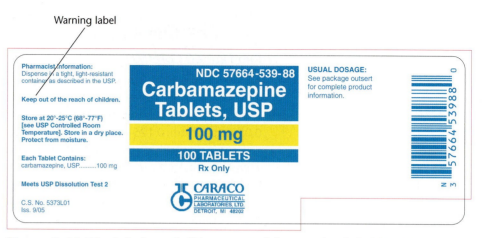

Figure 5-14 The label reads "Keep out of the reach of children."

Storage information

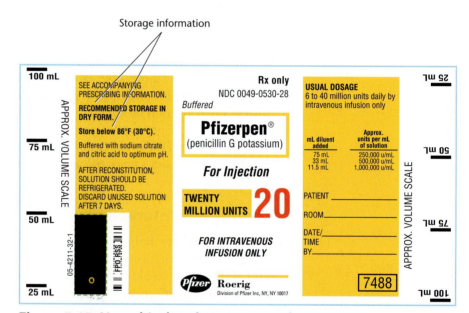

Figure 5-15 Note this drug has two sets of storage instructions.

Manufacturing Information

Pharmaceutical manufacturers are strictly regulated by the U.S. Food and Drug Administration (FDA). FDA regulations state that every drug label must include the name of the manufacturer, an NDC number, an expiration date (abbreviated EXP) after which the drug may no longer be used, and the lot number (see Figure 5-16). Controlled substances must have a controlled substance mark on the label to indicate the control schedule of a drug with a potential for abuse.

NDC (National Drug Code) Number

Drug manufacturers assign a specific identification number to each of their drug products, called an **NDC (National Drug Code) number.** Each NDC number has 10 digits and is divided into three groups of numbers. The first

NDC (National Drug Code) number: A specific identification number on the drug product.

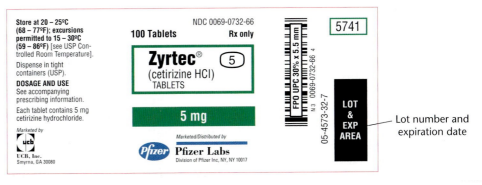

Figure 5-16 Lot number and EXP.

group of numbers identifies the manufacturer; the second group identifies the medication, its strength, and its dosage form; and the third group identifies the package size. If any the three groups of numbers begin with zeros, the manufacture may omit the zeros when printing the numbers on the product label. When ordering drugs and comparing NDC numbers on the drug label on the drug bottle all 10 digits are used (see Figure 5-17).

NDC number

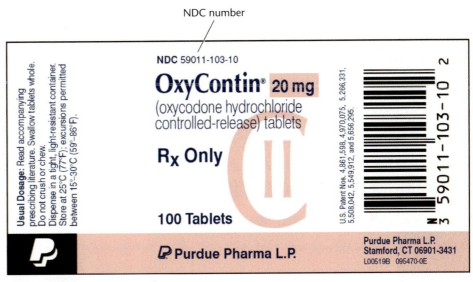

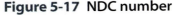

Figure 5-17 NDC number

* This drug is a controlled substance and has a controlled substance mark of C-II on the label.

Expiration Date

The expiration date indicates a specific date when a drug may no longer be used. It is listed in month/year format, for example, 12/09. The drug may be used up to the last day of the month listed in the year listed. Never use a drug after the expiration date has passed, as the drug properties change and the drug may no longer be reliable for its intended therapeutic use. Older drugs may become chemically unstable or altered. As a result, they may not provide the correct dosage strength. Worse, they could have an effect different from the intended one. Advise patients to check the expiration dates on all drug labels. If patients have not used a product by the date listed, they should discard it. At an inpatient setting, the medication may need to be returned to the pharmacy, depending on the facility's policy.

Lot Number

Medications are produced in batches, known as *lots*. The lot number is a code that indicates when and where a drug was produced. It allows the manufacturer to trace problems linked to a particular batch. If a manufacturer has to remove an entire lot from the market because of contamination, suspected tampering, or unexpected side effects, the lot number helps identify which batch to recall.

> **Super Tech . . .**
>
> Open the CD-ROM that accompanies your textbook and select Chapter 5, Exercise 5-3. Review the animation and example problems, and then complete the practice problems. Continue to the next section of the book once you have mastered the information presented.

✓ Review and Practice 5-1 Drug Labels and Package Inserts

In Exercises 1–6, refer to label A.

1. What is the trade name of the drug?

2. What is the generic name of the drug?

3. Does this container hold multiple doses or a unit dose?

4. What is the name of the manufacturer?

5. What is the dosage strength?

6. At what temperature should the drug be stored?

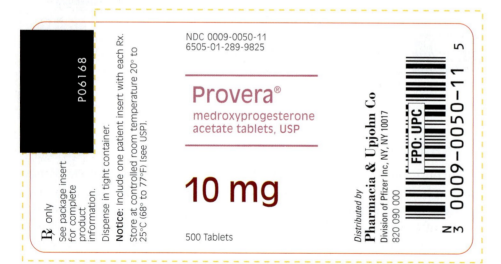

Label A

In Exercises 7–12, refer to label B.

7. What is the generic name of the drug?

8. What is the trade name of the drug?

9. What is the dosage strength?

10. What is the name of the manufacturer?

11. What is the NDC number?

12. What are the storage requirements for this drug?

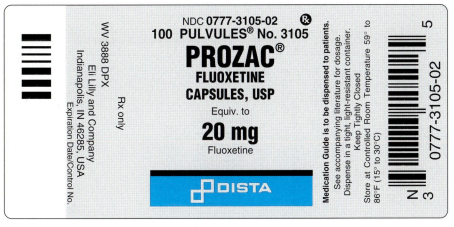

Label B

In Exercises 13–18, refer to label C.

13. What is the trade name of the drug?

14. What is the name of the manufacturer?

15. What is the dosage strength?

16. Does this container hold multiple doses or a unit dose?

17. How would you store this drug?

18. How should this drug be dispensed?

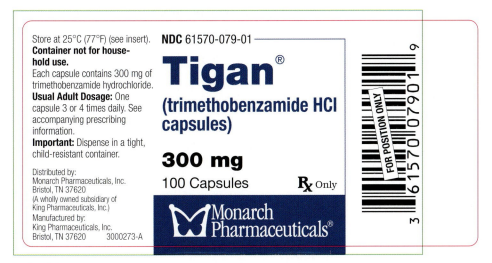

Label C

In Exercises 19–24, refer to label D.

19. What is the generic name of the drug?

20. By what route is this drug administered?

21. What is the usual dose information on the label?

22. What is the dosage strength?

23. If you had a drug order for 250 mg of Cefprozil, how many teaspoons would your patient take?

24. How long would two bottles of medication last if you administered 2 doses of 10 mL daily?

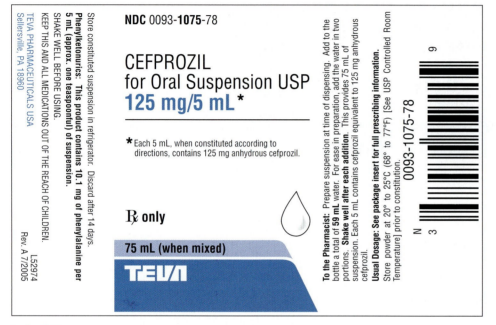

Label D

In Exercises 25–30, refer to label E.

25. What is the generic name of the drug?

26. What is the trade name of the drug?

27. By what route is this drug administered?

28. What special storage information is provided on the label?

29. How many tablets are in the container?

30. What is the drug strength?

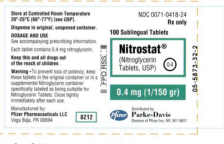

Label E

In Exercises 31–36, refer to label F.

31. What is the generic name of this drug?

32. How would you reconstitute this drug?

33. How much water should initially be added to the powder?

34. When it is reconstituted, what is the dosage strength?

35. What special storage information is provided on the label?

36. If the usual dose is 10 mL, how many doses are in this container?

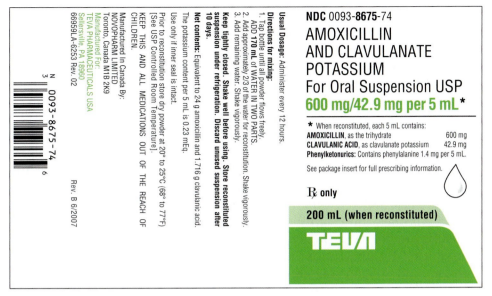

Label F

In Exercises 37–43, refer to label G.

37. What is the trade name of the drug?

38. What is the generic name of the drug?

39. What is the dosage strength?

40. What is the NDC number?

41. Through what route is this drug administered?

42. How many prescriptions could be filled from this bottle if each prescription's quantity was 30 tablets?

43. What is the name of the manufacturer?

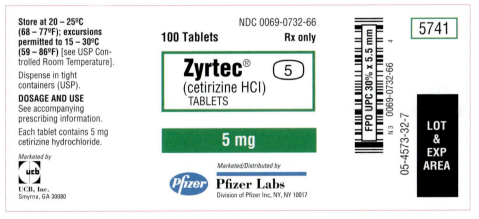

Label G

Reading Drug Labels

Oral Drugs

Oral medications are available in either solid (tablets and capsules) or liquid form. Tablets are the most common form. They may be unscored or scored, chewable, or enteric coated. Scored tablets can be broken into equal portions so that you can administer a partial dosage, if necessary. You may break tablets to give a partial dose *only* when the tablets are scored. Chewable tablets may indicate on the label that it must to be chewed to be effective; however, some chewable tablets may be swallowed or chewed. Enteric-coated tablets should be swallowed whole. Chewing them or dividing them breaks the seal provided by their coating, allowing the drug to be absorbed sooner than intended.

Capsules have a gelatin shell that contains the drug. In most cases, they should be swallowed whole. In some cases, capsules may be opened and mixed with food. Abbreviations such as CR, SR, and ER listed after the drug name indicate a special drug action. CR stands for *controlled-release capsules*, also called SR for *sustained-release capsules* or ER for *extended-release capsules;* these capsules release the drug over a long time. If these capsules are not swallowed whole, they may release too much of the drug too quickly for absorption. Enteric-coated, controlled-release, extended-release, and sustained-release medications should *never* be crushed or broken. These medications can not be divided to give a partial dose (see Figure 5-18).

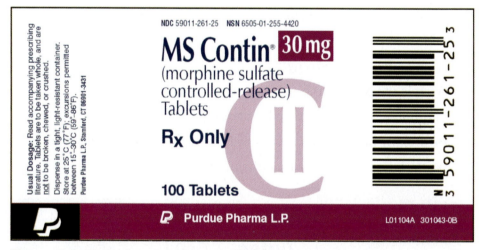

Figure 5-18 Enteric-coated, controlled-release, extended-release, and sustained-release medications are to be taken whole and are *not* to be broken, chewed, or crushed.

Liquid oral medications are described as oral solutions, syrups, elixirs, oral suspensions, and simply liquids (see Figures 5-19 and 5-20). In liquid medications, the dosage strength corresponds to a specific volume of the solution, for example, 250 mg/5 mL.

If a medication needs to be reconstituted, the instructions will be on the label. When you reconstitute a drug, you must write your initials as well as the time and date of reconstitution on the label. Oral liquids may be measured in droppers, calibrated spoons, medicine cups, or oral syringes. Calibrated cups and spoons are available at most pharmacies and sometimes come with the medication. Advise patients who take oral liquid medications at home to use a medicine cup or baking measuring spoon—not a household cup or spoon—if they do not have calibrated cups or spoons.

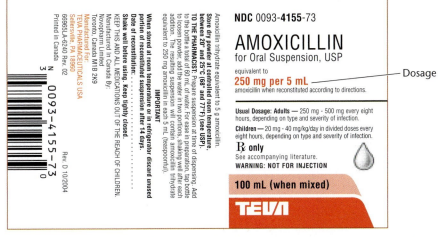

Figure 5-19 For liquid medications, the dosage strength corresponds to a number of milligrams per a specific volume of solution.

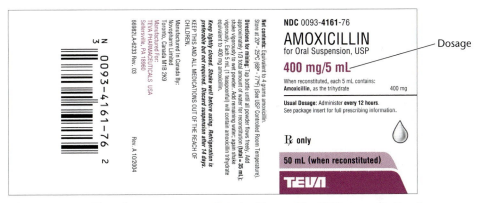

Figure 5-20 The dosage strength is indicated in 400 mg per 5 mL volume for this medication.

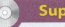

Super Tech . . .

Open the CD-ROM that accompanies your textbook and select Chapter 5, Exercise 5-4. Review the animation and example problems, and then complete the practice problems. Continue to the next section of the book once you have mastered the information presented.

Patient Education

Pharmacists educate patients about the proper way to take drugs at home. If you are authorized to assist the pharmacist with patient education, you should take the following steps:

1. Make sure the patient understands English. Otherwise, you may need to include an English-speaking member of the patient's household in the patient education process.

2. Be sure the patient or caretaker can read and understand the label. Some patients cannot see the fine print on labels. Others do not have the necessary literacy skills.

3. Ask the patient about drug allergies and any medications that he or she may be taking. Check the label or the package insert for drug interactions. Also check with the patient about any over-the-counter medications and herbal remedies being taken.

4. Review the dose, frequency, and length of time the drug is to be taken. Have the patient or caretaker repeat this information to you.

5. Review any special written instructions. Have the patient or caretaker repeat this to you.

6. Describe any adverse effects of the drug that are serious enough to warrant prompt medical attention. Encourage the patient to seek help immediately if these side effects occur. Also discuss side effects that are considered normal.

7. Remind the patient to refer to the label when needed. Emphasize that the patient should call the pharmacy or physician with any questions that cannot be answered from the label or additional written instructions that are provided by the pharmacy.

✔ Review and Practice 5-2 Reading Drug Labels

In Exercises 1–4, refer to label A.

1. What is the NDC number?

2. What is the dosage strength?

3. Can you store this drug on a shelf in the storeroom?

4. How many tablets are in the container?

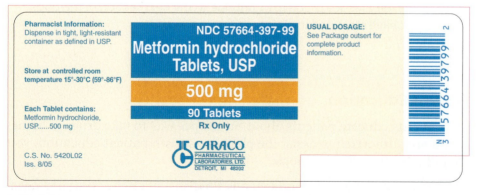

Label A

In Exercises 5–8, refer to label B.

5. What is the trade name of this drug?

6. Who is the manufacturer?

7. What is the dosage strength?

8. How many tablets are in the container?

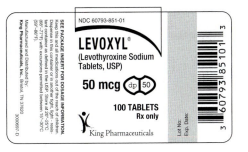

Label B

In Exercises 9–12, refer to label C.

9. What is the generic name of this drug?

10. How many tablets are in this container?

11. What is the dosage strength and type?

12. Can these tablets be broken or crushed?

Label C

In Exercises 13–16, refer to label D.

13. How many milliliters of water should be used to reconstitute this drug?

14. What is the dosage strength when the drug is reconstituted?

15. What is the total volume in the container when the drug is reconstituted?

16. How long can this drug be stored after it is reconstituted?

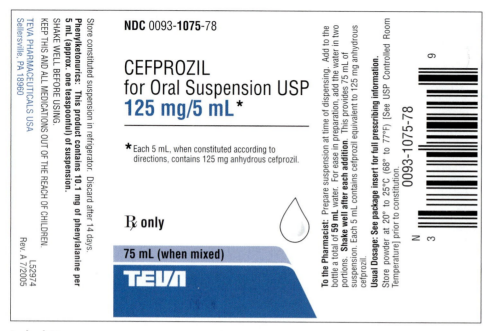

Label D

Parenteral Drugs

Parenteral: Medication administered by a route other than oral; medications that are delivered outside the digestive tract; most often referred to as injections.

Parenteral medications are medications that are delivered outside the digestive tract; most often referred to as injections. Parenteral drugs may be packaged in single-use ampules or vials, single-use prefilled syringes, or multiuse vials. These small containers have small labels that have limited space for providing comprehensive information. You must read these labels with extra care. You will often need to review the package insert to obtain complete drug information.

Most parenteral drugs can be injected intradermally (ID), intramuscularly (IM), intravenously (IV), or subcutaneously (Sub-Q). Inhalant medications are also considered parenteral. The drug label specifies the appropriate route. Depo-Provera® is made for IM (intramuscular) use only (see Figure 5-21). Furosemide is a drug that can be administered either intramuscularly or intravenously (see Figure 5-22). Figure 5-23 indicates that Camptosar® is for IV (intravenous) use only.

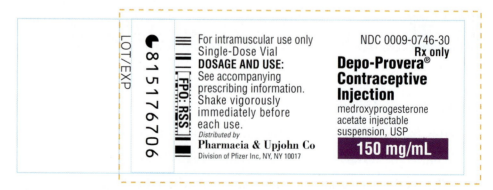

Figure 5-21 Depo-Provera® for intramuscular use only, single-dose vial, 150 mg/mL.

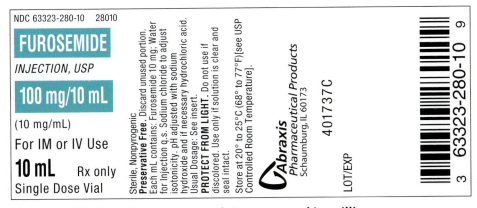

Figure 5-22 This dosage strength is expressed in milligrams per milliliter, 100mg/10mL.

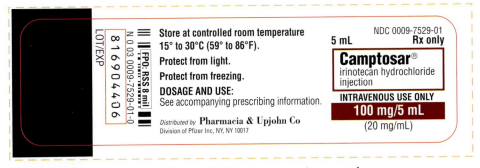

Figure 5-23 Camptosar® is for IV (Intravenous) use only.

On the label of parenteral medications the dosage strength may be labeled as a ratio in milligrams or in units. In some cases the label is marked with milligrams and micrograms. Dosage strength may also be expressed in milliequivalents per milliliter or as a percent, which is grams per 100 mL. *Remember,* the actual dosage strength is a ratio, which is an amount of medication found in an amount of liquid or solid, such as milligram per milliliter or grams per tablet.

Look at the labels for insulin in Figures 5-24 and 5-25. In addition to the standard components, these labels contain information about the origin of the medication and how quickly the insulin takes effect. Insulin can be made from human sources (recombinant DNA origin, or rDNA) or animal sources (beef or pork). Most animal-source insulin is being phased out in the United States. Different types of insulin take effect over different time periods. NPH insulin (Figure 5-24) is an intermediate-acting insulin. Regular insulin (Figure 5-25) is fast-acting.

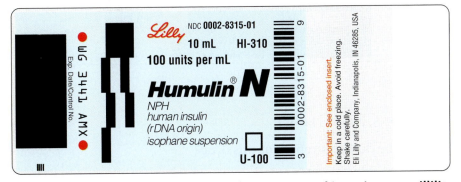

Figure 5-24 Insulin dosage strength is expressed in units per milliliter.

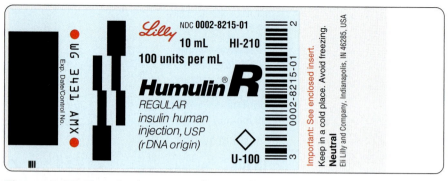

Figure 5-25 Fast-Acting Humulin R®; all insulin has dosage strength of 100 units/mL.

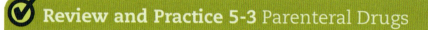

✔ Review and Practice 5-3 Parenteral Drugs

In Exercises 1–4, refer to label A.

1. What is the dosage strength?

2. By what route of administration is this drug given?

3. What other instructions does this label provide?

4. How long can this product be stored?

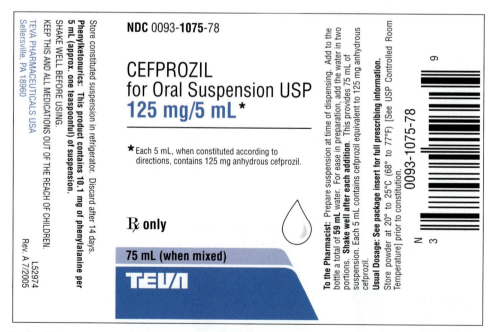

Label A

In Exercises 5–8, refer to label B.

5. What is the dosage strength of this drug?

6. What is the NDC number?

7. What is the generic name of this medication?

8. By what route of administration is this drug given?

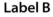

Store at or below 86°F (30°C).

DOSAGE AND USE
See accompanying prescribing information.

Constitute to 100 mg/mL* with
4.8 mL of Sterile Water For Injection.

Must be further diluted before use.
For appropriate diluents and storage
recommendations, refer to prescribing information.

*Each mL contains azithromycin dihydrate
equivalent to 100 mg of azithromycin,
76.9 mg of citric acid, and sodium hydroxide
for pH adjustment.

Rx only

NDC 0069-3150-83

Zithromax®
(azithromycin for injection)

*For **I.V.** infusion only*
STERILE
equivalent to
500 mg
of azithromycin
Distributed by
Pfizer **Pfizer Labs**
Division of Pfizer Inc, NY, NY 10017

05-5191-32-2

Lot No.
Exp. Date

Label B

In Exercises 9–12, refer to label C.

9. What are the storage requirements for this medication?

10. What is the dosage strength?

11. By what route of administration is this drug given?

12. What is the NDC number?

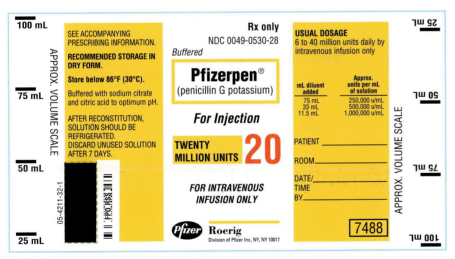

| 100 mL | | | |
| | | | 25 mL |

SEE ACCOMPANYING
PRESCRIBING INFORMATION.

**RECOMMENDED STORAGE IN
DRY FORM.**

Store below 86°F (30°C).

Buffered with sodium citrate
and citric acid to optimum pH.

AFTER RECONSTITUTION,
SOLUTION SHOULD BE
REFRIGERATED.
DISCARD UNUSED SOLUTION
AFTER 7 DAYS.

APPROX. VOLUME SCALE

Rx only
NDC 0049-0530-28
Buffered

Pfizerpen®
(penicillin G potassium)

For Injection

**TWENTY
MILLION UNITS** **20**

**FOR INTRAVENOUS
INFUSION ONLY**

Pfizer **Roerig**
Division of Pfizer Inc, NY, NY 10017

USUAL DOSAGE
6 to 40 million units daily by
intravenous infusion only

mL diluent added	Approx. units per mL of solution
75 mL	250,000 u/mL
33 mL	500,000 u/mL
11.5 mL	1,000,000 u/mL

PATIENT _____
ROOM_____
DATE/_____
TIME
BY_____

7488

APPROX. VOLUME SCALE

75 mL

50 mL

50 mL

75 mL

25 mL

100 mL

05-4211-32-1

Label C

In Exercises 13–16, refer to label D.

13. What is the origin of this insulin?

14. What is the dosage strength of the insulin?

15. Who is the manufacturer?

16. If the usual dose is 10 units, how many doses are in this container?

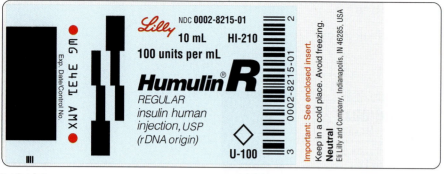

Label D

In Exercises 17–20, refer to label E.

17. What is the dosage strength?

18. What is the generic name of this medication?

19. Does this container hold multiple doses or a unit dose?

20. Who is the manufacturer?

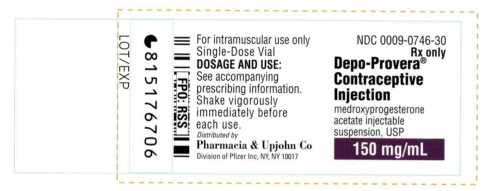

Label E

Drugs Administered by Other Routes

Although many drugs use oral and parenteral routes of administration, other routes exist. They include *sublingually* (under the tongue), *buccally* (between the tongue and cheek), *rectally,* and *vaginally*. Drugs may also be administered as topical ointments (used on the skin); and in **transdermal** form, where the medication is administered through the skin, typically via a patch.

The dosage strength is expressed slightly differently on these labels. In Figure 5-26, the dosage strength is the percentage that the active ingredient, becaplermin, makes up of the entire lotion. The total amount of lotion is given in grams. In Figure 5-27, the dosage rate is given as 100mcg/h fentanyl for 72 hours; this drug is absorbed over time through the skin. Thus the dosage rate indicates 100 mcg are delivered each hour.

Transdermal: Medication administered through the skin, typically via a patch.

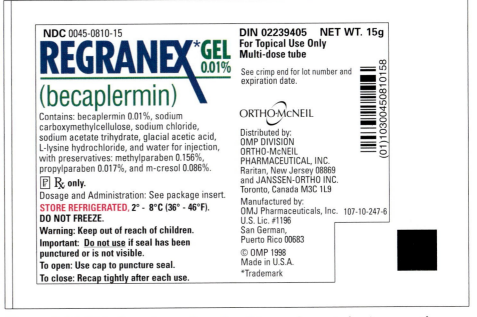

Figure 5-26 This drug is used on the skin, or dermatologic use only.

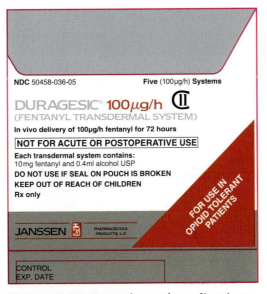

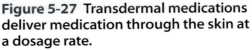

Figure 5-27 Transdermal medications deliver medication through the skin at a dosage rate.

> ⚠️ **Caution!**
>
> Cortisporin® is an anti-inflammatory medication that is available in a variety of forms, including an antibacterial suspension for otic (ear) use and an antimicrobial suspension for ophthalmic (eye) use. The usual dosage of the otic suspension is 4 drops instilled 3 to 4 times a day into the affected ear. The usual dosage of the ophthalmic suspension is 1 or 2 drops instilled into the affected eye every 3 or 4 h. If you were to dispense the otic suspension for the patient's eye, you would not only fail to provide appropriate care for the eye, but also cause considerable irritation to the eye. *The bottom line: do not administer drugs by any route other than intended, as described on the drug label and on the order.* Remember, this is one of the rights of medication administration.

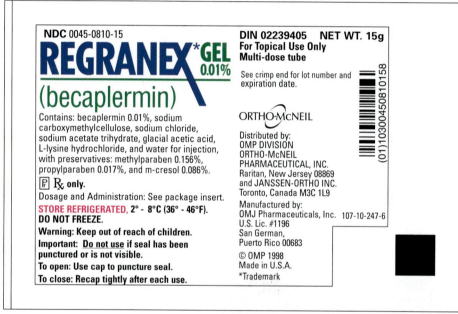

Super Tech . . .

Open the CD-ROM that accompanies your textbook and select Chapter 5, Exercise 5-5. Review the animation and example problems, and then complete the practice problems. Continue to the next section of the book once you have mastered the information presented.

✓ Review and Practice 5-4 Drugs Administered by Other Routes

In Exercises 1–4, refer to label A.

1. What is the generic name?

2. What is the dosage strength?

3. What is the route of administration?

4. How would this medication be stored?

NDC 0045-0810-15

REGRANEX *GEL 0.01%
(becaplermin)

DIN 02239405   NET WT. 15g
For Topical Use Only
Multi-dose tube

See crimp end for lot number and expiration date.

ORTHO·McNEIL

Distributed by:
OMP DIVISION
ORTHO-McNEIL
PHARMACEUTICAL, INC.
Raritan, New Jersey 08869
and JANSSEN-ORTHO INC.
Toronto, Canada M3C 1L9

Contains: becaplermin 0.01%, sodium carboxymethylcellulose, sodium chloride, sodium acetate trihydrate, glacial acetic acid, L-lysine hydrochloride, and water for injection, with preservatives: methylparaben 0.156%, propylparaben 0.017%, and m-cresol 0.086%.

℞ only.
Dosage and Administration: See package insert.
STORE REFRIGERATED, 2° - 8°C (36° - 46°F).
DO NOT FREEZE.
Warning: Keep out of reach of children.
Important: Do not use if seal has been punctured or is not visible.
To open: Use cap to puncture seal.
To close: Recap tightly after each use.

Manufactured by:
OMJ Pharmaceuticals, Inc. 107-10-247-6
U.S. Lic. #1196
San German,
Puerto Rico 00683
© OMP 1998
Made in U.S.A.
*Trademark

(01)10300450810158

Label A

In Exercises 5–8, refer to label B.

5. By what route is this drug to be administered?

6. What is the NDC number?

7. What is the dosage strength?

8. How many doses are in this box?

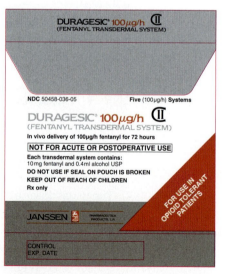

Label B

In Exercises 9–12, refer to label C.

9. What is the route of administration?

10. What is the generic name?

11. How many metered sprays are in this container?

12. Can this spray be delivered through more than one route?

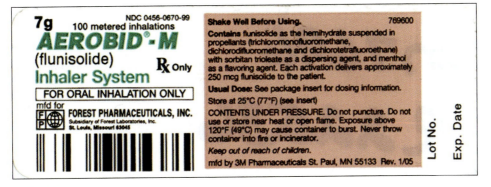

Label C

Super Tech . . .

Open the CD-ROM that accompanies your textbook and select Chapter 5, Exercise 5-6. Review the animation and example problems, and then complete the practice problems. Continue to the next section of the book once you have mastered the information presented.

⚠ Caution!

Suppose the drug order reads Biaxin® 250 mg po b.i.d. Biaxin®, an antibiotic, is available in 250-mg tablets and as an oral suspension with a reconstituted dosage strength of 125 mg/5 mL. (An *oral suspension* is a liquid that contains solid particles of medication. You shake the medication before administering it, suspending the particles.)

It may seem logical to fill the order with one tablet. Yet the age or health of the patient may make a liquid the better choice, especially for children or patients who have difficulty swallowing. If you see a situation in which another form of a drug may work better, consult the physician or pharmacist about changing the form of the drug.

Package Inserts

Package inserts provide complete and authoritative information about a medication. The information in package inserts can also be found in the PDR and other guides. Figure 5-28 shows a portion of a package insert. Table 5-1 summarizes the sections of a package insert.

ARICEPT®
(Donepezil Hydrochloride Tablets)

DESCRIPTION

ARICEPT® (donepezil hydrochloride) is a reversible inhibitor of the enzyme acetylcholinesterase, known chemically as (±)-2,3-dihydro-5,6-dimethoxy-2-[[1-(phenylmethyl)-4-piperidinyl]methyl]-1H-inden-1-one hydrochloride. Donepezil hydrochloride is commonly referred to in the pharmacological literature as E2020. It has an empirical formula of $C_{24}H_{29}NO_3HCl$ and a molecular weight of 415.96. Donepezil hydrochloride is a white crystalline powder and is freely soluble in chloroform, soluble in water and in glacial acetic acid, slightly soluble in ethanol and in acetonitrile and practically insoluble in ethyl acetate and in n-hexane.

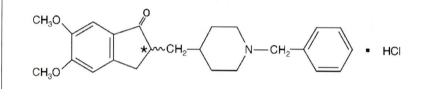

ARICEPT® is available for oral administration in film-coated tablets containing 5 or 10 mg of donepezil hydrochloride. Inactive ingredients are lactose monohydrate, corn starch, microcrystalline cellulose, hydroxypropyl cellulose, and magnesium stearate. The film coating contains talc, polyethylene glycol, hypromellose and titanium dioxide. Additionally, the 10 mg tablet contains yellow iron oxide (synthetic) as a coloring agent.

CLINICAL PHARMACOLOGY

Current theories on the pathogenesis of the cognitive signs and symptoms of Alzheimer's Disease attribute some of them to a deficiency of cholinergic neurotransmission.

Figure 5-28 Top portion of a typical package insert.

Table 5-1 Components of a Package Insert: Section, Description, and Example Information

Section	Description	Example Information
Description	Chemical and physical description of the drug	Aricept® (donepezil hydrochloride) is a reversible of the drug inhibitor of the enzyme acetylcholinesterase, known chemically as (±)-2, 3-dihydro-5, 5-dimethoxy-2-[[1-(phenylmethyl)-4 -piperidinyl] methyl]-1*H*-inden-1-one hydrochloride.
Clinical pharmacology	Description of the actions of the drug	Current theories on the pathogenesis of the cognitive signs and symptoms of Alzheimer's Disease attribute some of them to a deficiency of cholinergic neurotransmission.
Indications and usage	Medical conditions in which the drug is safe and effective; instructions for use	Aricept® is indicated for the treatment of mild to moderate dementia of the Alzheimer's type.
Contraindications	Conditions and situations under which the drug should not be administered	Aricept® is contraindicated in patients with known hypersensitivity to donepezil hydrochloride or to piperidine derivatives.
Warnings	Information about serious, possibly fatal, side effects	*Gastrointestinal conditions:* Through their primary action, cholinesterase inhibitors may be expected to increase gastric acid secretion due to increased cholinergic activity.
Precautions	Information about drug interactions and other conditions that may cause unwanted side effects	*Use with anticholinergics:* Because of their mechanism of action, cholinesterase inhibitors have the potential to interfere with the activity of anticholinergic medications.
Adverse reactions	Less serious, anticipated side effects that can be caused by the drug	These include nausea, diarrhea, insomnia, vomiting, muscle cramps, fatigue, and anorexia. These adverse events were often of mild intensity and transient, resolving during continued Aricept® treatment without the need for dose modification.
Overdosage	Effects of overdoses and instructions for treatment	As in any case of overdose, general supportive measures should be utilized. Overdosage with cholinesterase inhibitors can result in cholinergic crisis characterized by severe nausea, vomiting, salivation, sweating, bradycardia, hypotension, respiratory depression, collapse, and convulsions.
Dosage and administration	Recommended dosages under various conditions and recommendations for administration routes	The dosages of Aricept® shown to be effective in controlled clinical trials are 5 mg and 10 mg administered once per day.
Preparation for administration	Directions for reconstituting or diluting the drug, if necessary	Aricept® should be taken in the evening, just prior to retiring. Aricept® can be taken with or without food.
Manufacturer supply	Information on dosage strengths and forms of the drug available	Aricept® is supplied as film-coated, round tablets containing either 5 mg or 10 mg of donepezil hydrochloride.

✔ Review and Practice 5-5 Package Inserts

Using Table 5-1, answer the following questions.

1. List five section types of a package insert.

2. What type of information can be found in the description area of a package insert?

3. What type of information can be found in the Example Information area of a package insert?

✔ Chapter 5 Review

Test Your Knowledge

Answer the following questions.

_____ 1. Distinguish a drug's trade name from its generic name.

_____ 2. Explain the difference between IM and IV.

_____ 3. List the types of tablets that cannot be divided, broken, or crushed to give a partial dose and explain why.

_____ 4. Explain the importance of a lot number.

_____ 5. Based on the expiration date of 12/09, when is the last day this drug can be used?

_____ 6. What do the three groups of numbers indicate in an NDC number?

Practice Your Knowledge

In Exercises 7–10, refer to label A.

7. What name would be used in writing a drug order for this medication?

8. What is the total number of tablets in this container?

9. What is the name of the manufacturer of this drug?

10. What is the dosage strength?

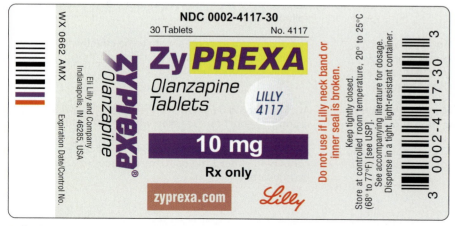

Label A

In Exercises 11–14, refer to label B.

11. What is the generic name of this drug?

12. How is this drug stored?

13. What is the dosage strength?

14. How many doses are in the container?

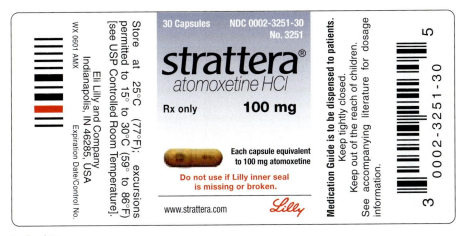

Label B

In Exercises 15–18, refer to label C.

15. Can this medication be divided, broken, or crushed to give a partial dose?

16. What is the dosage strength?

17. What is the generic name?

18. How many tablets are in the container?

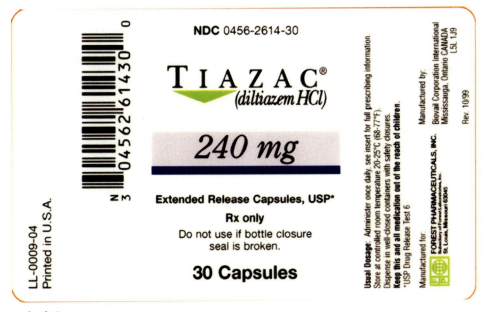

Label C

In Exercises 19–22, refer to label D.

19. What is the origin of this insulin?

20. How many milliliters are in the vial?

21. How is this drug administered?

22. What is the dosage strength?

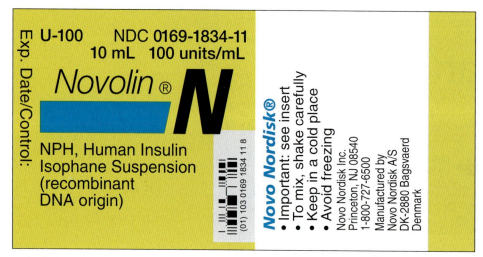

Label D

Apply Your Knowledge

Which is right?

You are the pharmacy technician working in a retail pharmacy. The pharmacist receives a faxed drug order for erythromycin for a 3-year-old patient. The prescribed dose is available in tablet and liquid forms. The drug order does not list which form to dispense.

Answer the following questions:

1. On the basis of the patient's age, what form should be dispensed?

_____

2. If the patient is healthy and 27 years old, what form should be dispensed?

_____

3. If the patient is 96 years old and has difficulty swallowing, what form should be dispensed?

_____

Internet Activity

Mr. Neads is about to be discharged from the hospital with instructions to take Coumadin® 1 mg bid. Mr. Neads is an elderly, easily confused man who will be cared for by his daughter. Although you have reviewed his medication instructions with him several times, you are not completely confident he understands that he should not drink alcohol or take any self-prescribed, over-the-counter medications or herbal cures while he is taking Coumadin®.

Assignment: Conduct an Internet search to find information in plain language regarding the importance of not taking any over-the-counter medications while taking Coumadin®.

Super Tech . . .

Open the CD-ROM that accompanies your textbook, and complete a final review of the rules, practice problems, and activities presented for this chapter. For a final evaluation, take the chapter test and email or print your results for your instructor. A score of 95 percent or above indicates mastery of the chapter concepts.

6

Dosage Calculation

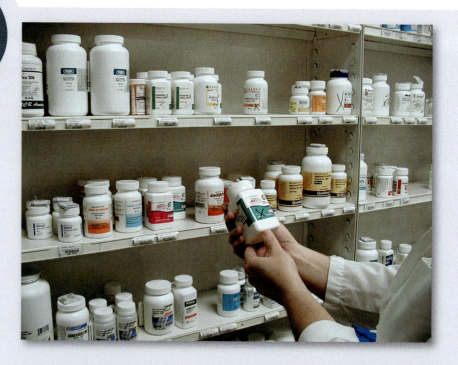

Learning Outcomes

When you have successfully completed Chapter 6, you will have mastered skills to be able to:

▶ Identify the information on a medication order and drug label needed to calculate the *desired dose*.

▶ Convert the *dosage order* to the *desired dose*.

▶ Calculate the *amount to dispense* of a drug.

▶ Recognize common errors that occur during dose calculation.

▶ Calculate estimated days supply.

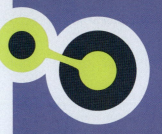

Introduction

Performing dosage calculations is a large part of the pharmacy technician's daily responsibilities. Now that you have learned basic math skills, how to interpret information from the physician's order and drug labels, and methods of converting quantities from one unit of measurement to another, it is time to put all of those skills together to learn how to calculate the amount of medication to be administered to a patient.

Do not hesitate to refer to previous chapters to help you solve the problems presented here. It is important to always use any resources available to you when performing dosage calculations.

Critical Thinking in the Pharmacy
What Is the Dosage Ordered?

You are the pharmacy technician working in a retail pharmacy when the following prescription comes in: "Valium 7.5 mg PO tid for 7 days." The drug is available in 2-mg scored tablets, 5-mg scored tablets, and 10-mg scored tablets, and you have all three strengths on hand for filling this prescription. What is the desired dose and amount to dispense?

When you have completed Chapter 6 you will be able determine if a drug order is correct and complete in order to be able to calculate the desired dose and amount to be administered to the patient.

PTCB Correlations

When you have completed this chapter you will have the mathematical building block of knowledge needed to assist you in performing dosage calculations.

▶ Knowledge of pharmacy calculations (Statement I-50).

▶ Knowledge of dosage forms (Statement II-4).

Doses and Dosages

Desired dose: The amount of the drug that the patient is to take a single time.

Dosage ordered: The amount of drug the physician has ordered and the frequency that it should be taken or given.

Dosage strength: The amount of drug per dosage unit.

Dose on hand: Amount of drug contained in each dosage unit.

Dose unit: The unit by which the drug will be measured when taken by or given to the patient.

Before you can calculate how much medication to dispense to a patient, you must first find the **desired dose**—the amount of the drug that the patient is to take at a single time. To determine the desired dose, you need to know the following information: the *dosage ordered* and the *dose on hand*.

The **dosage ordered** is the amount of drug the physician has ordered and the frequency that it should be taken or given. This information is found on the physician's medication order or prescription, and in inpatient settings, on the medication administration record (MAR).

The **dosage strength** measures the amount of drug per dosage unit. Many medications are available in different dosage strengths. For example, a medication may be produced in two different strengths, 75 mg per tablet and 100 mg per tablet.

Once you have determined the dosage strength, you need to know two other key terms—the *dose on hand* and the *dosage unit*. The **dose on hand** is the amount of drug contained in a dosage unit. In this example, the dose on hand for the first tablet is 75 mg. The dose on hand for the second tablet is 100 mg. For both strengths, the **dosage unit** is the unit by which the drug will be measured when taken by or given to the patient, for example, a single tablet or a teaspoonful. With all medication you have available, you can read the drug label to determine the dose on hand and the dosage unit. To summarize, the dosage strength is the dose on hand per dosage unit.

Conversion Factors

Conversion factors are expressions that allow you to switch from one unit of measurement to another. With some medications the *dosage ordered* and the *dose on hand* have the same unit of measurement. In these cases, since the desired dose is already in the same unit of measurement as the dosage ordered, no conversion is necessary. Frequently, however, the dosage ordered and the dose on hand are expressed in different units of measurement. In these cases, you have to convert the dosage ordered so that it has the same unit of measurement as the dose on hand. As a pharmacy technician you need to be able to convert between units in the same system of measurement; such as using conversion factors of milligrams and micrograms. You will also need to convert between different systems of measurement using conversion factors such as the household measurement of teaspoons and the metric measurement of milliliters. An example would be if the medication order were for 5 mL qid. We know that 1 teaspoon is equal to 5 mL, so the patient is to take 1 teaspoonful, 4 times a day. This conversion leads you to the *desired dose*.

See Table 6-1 for a summary of the language of dosage calculations. Refer to Figure 6-1 for an illustration of the Examples column of Table 6-1.

Table 6-1   The Language of Dosage Calculations

Term	Abbreviation	Definition	Examples: Refer to Figure 6-1
Dosage ordered	O	The amount of drug to be given to the patient and how often it is to be given. *This value will be found on the drug order or prescription.*	40 mg daily
Desired dose	D	The amount of drug to be given at a single time. *The unit of measurement must be the same as the dose on hand. The drug order and the drug label must be consulted.*	This amount must be calculated when the dosage ordered is a different unit of measurement from the dose on hand. In this example a calculation will not be necessary.
Dosage unit	Q	The units by which the drug will be measured when it is administered. *This value will be found on the drug label.*	In Figure 6-1 this is in capsules. Other examples include: tablets 1 mL, 5 mL, drops, or units.
Dose on hand	H	The amount of a drug contained in each dosage unit. *This value is found on the drug label.*	In Figure 6-1 this is 20 mg.
Amount to dispense	A	The volume of a liquid or the number of solid dosage units that contain the desired dose. *This value is found with a calculation.*	If the desired dose is 40 mg and the dosage strength is 20 mg per capsule, the amount to dispense is 2 capsules.
Dosage strength	$\frac{H}{Q}$	Dose on hand per dosage unit. *This value can be determined from the drug label.*	In Figure 6-1 this is 20 mg per capsule.

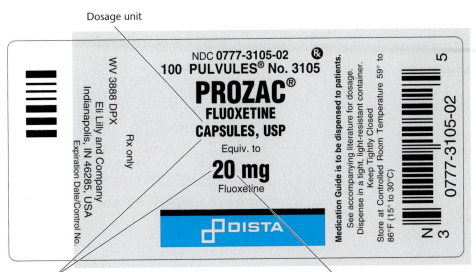

Figure 6-1 Prozac® 20 mg

Calculating the Desired Dose

Before you calculate the *amount to dispense*, it is first necessary to determine the desired dose. As stated in Table 6-1, the desired dose D (the amount of drug given at one time) must have the same unit of measurement as the dose on hand H (found on the drug label). Unfortunately, the dosage ordered O will not always be written in the same units as are found on the drug label. For example, an order may be written in grams while the drug is labeled in milligrams. When this occurs, it is necessary to convert the dosage ordered to a desired dose having the same units as the dose on hand.

In this section you will work with three different methods that can be used to calculate the desired dose. You may choose to use the fraction proportion method or the ratio proportion method; we will also introduce the dimensional analysis method. Each method will give you the same result, and the method you use is a matter of personal preference. Once you identify the method you prefer, follow the color coding of that method. Regardless of the method that you choose, you will want to become familiar with the terms contained in Table 6-1 before you proceed.

The first step in calculating the desired dose D is making sure that the unit of measurement for the desired dose D is the same as the unit of measurement of the dose on hand H. This must be done before the amount to dispense can be calculated. This is calculated by converting the dosage ordered O into the same unit of measurement as the dose on hand H; once converted, it becomes the desired dose D.

EXAMPLE ▶ The physician has ordered the patient to receive 0.1 mg of medication. This is the dosage ordered O. On the label of the bottle of medication (see Figure 6-2), the dosage strength is 50 mcg/1 tablet, making the unit of measure of the dose on hand (H) micrograms (mcg). *Recall the dosage strength is the dose on hand per dosage unit*.

Since the medication comes in micrograms and the order is for milligrams, you must convert the dosage ordered (O) (0.5mg) to the same unit of measurement as the dose on hand (H) (micrograms) to obtain the desired dose. You will see this calculated by three different methods in the following examples.

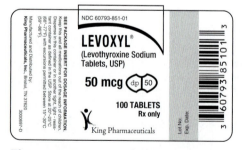

Figure 6-2 Levoxyl® 50 mcg

Using Conversion Factors

Fraction Proportion Method

You can use fraction proportions to convert from one unit of measure to another. Use the following procedure check list to work your conversion.

Procedure Checklist 6-1

Converting by the Fraction Proportion Method

1. Write a conversion factor with the units that you are converting to in the numerator and the units you are converting from in the denominator.
2. Write a fraction with the unknown as the numerator and the number that you need to convert as the denominator. (*The unknown is the desired dose D. The number you need to convert is the dosage ordered O.*)
3. Set up the two fractions as a proportion.
4. Cancel units.
5. Cross-multiply and then solve for the unknown value.

EXAMPLE 1 ▶   The dosage ordered is 0.1 mg once a day.

The dosage strength is 50 mcg per tablet.
Find the desired dose.
In this case, the drug is measured in milligrams on the drug order and micrograms on the drug label. The units for the desired dose must match those found on the drug label, which means that we must convert 0.1 mg to micrograms.

Follow the steps of Procedure Checklist 6-1.

1. Since we are converting to micrograms, micrograms must appear in the numerator of our conversion factor. Our conversion factor is $\frac{1000 \text{ mcg}}{1 \text{ mg}}$.
2. The other fraction for our proportion has the unknown D for a numerator. The value that is being converted, 0.1 mg, or the dosage ordered, must appear as the denominator. Our conversion factor is $\frac{D}{0.1 \text{ mg}}$.
3. Setting the two fractions into a proportion gives us the following equation:

$$\frac{D}{0.1 \text{ mg}} = \frac{1000 \text{ mcg}}{1 \text{ mg}}$$

4. Cancel units.

$$\frac{D}{0.1 \text{ m\cancel{g}}} = \frac{1000 \text{ mcg}}{1 \text{ m\cancel{g}}}$$

5. Cross-multiply and then solve for the unknown.

$$1 \times D = 1000 \text{ mg} \times 0.1$$
$$D = 100 \text{ mcg} = \text{desired dose}$$

EXAMPLE 2 ▶   The order reads "aspirin gr v PO daily."

The drug label indicates 325-mg tablets.
Find the desired dose.
Again, the drug order and the drug label use different units. In this case, we must convert the dosage ordered (O) (5 grains) to milligrams to find the desired dose (D).

Follow the steps of Procedure Checklist 6-1.

1. Since we are converting to milligrams, our conversion factor is

$$\frac{65 \text{ mg}}{1 \text{ gr}}$$

Note: For this medication, 65 mg per 1 gr is used; note that 60 mg per 1 grain can also be used.

2. The other fraction for our proportion is $\frac{D}{5 \text{ gr}}$.
3. Setting the two fractions into a proportion gives the following equation:

$$\frac{D}{5 \text{ gr}} = \frac{65 \text{ mg}}{1 \text{ gr}}$$

4. Cancel units.

$$\frac{D}{5 \text{ g\!r}} = \frac{65 \text{ mg}}{1 \text{ g\!r}}$$

5. Cross-multiply and then solve for the unknown.

$$1 \times D = 65 \text{ mg} \times 5$$
$$D = 325 \text{ mg} = \text{desired dose}$$

Super Tech . . .

Open the CD-ROM that accompanies your textbook and select Chapter 6, Exercise 6-1. Review the animation and example problems, and then complete the practice problems. Continue to the next section of the book once you have mastered the information presented.

⚠ Caution!

In a fraction proportion, units from the two fractions can be canceled *only* when they are in the same portion of the fraction. Units in the denominator of one fraction cannot be canceled with units found in the numerator of the other.

If you set up a proportion with mismatched units, you will calculate the desired dose incorrectly. In an earlier example, the dosage ordered was in grains, and the dosage strength was measured in milligrams. Suppose that you had used the conversion factor $\frac{1 \text{ gr}}{65 \text{ mg}}$ instead of $\frac{65 \text{ mg}}{1 \text{ gr}}$. Your incorrect proportion would then have been $\frac{D}{5 \text{ gr}} = \frac{1 \text{ gr}}{65 \text{ mg}}$.

Here, the units are mismatched and cannot be canceled. You should immediately realize that the conversion factor is incorrect because the units in the denominators of the proportion do not match. If you had not included the units when setting up the proportion, the error may have gone unnoticed. *Always include the units when you perform calculations*.

Using Conversion Factors

Ratio Proportion Method
Procedure Checklist 6-2

Converting by the Ratio Proportion Method
When setting up a ratio proportion, write it in the following format, A:B::C:D. For these equations, you will set your proportions up using the appropriate abbreviations, units of measurement, and numbers.

1. Write the conversion factor as a ratio using the appropriate values for $O:H$ so that O has the units of the value that you are converting (the dosage ordered) and H has the unit of value of the dose on hand.
2. Write a second ratio using the appropriate values for $D:O$ so that D is the missing value (desired dose) and O is the number that is being converted (the dosage ordered).
3. Write the proportion in the form $O:H::D:O$. *Note: When you are using the ratio proportion method to calculate the desired dose, D indicates the unknown value (desired dose).*
4. Cancel units.
5. Solve the proportion by multiplying the means and extremes.

EXAMPLE 1 ▶ The dosage ordered is 0.1 mg once a day.

The dosage strength is 50 mcg per tablet.
Find the desired dose.
The drug is measured in milligrams on the drug order and micrograms on the drug label. The units for the desired dose must match those found on the drug label, which means that we must determine how many micrograms are equivalent to 0.1 mg.

Follow the steps of Procedure Checklist 6-2.

1. Since we are converting to micrograms (dose on hand H), micrograms must appear at the beginning of our conversion ratio. We are converting from milligrams (dosage ordered O), which must appear at the end of our conversion ratio. Our conversion ratio is

$$1000 \text{ mcg} : 1 \text{ mg}$$

2. The second ratio in our proportion will be $D:0.1$ mg, with D being the unknown value or desired dose and 0.1 mg being the dosage ordered, or the number that is being converted.
3. Our proportion is

$$1000 \text{ mcg} : 1 \text{ mg} :: D : 0.1 \text{ mg}$$

4. Cancel units.

$$1000 \text{ mcg}:1 \text{ mg}::D:0.1 \text{ mg}$$

5. Multiply the means and extremes, and then solve for the missing value.

$$1 \times D = 1000 \text{ mcg} \times 0.1$$
$$D = 100 \text{ mcg} = \text{desired dose}$$

EXAMPLE 2 ▶ The order reads "aspirin gr v PO daily."

The drug label indicates 325-mg tablets.
Find the desired dose.
Again, the drug order and the drug label use different units. In this case, we must convert the dosage ordered (5 grains) to milligrams to find the desired dose.

Follow the steps of Procedure Checklist 6-2.

1. Since we are converting to milligrams, our conversion ratio is

$$65 \text{ mg}:1 \text{ gr}$$

Note: For this medication 65 mg per 1 gr is used.

2. Our second ratio will be $D:5$ gr.
3. Our proportion is

$$65 \text{ mg}:1 \text{ gr}::D:5 \text{ gr}$$

4. Cancel units.

$$65 \text{ mg}:1 \text{ gr}::D:5 \text{ gr}$$

5. Multiply the means and extremes, and then solve for the missing value.

$$1 \times D = 65 \text{ mg} \times 5$$
$$D = 325 \text{ mg} = \text{desired dose}$$

 Super Tech . . .

Open the CD-ROM that accompanies your textbook and select Chapter 6, Exercise 6-2. Review the animation and example problems, and then complete the practice problems. Continue to the next section of the book once you have mastered the information presented.

⚠ Caution!

In a ratio proportion, units can be canceled *only* when they are found in the same part of each of the ratios.

In an earlier example, the dosage ordered was in milligrams, and the dosage strength was measured in micrograms. Suppose that you had used the conversion ratio 1 mg : 1000 mcg instead of 1000 mcg : 1 mg. Your incorrect proportion would then have been 1 mg : 1000 mcg : : D : 0.1 mg.

The common unit in the two ratios is not found in the same part of the ratios—grams are found at the beginning of the first and at end of the second ratio. Therefore, the units cannot be canceled. You should immediately realize that the conversion ratio is incorrect because the units cannot be canceled. If you had not included the units when setting up the proportion, the error might have gone unnoticed. *Always include the units when you are performing calculations.*

Using Conversion Factors

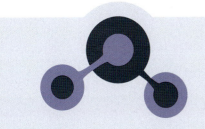

Dimensional Analysis

The dimensional analysis (DA) method is a modification of the fraction proportion and ratio proportion methods. When we are using DA, the unknown value stands alone on one side of an equation. In this case, the unknown is the desired dose D. The conversion factor is placed on the other side of the equation, and the number being converted is placed over 1.

Procedure Checklist 6-3

Converting Using the Dimensional Analysis (DA) Method

1. Determine the unit of measure for the answer, and place it as the unknown on one side of the equation.
2. On the other side of the equation, write a conversion factor with the units of measure for the answer on top as the numerator and the units you are converting from on the bottom as the denominator.
3. Multiply the conversion factor by the number that is being converted over 1.
4. Cancel units on the right side of the equation. The remaining unit of measure on the right side of the equation should match the unknown unit of measure on the left side of the equation.
5. Solve the equation.

EXAMPLE 1 ▶ The dosage ordered is 0.1 mg once a day.

The dosage strength is 50 mcg per tablet.
Find the desired dose.
The drug is measured in milligrams on the drug order and in micrograms on the drug label. The units for the desired dose must match the units of the dose on hand. We must determine how many micrograms are equivalent to 0.1 mg.

Follow the steps of Procedure Checklist 6-3.

1. The unit of measure for the answer is micrograms. Place this on the left side of the equation.

$$D \text{ mcg} =$$

(*D* represents the desired dose, which is the unknown.)

2. Since we are converting to micrograms, micrograms must appear in the numerator of our conversion factor. Our conversion factor is

$$\frac{1000 \text{ mcg}}{1 \text{ mg}}$$

This will go on the other side of the equation.

3. Multiply the numerator of the conversion factor by the number that is being converted (the dosage ordered over 1).

$$D \text{ mcg} = \frac{1000 \text{ mcg}}{1 \text{ mg}} \times \frac{0.1 \text{ mg}}{1}$$

4. Cancel units. The remaining unit on both sides is micrograms.

$$D \text{ mcg} = \frac{1000 \text{ mcg}}{1 \text{ mg}} \times \frac{0.1 \text{ mg}}{1}$$

5. Solve the equation.

$$D \text{ mcg} = 1000 \text{ mcg} \times 0.1 = 100 \text{ mcg} = \text{desired dose}$$

EXAMPLE 2 ▶ The order reads "aspirin gr v PO daily."

The drug label indicates 325-mg tablets.
Find the desired dose.
Again, the drug order and the drug label use different units. In this case, we must convert the dosage ordered (5 grains) into milligrams (mg) to find the desired dose.

Follow the steps of Procedure Checklist 6-3.

1. The unit of measure for the answer is milligrams. Place this on the left side of the equation.

$$D \text{ mg} =$$

(*D* represents the desired dose, which is the unknown.)

2. Since we are converting to milligrams, our conversion factor is

$$\frac{65 \text{ mg}}{1 \text{ gr}}$$

Note: For this medication 65 mg per 1 gr is used.

3. Multiply the numerator of the conversion factor by the number being converted (dosage ordered over 1).

$$D = \frac{65 \text{ mg}}{1 \text{ gr}} \times \frac{5 \text{ gr}}{1}$$

4. Cancel units.

$$D = \frac{65 \text{ mg}}{1 \text{ gr}} \times \frac{5 \text{ gr}}{1}$$

5. Solve the equation.

$$D = 65 \text{ mg} \times 5 = 325 \text{ mg} = \text{desired dose}$$

Super Tech . . .

Open the CD-ROM that accompanies your textbook and select Chapter 6, Exercise 6-3. Review the animation and example problems, and then complete the practice problems. Continue to the next section of the book once you have mastered the information presented.

⚠ Caution!

In dimensional analysis, units can be canceled *only* when they are found in both the numerator and the denominator of the fraction.

In an earlier example, the dosage ordered was in milligrams and the dosage strength was measured in micrograms. Suppose that you had used the conversion factor $\frac{1 \text{ mg}}{1000 \text{ mcg}}$ instead of $\frac{1000 \text{ mcg}}{1 \text{ mg}}$. Your incorrect equation would then have been $D = \frac{1 \text{ mg}}{1000 \text{ mcg}} \times \frac{0.1 \text{ mg}}{1}$.

You may cancel units within a fraction only when they are found in both the numerator and the denominator. Here, the common unit (grams) is found in the numerator only and cannot be canceled. You should immediately realize that the conversion factor is incorrect because the units cannot be canceled. If you had not included the units when setting up the equation, the error might have gone unnoticed. *Always include the units when you are performing calculations.*

✓ Review and Practice 6-1 Doses and Dosages

In Exercises 1–18, using your method of choice, convert the dosage ordered to the same unit as that of the dose on hand or measuring device and determine how many times a day the patient will take each medication.

1. Ordered: Amoxicillin 0.25 g qid for 10 days   Desired dose: _____
   On hand: Amoxicillin 125-mg capsules

   How many times per day will the patient take this medication?   _____

2. Ordered: Erythromycin 0.5 g bid for 7 days
   On hand: Erythromycin 500-mg tablets

   How many times per day will the patient take this medication?

   Desired dose: _____

   _____

3. Ordered: Phenobarbital gr ss po daily
   On hand: Phenobarbital 15-mg tablets

   How many times per day will the patient take this medication?

   Desired Dose: _____

   _____

4. Ordered: Penicillin VK 0.25 g tid for 10 days
   On hand: Penicillin VK 500 mg

   How many times per day will the patient take this medication?

   Desired dose: _____

   _____

5. Ordered: Levoxyl® 0.15 mg po daily
   On hand: Levoxyl® 300-mcg tablets

   How many times per day will the patient take this medication?

   Desired dose: _____

   _____

6. Ordered: Duratuss® HD 5 mL po q 6 hours prn
   Available measuring device is marked in teaspoons.

   How many times per day will the patient take this medication?

   Desired dose: _____

   _____

7. Ordered: Robitussin® DM 2 tsp po q 4 to 6 hours prn
   Available measuring device is marked in mL.

   How many times per day will the patient take this medication?

   Desired dose: _____

   _____

8. Ordered: Keppra® 1 g PO daily
   On hand: Keppra® 500 mg tablets

   How many times per day will the patient take this medication?

   Desired dose: _____

   _____

9. Ordered: Morphine $\frac{1}{4}$ gr q 12 hours prn severe pain
   On hand: Morphine sulfate 15 mg immediate-release tablets

   How many times per day will the patient take this medication?

   Desired dose: _____

   _____

10. Ordered: Synthroid® 0.05 mg po daily
    On hand: Synthroid® 50 mcg

    How many times per day will the patient take this medication?

    Desired dose: _____

    _____

11. Ordered: Synthroid® 0.088 mg PO daily
    On hand: Synthroid® 88 mcg

    How many times per day will the patient take this medication?

    Desired dose: _____

    _____

12. Ordered: Depakote® 0.5 g PO q am
    On hand: Depakote® 125 mg tablets

    How many times per day will the patient take this medication?

    Desired dose: _____

    _____

13. Ordered: Levsin® 250 mcg PO daily
    On hand: Levsin® 0.125 mg

    How many times per day will the patient take this medication?

    Desired dose: _____

    _____

14. Ordered: 1½ teaspoon Zithromax® 200 mg/ 5 mL PO q6h   Desired dose: _____
    On hand: Zithromax® 200 mg/5 mL
    Available measuring device is marked in mL.

    How many times per day will the patient take this medication?   _____

15. Ordered: 7.5 mL clarithromycin PO q4h   Desired dose: _____
    On hand: clarithromycin 125mg / 5 mL
    Only available measuring device is a teaspoon.

    How many times per day will the patient take this medication?   _____

16. Ordered: Levothroid® 0.137 mg PO daily   Desired dose: _____
    On hand: Levothroid® 137 mcg

    How many times per day will the patient take this medication?   _____

17. Ordered: Risperdal® 250 mcg PO daily   Desired dose: _____
    On hand: Risperdal® 0.5 mg

    How many times per day will the patient take this medication?   _____

18. Ordered: Metformin 1 g po qd   Desired dose: _____
    On hand: Metformin 500 mg

    How many times per day will the patient take this medication?   _____

Calculating the Amount to Dispense

Once you have determined the desired dose, you still have one more step that must be completed. While the desired dose tells you how many grams, milligrams, or grains of a drug the patient is to receive, you will need to know how many tablets, capsules, teaspoons, or milliliters of the medication must be given to deliver the desired dose. You must calculate an **amount to dispense,** which is the volume of liquid or number or solid dosage units that contain the desired dose.

In this section, you will be presented with four methods for calculating the *amount to dispense*. As with previous calculations, you may choose to use fraction proportion, ratio proportion, or dimensional analysis. We will also introduce the formula method. Again, the method that you choose to use is up to you—each will give you the same result.

To calculate the amount to dispense *A*, the following information must be known:

Amount to dispense: The volume of liquid or number or solid dosage units that contain the desired dose.

- The desired dose *D*, or the amount of drug to be given at a single time. This is the dosage ordered converted to the same units as those of the dose on hand, if necessary.
- The dosage strength of the dose on hand *H* per dosage unit *Q*. Recall, the dose on hand *H* is the amount of drug contained in a dosage unit. The dosage unit *Q* is the unit by which you will measure the medication—tablets, capsules, milliliters, teaspoons, etc. This is obtained from the medication label.

EXAMPLE ▶ Ordered: Famvir® 500 mg PO q8h.

On hand: 250-mg tablets

In this case the dose on hand is 250 mg and the dosage unit is tablets. You determine that the dose on hand is 250 mg and the dose ordered is 500 mg. In this case you do not need to convert the dose ordered because it is already in the same unit of measurement as that of the dose on hand. You have all the necessary information to calculate the amount to dispense.

- D = desired dose = 500 mg
- H = dose on hand = 250 mg
- Q = dosage unit = 1 tablet

Calculating the Amount to Dispense

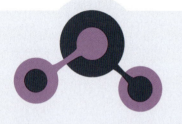

Fraction Proportion Method
Procedure Checklist 6-4

Calculating the Amount to Dispense by Fraction Proportion Method

1. Set up the proportion as follows:

$$\frac{\text{Dosage unit}}{\text{Dose on hand}} = \frac{\text{amount to dispense}}{\text{desired dose}} \quad \text{or} \quad \frac{Q}{H} = \frac{A}{D}$$

2. Cancel units.
3. Cross-multiply and then solve for the unknown value.

EXAMPLE 1 ▶ Find the amount to dispense. See Figure 6-3.

Ordered Famvir® 500 mg PO q8h
On hand: 250 mg tablets

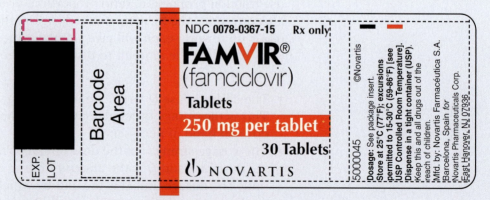

Figure 6-3 Famvir® 250-mg Tablets

The drug is ordered in milligrams, which is the same unit used on the label. Therefore, the dosage ordered is the same as the desired dose (500 mg). By reading the label we find that the dosage unit is 1 tablet and the dose on hand is 250 mg.

Therefore,

D = 500 mg
Q = 1 tablet
H = 250 mg

Follow the Procedure Checklist 6-4.

1. Fill in the proportion.
   (Think: If 1 tablet equals 250 mg, then how many tablets equal 500 mg?)

$$\frac{1 \text{ tablet}}{250 \text{ mg}} = \frac{A}{500 \text{ mg}}$$

2. Cancel units.

$$\frac{1 \text{ tablet}}{250 \text{ mg}} = \frac{A}{500 \text{ mg}}$$

3. Cross-multiply and solve for the unknown.

$$250 \times A = 1 \text{ tablet} \times 500$$

$$A = \frac{500}{250} \text{ tablets}$$

$$A = 2 \text{ tablets} = \text{amount to dispense}$$

EXAMPLE 2 ▶ Ordered: Metformin 2 g PO daily. See Figure 6-4.

On hand: 1000-mg tablets

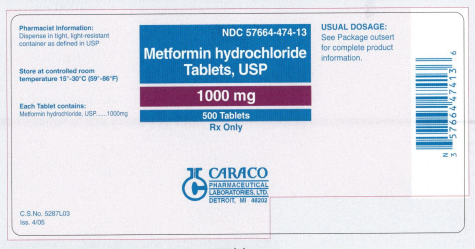

Figure 6-4 Metformin 1000-mg Tablets

In this case, the order is written in grams, and the drug is labeled in milligrams. Before we can determine the amount to dispense, we must calculate a desired dose that is in milligrams.

Follow the Procedure Checklist 6-1.

1. Recall that 1 g = 1000 mg. Since we are converting to milligrams, our conversion factor is

$$\frac{1000 \text{ mg}}{1 \text{ g}}$$

2. The other fraction for our proportion is $\frac{D}{2 \text{ g}}$.
3. Set up the fraction proportion equation:

$$\frac{D}{2 \text{ g}} = \frac{1000 \text{ mg}}{1 \text{ g}}$$

4. Cancel units.

$$\frac{D}{2 \, \cancel{g}} = \frac{1000 \text{ mg}}{1 \, \cancel{g}}$$

5. Solve for the unknown.

$$1 \times D = 1000 \text{ mg} \times 2$$
$$D = 2000 \text{ mg} = \text{desired dose}$$

We now have the three necessary pieces of information: The desired dose is 2000 mg, the dosage unit is 1 tablet, and the dose on hand is 1000 mg.

Follow the Procedure Checklist 6-4.

1. Fill in the proportion.
   (Think: *If 1 tablet has 1000 mg, then how many tablets will have 2000 mg?*)

$$\frac{1 \text{ tablet}}{1000 \text{ mg}} = \frac{A}{2000 \text{ mg}}$$

2. Cancel units.

$$\frac{1 \text{ tablet}}{1000 \, \cancel{\text{mg}}} = \frac{A}{2000 \, \cancel{\text{mg}}}$$

3. Cross-multiply and solve for the unknown.

$$1000 \times A = 1 \text{ tablet} \times 2000 \qquad \text{(divide both sides by 1000)}$$

$$A = \frac{2000}{1000} = 2 \text{ tablets} = \text{amount to dispense}$$

Super Tech . . .

Open the CD-ROM that accompanies your textbook and select Chapter 6, Exercise 6-4. Review the animation and example problems, and then complete the practice problems. Continue to the next section of the book once you have mastered the information presented.

Tech Check

When in Doubt, Double Check Your Work!

Always use critical thinking skills to evaluate your answer before you administer a drug. For example, in Example 2 the medication ordered is 2 g, and the medication comes in bottles of 1000-mg tablets. If you set up the problem incorrectly, you may get the answer $\frac{1}{2}$. Here is how.

First you determine that the desired dose is 2000 mg, and then you set up the problem, reversing the dose on hand with the desired dose.

$$\frac{1 \text{ tablet}}{2000 \text{ mg}} = \frac{A}{1000 \text{ mg}}$$

$$\frac{1 \text{ tablet}}{2000 \text{ mg}} = \frac{A}{1000 \text{ mg}}$$

(Canceling the units makes the problem appear correct.)
When you cross-multiply, you come up with the following.

$$2000 \times A = 1 \text{ tablet} \times 1000 \text{ (Divide both sides by 2000)}$$

$$A = \frac{1000}{2000} = \frac{1}{2}$$

Think Before You Act

If 1 tablet of Metformin is 1000 g and you need to give the patient 2000 g, you realize that you need to give more than $\frac{1}{2}$ tablet. With critical thinking you would determine that the answer appears incorrect and you should recalculate. *Never administer a medication if you are uncertain or uncomfortable with the answer you obtain.*

Calculating the Amount to Dispense

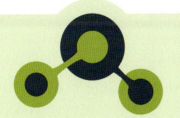

Ratio Proportion Method

Procedure Checklist 6-5

Calculating Amount to Dispense by Ratio Proportion Method

1. The proportion will be set up as follows:
   Dosage unit : dose on hand :: amount to dispense : desired dose, or
   $Q:H::A:D$
2. Cancel units.
3. Multiply the means and extremes and then solve for the missing value.

EXAMPLE 1 ▶   Ordered: Famvir® 500 mg PO q8h

On hand: Famvir® 250 mg per/tablet (see Figure 6-3 on page 168).
Find the amount to dispense.

The drug is ordered in milligrams, which is the same unit used on the label. Therefore, the desired dose is 500 mg. Reading the label tells us that the dosage unit is 1 tablet and the dose on hand is 250 mg.

Follow Procedure Checklist 6-5.

1. Fill in the proportion.
   (Think: *If 1 tablet is 250 mg, then how many tablets make 500 mg?*)

$$1 \text{ tablet}:250 \text{ mg}::A:500 \text{ mg}$$

2. Cancel units.

$$1 \text{ tablet}:250 \text{ mg}::A:500 \text{ mg}$$

3. Multiply the means and extremes, and then solve for the missing value.

$$250 \times A = 1 \text{ tablet} \times 500$$
$$\frac{250}{250} \times A = 1 \text{ tablet} \times \frac{500}{250}$$
$$A = 2 \text{ tablets} = \text{amount to dispense}$$

EXAMPLE 2 ❯ Ordered: Metformin 2 g PO daily.

On hand: Metformin hydrochloride 1000 mg (see Figure 6-4 on page 169) Calculate the amount to dispense.

In this case, the order is written in grams, and the drug is labeled in milligrams. Before we can determine the amount to dispense, we must calculate a desired dose that is in milligrams.

Follow Procedure Checklist 6-2.

1. Recall that 1 g = 1000 mg. Since we are converting to milligrams, our conversion factor is 1000 mg:1 g
2. The other ratio in our proportion is:

$$D:2 \text{ g}$$

3. Set up the ratio proportion equation:

$$1000 \text{ mg}:1 \text{ g}::D:2 \text{ g}$$

4. Cancel units.

$$1000 \text{ mg}:1 \text{ g}::D:2 \text{ g}$$

5. Multiply the means and extremes, and solve the equation.

$$1 \times D = 1000 \text{ mg} \times 2$$
$$D = 2000 \text{ mg} = \text{desired dose}$$

We now have the three necessary pieces of information: The desired dose is 2000 mg, the dosage unit is 1 tablet, and the dose on hand is 1000 mg.

$$D = 2000 \text{ mg}$$
$$Q = 1 \text{ tablet}$$
$$H = 1000 \text{ mg}$$

Follow Procedure Checklist 6-5.

1. Fill in the ratio proportion. (Think: *If 1 tablet equals 1000 mg, then how many tablets equal 2000 mg?*)

$$1 \text{ tablet} : 1000 \text{ mg} :: A : 2000 \text{ mg}$$

2. Cancel units.

$$1 \text{ tablet} : 1000 \text{ m\!g} :: A : 2000 \text{ m\!g}$$

3. Multiply the means and extremes, and solve for the unknown.

$$1000 \times A = 2000 \times 1 \text{ tablet} \qquad \text{(Divide both sides by 1000)}$$
$$A = 2 \text{ tablets} = \text{amount to dispense}$$

Super Tech . . .

Open the CD-ROM that accompanies your textbook and select Chapter 6, Exercise 6-5. Review the animation and example problems, and then complete the practice problems. Continue to the next section of the book once you have mastered the information presented.

Calculating the Amount to Dispense

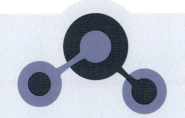

Dimensional Analysis
Procedure Checklist 6-6

Calculating the Amount to Dispense by the Dimensional Analysis Method

With dimensional analysis, you will not need to calculate the desired dose and amount to dispense separately. You will place your unknown (amount to dispense) on one side of the equation and then multiply a series of factors on the right side of the equation. Canceling units will help you determine that the equation has been set up correctly.

1. Determine the unit of measure for the answer, and place it as the unknown on one side of the equation. (In this case the answer would be the amount to dispense. The unit of measure will be the same unit of measure as that of the dosage unit.)
2. On the right side of the equation, write a conversion factor with the unit of measure for the desired dose on top and the unit of measure for the dosage ordered on the bottom. (*This is necessary if the dose ordered is in a different unit of measurement than the dose on hand.*)
3. Multiply the conversion factor by a second factor—the dosage unit over the dose on hand.
4. Multiply by a third factor—dose ordered over the number 1
5. Cancel units on the right side of the equation. The remaining unit of measure on the right side of the equation should match the unknown unit of measure on the left side of the equation.
6. Solve the equation.

EXAMPLE 1 ▶ Ordered: Famvir® 500 mg PO q8h

On hand: Famvir® 250 mg per tablet (see Figure 6-3 on page 168)
Find the amount to dispense.

Follow Procedure Checklist 6-6.

1. The unit of measure for the amount to dispense will be tablets. This is the dosage unit.

$$A \text{ tablets} =$$

2. Since the unit of measurement for the dosage ordered is the same as the dose on hand, no conversion factor is necessary.
3. The dosage unit is 1 tablet. The dosage strength is 250 mg. This is our first factor.

$$\frac{1 \text{ tablet}}{250 \text{ mg}}$$

4. The dose ordered is 500 mg. Place this quantity over the number 1 for the next factor.

$$A \text{ tablet} = \frac{1 \text{ tablet}}{250 \text{ mg}} \times \frac{500 \text{ mg}}{1}$$

5. Cancel the units.

$$A \text{ tablet} = \frac{1 \text{ tablet}}{250 \text{ m\!g}} \times \frac{500 \text{ m\!g}}{1}$$

6. Solve the equation.

$$A \text{ tablet} = 1 \text{ tablet} \times \frac{500}{250}$$

$$A = 2 \text{ tablets} = \text{amount to dispense}$$

EXAMPLE 2 ▶ Ordered: Metformin 2 g PO daily

On hand: Metformin hydrochloride 1000 mg (see Figure 6-4 on page 169)
Find the amount to dispense.

Follow Procedure Checklist 6-6.

1. The unit of measure for the amount to dispense will be tablets.

$$A \text{ tablets} =$$

2. The unit of measure for the dosage ordered is grams. The unit of measure for the desired dose is milligrams. Recall the conversion factor 1 g = 1000 mg. We will be converting to milligrams.

$$\frac{1000 \text{ mg}}{1 \text{ g}}$$

3. The dosage unit is 1 tablet, and the dose on hand is 1000 mg. This is our second factor.

$$\frac{1000 \text{ mg}}{1 \text{ g}} \times \frac{1 \text{ tablet}}{1000 \text{ mg}}$$

4. The dose ordered is 2 g. Place this over 1:

$$A \text{ tablet} = \frac{1000 \text{ mg}}{1 \text{ g}} \times \frac{1 \text{ tablet}}{1000 \text{ mg}} \times \frac{2 \text{ g}}{1}$$

5. Cancel units.

$$A \text{ tablet} = \frac{1000 \text{ m\cancel{g}}}{1 \text{ \cancel{g}}} \times \frac{1 \text{ tablet}}{1000 \text{ m\cancel{g}}} \times \frac{2 \text{ \cancel{g}}}{1}$$

6. Solve the equation.

$$A \text{ tablet} = \frac{2000}{1000} \qquad \text{(Reduce the fraction to lowest terms)}$$

$$A = 2 \text{ tablets} = \text{amount to dispense}$$

Super Tech . . .

Open the CD-ROM that accompanies your textbook and select Chapter 6, Exercise 6-6. Review the animation and example problems, and then complete the practice problems. Continue to the next section of the book once you have mastered the information presented.

Calculating the Amount to Dispense

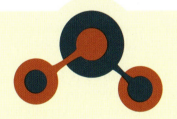

Formula Method

Procedure Checklist 6-7

Calculating the Amount to Dispense by the Formula Method

1. Determine the desired dose. Calculate it using the fraction proportion, ratio proportion, or dimensional analysis method. Determine the dose on hand H and dosage unit Q.
2. Fill in the formula:

$$\frac{D}{H} \times Q = A$$

where

D = desired dose—this is the dose ordered changed to the same unit of measure as the dose on hand
H = dose on hand—the amount of drug contained in each unit
Q = dosage unit—how the drug will be administered, such as tablets or milliliters
A = amount to dispense (unknown).

3. Cancel the units.
4. Solve for the unknown.

EXAMPLE 1 ▶ Ordered: Famvir® 500 mg PO q8h

On hand: Famvir® 250 mg per tablet (see Figure 6-3 on page 168)
Find the amount to dispense.

Follow Procedure Checklist 6-7.

1. The drug is ordered in milligrams, which is the same unit used on the label. Therefore, the desired dose is 500 mg. Reading the label tells us that the dosage unit is 1 tablet and the dose on hand is 250 mg. Therefore,

$$D = 500 \text{ mg}$$
$$Q = 1 \text{ tablet}$$
$$H = 250 \text{ mg}$$

2. Fill in the formula.

$$\frac{500 \ mg}{250 \ mg} \times 1 \ tablet = A$$

3. Cancel units.

$$\frac{500 \ \cancel{mg} \times 1 \ tablet}{250 \ \cancel{mg}} = A$$

4. Solve for the unknown.

$$\frac{500}{250} \times 1 \text{ tablet} = A$$

$$A = 2 \text{ tablets} = \text{amount to dispense}$$

EXAMPLE 2 ▶ Ordered: Metformin 2 g PO daily

On hand: Metformin hydrochloride 1000 mg (see Figure 6-4 on page 169)
Calculate the amount to dispense.
In this case, the order is written in grams, and the drug is labeled in milligrams. Before we can determine the amount to dispense, we must calculate a desired dose that is in milligrams. (In this example we will use the ratio proportion method Procedure Checklist 6-2.)

1. Recall that 1 g = 1000 mg. Since we are converting to milligrams, our conversion factor is:

$$1000 \text{ mg} : 1 \text{ g}$$

2. The other ratio in our proportion is:

$$D : 2 \text{ g}$$

3. Set up the ratio proportion equation.

$$1000 \text{ mg} : 1 \text{ g} :: D : 2 \text{ g}$$

4. Cancel units.

$$1000 \text{ mg} : 1 \cancel{g} :: D : 2 \cancel{g}$$

5. Multiply the means and extremes and solve the equation.

$$1 \times D = 1000 \text{ mg} \times 2$$

$$D = 2000 \text{ mg} = \text{desired dose}$$

Follow Procedure Checklist 6-7.

1. The three necessary pieces to complete the formula are the desired dose of 2000 mg, the dosage unit of 1 tablet, and the dose on hand of 1000 g.

$$D = 2000 \text{ mg}$$

$$Q = 1 \text{ tablet}$$

$$H = 1000 \text{ mg}$$

2. Insert the numbers and units into the formula.

$$\frac{2000 \text{ g}}{1000 \text{ g}} \times 1 \text{ tablet} = A$$

3. Cancel units.

$$\frac{2000 \cancel{g}}{1000 \cancel{g}} \times 1 \text{ tablet} = A$$

4. Solve for the unknown.

$$\frac{2000}{1000} \times 1 \text{ tablet} = A$$

$$A = 2 \text{ tablets} = \text{amount to dispense}$$

⊙ Super Tech . . .

Open the CD-ROM that accompanies your textbook and select Chapter 6, Exercise 6-7. Review the animation and example problems, and then complete the practice problems. Continue to the next section of the book once you have mastered the information presented.

✔ Review and Practice 6-2 Calculating the Amount to Dispense

In Exercises 1–14, calculate the amount to dispense and write out the full drug order.

Example: Ordered: Ritalin® 15 mg PO bid ac
      On Hand: Ritalin® 5 mg
      Amount to dispense = 3 tablets
      Drug order: Take 3 tablets by mouth two times per day with meals

1. Ordered: Thorazine® 20 mg PO tid
   On hand: Thorazine® 10 mg tablets

Amount to dispense: _____

Drug order: _____

2. Ordered: Ranitidine hydrochloride 150 mg PO bid
   On hand: Zantac® syrup 15 mg ranitidine hydrochloride per mL

   Amount to dispense: _____

   Drug order: _____

3. Ordered: Ceclor® 0.375 g PO bid
   On hand: Ceclor® Oral Suspension 187 mg per 5 mL

   Amount to dispense: _____

   Drug order: _____

4. Ordered: Nitroglycerin gr 1/100 SL stat
   On hand: Nitroglycerin 0.3-mg tablets

   Amount to dispense: _____

   Drug order: _____

5. Ordered: Amoxicillin 250 mg PO tid
   On hand: Amoxicillin 250 mg/5 mL

   Amount to dispense: _____

   Drug order: _____

6. Ordered: Tricor® 108 mg PO daily
   On hand: Tricor® 54 mg tablets

   Amount to dispense: _____

   Drug order: _____

7. Ordered: Procardia® 20 mg PO tid
   On hand: Procardia® 10 mg capsules

   Amount to dispense: _____

   Drug order: _____

8. Ordered: Moexipril hydrochloride 15 mg PO q.d. a.c.
   On hand: Moexipril hydrochloride 7.5 mg tablets

   Amount to dispense: _____

   Drug order: _____

9. Ordered: Synthroid® 0.3 mg PO q.d.
   On hand: Synthroid® 150 mcg

   Amount to dispense: _____

   Drug order: _____

10. Ordered: Wellbutrin® 0.2 g PO bid
    On hand: Wellbutrin® 100 mg

    Amount to dispense: _____

    Drug order: _____

11. Ordered: Keflex® 500 mg PO q12h
    On hand: Keflex® 250 mg per 5 mL

    Amount to dispense: _____

    Drug order: _____

12. Ordered: Decadron® 6 mg IM q.i.d.
    On hand: Decadron® 4 mg per mL

    Amount to dispense: _____

    Drug order: _____

13. Ordered: Ketoconazole 100 mg PO qd
    On hand: Ketoconazole 200-mg scored tablets

    Amount to dispense: _____

    Drug order: _____

14. Ordered: Erythromycin oral suspension 150 mg PO bid
    On hand: Erythromycin oral suspension 200 mg per mL

    Amount to dispense: _____

    Drug order: _____

Estimated Days Supply

Estimated days supply: How long the medication will last the patient if taken correctly.

As a pharmacy technician you may need to determine the **estimated days supply** of a prescription, which is how long the medication will last the patient if taken correctly. If the physician orders Zocor 20 mg tablets #90 i po daily, the prescription will last the patient 90 days. To determine estimated days supply you will multiply amount of medication to dispense by days needed over the number of dosage units per day.

$$\frac{\text{Amount to dispense}}{\text{Dosage units per day}} = \text{Estimated days supply}$$

EXAMPLE 1 ▶ The physician orders Motrin® 600 mg tablets #20 i po bid.

$$\frac{20 \text{ tablets}}{2} = 10 \text{ days}$$

The prescription should last the patient 10 days.

EXAMPLE 2 ▶ The physician orders Robitussin® AC 240 mL ii tsp tid.

The patient is to receive 10 mL (2 tsp) three times per day. So, the patient should take 30 mL per day.

$$\frac{240 \text{ mL}}{30 \text{ mL}} = 8 \text{ days}$$

The prescription should last the patient 8 days.

You will get additional practice calculating estimated days supply for the different routes of administration in Chapter 7.

Super Tech . . .

Open the CD-ROM that accompanies your textbook and select Chapter 6, Exercise 6-8. Review the animation and example problems, and then complete the practice problems. Continue to the next section of the book once you have mastered the information presented.

✓ Review and Practice 6-3 Estimated Days Supply

In Exercises 1-5 calculate the estimated days supply.

1. Procardia® 20 mg tablets # 180 i PO tid

2. Keflex® 500 mg capsules # 20 i PO q12h

3. Synthroid® 0.3 mg tablets # 30 i PO q.d.

4. Amoxicillin 250 mg/5 mL Disp 210 mL take i tsp PO tid

5. Thorazine® 20 mg # 90 i PO tid

✓ Chapter 6 Review

Test Your Knowledge

Multiple Choice

Select the best answer and write the letter on the line.

_____ 1. What is the abbreviation for dosage ordered?
  A. *H*
  B. *Q*
  C. *D*
  D. *O*
  E. *A*

_____ 2. What is the abbreviation for desired dose?
  A. *H*
  B. *Q*
  C. *D*
  D. *O*
  E. *A*

_____ 3. What is the abbreviation for dosage unit?
  A. *H*
  B. *Q*
  C. *D*
  D. *O*
  E. *A*

_____ 4. What is the abbreviation for dose on hand?
  A. *H*
  B. *Q*
  C. *D*
  D. *O*
  E. *A*

_____ 5. What is the abbreviation for amount to dispense?
  A. *H*
  B. *Q*
  C. *D*
  D. *O*
  E. *A*

Practice Your Knowledge

Check Up

In Exercises 1–18, calculate the desired dose. Then calculate the amount to dispense.

1. Ordered: Valium® 5 mg PO tid
   On hand: Valium® 2-mg scored tablets

   Desired dose: _____ Amount to dispense: _____

2. Ordered: Atacand® 16 mg PO bid
   On hand: Atacand® 8-mg tablets

   Desired dose: _____ Amount to dispense: _____

3. Ordered: Cimetidine 400 mg PO qid
   On hand: Tagamet® 200 mg tablets

   Desired dose: _____ Amount to dispense: _____

4. Ordered: Noroxin® 800 mg PO qd ac
   On hand: Noroxin® 400-mg tablets

   Desired dose: _____ Amount to dispense: _____

5. Ordered: Pergolide mesylate 100 mcg PO tid
   On hand: Pergolide mesylate 0.05-mg tablets

   Desired dose: _____ Amount to dispense: _____

6. Ordered: Zyloprim® 0.25 g PO bid
   On hand: Zyloprim® 100-mg scored tablets

   Desired dose: _____ Amount to dispense: _____

7. Ordered: Zaroxolyn® 7.5 mg PO daily
   On hand: Zaroxolyn® 2.5-mg tablets

   Desired dose: _____ Amount to dispense: _____

8. Ordered: Ciprofloxacin hydrochloride 500 mg PO q12h
   On hand: Ciprofloxacin hydrochloride 250 mg tablets

   Desired dose: _____ Amount to dispense: _____

9. Ordered: Lexapro® 20 mg PO daily
   On hand: Lexapro® 10 mg tablets

   Desired dose: _____ Amount to dispense: _____

10. Ordered: Toprol® XL 100 mg PO bid
    On hand: Toprol® XL 25 mg extended-release tablets

    Desired dose: _____ Amount to dispense: _____

11. Ordered: Depakene® 250 mg PO bid
    On hand: Depakene® 250 mg capsules

    Desired dose: _____ Amount to dispense: _____

12. Ordered: Dilantin® 60 mg PO daily
    On hand: Dilantin® 30 mg capsules

    Desired dose: _____ Amount to dispense: _____

13. Ordered: Lisinopril 40 mg PO daily
    On hand: Lisinopril 20 mg tablets

    Desired dose: _____ Amount to dispense: _____

14. Ordered: Biaxin® 125 mg PO tid
    On hand: Biaxin® 250 mg per 5mL oral suspension

    Desired dose: _____ Amount to dispense: _____

15. Ordered: Augmentin® 1 gram PO bid
    On hand: Augmentin® 400 mg/ 5 mL

    Desired dose: _____ Amount to dispense: _____

16. Ordered: Singulair® 5 mg PO daily
    On hand: Singulair® 5 mg chewable tablets

    Desired dose: _____ Amount to dispense: _____

17. Ordered: Augmentin® 200 mg PO q8h
    On hand: Augmentin® 125 mg/ 5 mL suspension

    Desired dose: _____ Amount to dispense: _____

18. Ordered: Valtrex® 0.5 g PO daily
    On hand: Valtrex® 500 mg caplets

    Desired dose: _____ Amount to dispense: _____

Apply Your Knowledge

What Is the Dosage Ordered?

You are the pharmacy technician working in a retail pharmacy. You are working in a pharmacy when the following prescription comes in: Valium® 7.5 mg PO tid for 7 days. The drug is available in 2-mg scored tablets, 5-mg scored tablets, and 10-mg scored tablets, and you have all three strengths on hand for filling this prescription.

Answer the following questions:

1. What is the desired dose?

   _____

2. What is the amount to dispense?

   _____

Internet Activity

Many times medications come in different dosage strengths. (Recall the dosage strength is the dose on hand per dosage unit.) If you do not look at the label carefully, you can easily select the wrong medication and/or calculate the amount to dispense incorrectly. Search the Internet for at least three medications that come in different dosage strengths. List each medication and its various dosage strengths. You may want to focus on the top 200 medications at www.rxlist.com.

Super Tech . . .

Open the CD-ROM that accompanies your textbook, and complete a final review of the rules, practice problems, and activities presented for this chapter. For a final evaluation, take the chapter test and email or print your results for your instructor. A score of 95 percent or above indicates mastery of the chapter concepts.

7

Oral Medications and Parenteral Dosages

Key Terms

Caplet
Capsule
Enteric-coated
Estimated days supply
Gelcap
Inhalant
Intradermally
Intramuscular
Intravenous
Parenteral
Rectal
Scored
Spansules
Sustained release
Subcutaneous
Tablet
Topical
Transdermal
Vaginal

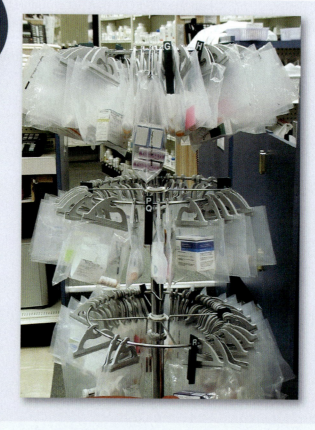

Learning Outcomes

When you have successfully completed Chapter 7, you will have mastered skills to be able to:

▶ Distinguish between different types of oral medications.

▶ Recognize the types of solid oral medications that may not be altered by crushing or opening them.

▶ Calculate the amount of oral and parenteral medication to administer.

▶ Select the appropriate syringe.

▶ Correctly reconstitute powdered medications.

▶ Calculate the amount of reconstituted medications to administer.

▶ Accurately calculate doses of inhalant, topical, transdermal, ophthalmic, otic, rectal, and vaginal medications.

▶ Identify errors that occur in calculating and preparing parenteral doses.

▶ Calculate estimated days supply.

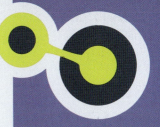

Introduction

So far you have learned the fraction proportion, ratio proportion, formula, and dimensional analysis methods for simple calculations. In this chapter you will apply these methods to oral and parenteral dosages. **Parenteral** medications are medications that are delivered outside of the digestive tract; the term most often refers to injections. The various types of injections used to deliver medications include:

- **Intramuscular (IM)** medication administered into a muscle by injection,
- **Subcutaneous (sub-Q)** medication administered under the skin by injection,
- **Intradermal (ID)** medication administered between the layers of skin, and
- **Intravenous (IV)** medication delivered directly to the bloodstream through a vein.

This chapter will focus on dosage calculations for oral and parenteral medications with the exception of intravenous and insulin administration, which will be covered in later chapters. By now you may have chosen one method with which you are most comfortable. If so, follow that method throughout this chapter, using the corresponding color coding in the examples given; then complete the practice problems, using your method of choice. While you are practicing these problems, remember that excellence is a *must* with dosage calculations.

PTCB Correlations

When you have completed this chapter you will have the mathematical building block of knowledge needed to assist you in performing dosage calculations.

- Knowledge of procedures to prepare reconstituted injectable and noninjectable medications. (Statement I-58).

- Knowledge of procedures to prepare oral dosage forms in unit-dose or non–unit-dose packaging. (Statement I-61).

Parenteral: Route of administration; medications that are delivered outside of the digestive tract; most often refers to injections.

Intramuscular (IM): Medication administered into a muscle by injection.

Subcutaneous (Sub-Q): Medication administered under the skin by injection.

Intravenous (IV): Medication delivered directly to the bloodstream through a vein.

Intradermal (ID): Medication administered between the layers of skin.

Critical Thinking in the Pharmacy
How Much Medication Needs to Be Dispensed?

You are the pharmacy technician working in a retail pharmacy. You are working in the pharmacy when the following prescription comes in: Biaxin® 187.5 mg PO qid for 5 days, qsad. On hand: Biaxin® 125 mg per 5 mL, 100 mL when mixed with 55 mL of water.

When you have completed Chapter 7 you will be able to determine how much medication to dispense as well as how many milliliters the patient will take per dose and in a 24-hour period.

1. How many milliliters need to be dispensed to fill the prescription?
2. How many milliliters will the patient take per dose?
3. How many milliliters will the patient take in 24 hours?

Tablets and Capsules

Solid oral medications come in several forms, including tablets, caplets, capsules, and gelcaps (see Figure 7-1).

A **tablet** is a solid disk or cylinder that contains a drug plus inactive ingredients. The tablet is the most common form of solid oral medication. It combines an amount of drug with inactive ingredients such as starch or talc to form a solid disk or cylinder that is convenient for swallowing. Certain tablets are specially designed to be administered sublingually (under the tongue) or buccally (between the cheek and gum). Sublingual and buccal tablets release medication into an area rich in blood vessels, where it can be quickly absorbed for rapid action. Some tablets are designed to be chewed; others dissolve in water to make a liquid that the patient can drink. Always check the drug label to determine how a tablet is meant to be administered.

Tablet: A solid disk or cylinder that contains a drug plus inactive ingredients.

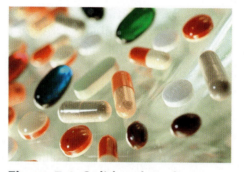

Figure 7-1 Solid oral medications including tablets, caplets, capsules, and gelcaps.

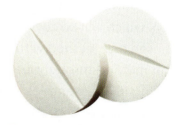

Figure 7-2 Scored tablets.

Caplets are oval-shaped pills similar to a tablet. Caplets have a special coating that makes them easy to swallow. **Capsules** are usually oval-shaped gelatin shells that contain medication in powder or granule form. The gelatin shell usually has two pieces that fit together. These pieces often may be separated to remove the medication when the patient cannot swallow a pill. **Gelcaps** consist of medication, usually liquid, in gelatin shells that are not designed to be opened.

Caplet: Oval-shaped pill similar to a tablet but having a coating for easy swallowing.

Capsule: Oval-shaped gelatin shell, usually in two pieces, that contains powder or granules.

Gelcap: Medication, usually liquid in a gelatin shell; not designed to be opened.

Calculating Dosages for Tablets and Capsules

Tablets are often **scored,** having indented lines indicating where they may be broken or divided when smaller doses are ordered. Most often, scored tablets divide into halves (see Figure 7-2), but some are scored to divide into thirds or quarters. The medication in scored tablets is evenly distributed throughout the tablet, allowing the dose to be divided evenly when the tablet is broken. Tablets may be broken into parts *only if they are scored,* and they must be broken only along the line of the scoring. Unscored tablets **must not** be broken into parts. Remember, breaking scored tablets to administer an ordered dosage is permitted but not optimal. Determine if a different dosage strength is available before you break scored tablets.

Always question and/or verify when your calculation indicates giving a portion of a capsule or a tablet when the tablet is not scored.

Scored: Medication tablets having indented lines indicating where they may be broken or divided.

EXAMPLE 1 ▶ Do not dispense $\frac{1}{2}$ of a capsule or unscored tablet.

EXAMPLE 2 ▶ Do not dispense $\frac{1}{3}$ or $\frac{3}{4}$ of a tablet scored for division in two pieces.

Question and recheck any calculation that indicates that you should dispense more than 3 tablets or capsules.

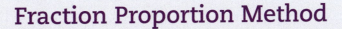

Super Tech...

Open the CD-ROM that accompanies your textbook and select Chapter 7, Exercise 7-1. Review the animation and example problems, and then complete the practice problems. Continue to the next section of the book once you have mastered the information presented.

To calculate the *amount per dose and the amount to dispense,* you must know the *desired dose,* the *dose on hand,* and the *dosage unit.* The desired dose and the dose on hand must be in the same unit of measurement. Generally, the dosage unit for solid oral medications will be 1, such as 1 tablet, 1 caplet, 1 capsule, or 1 gelcap.

Follow these steps when you are determining the amount of oral medication to be administer to or taken by a patient.

1. If necessary, convert the *dosage ordered O* to the *desired dose D* that has the same unit of measure as the *dose on hand H.*
2. Calculate the *amount to be administered* by the method of your choice:

   a. The fraction proportion method
   b. The ratio proportion method
   c. Dimensional analysis
   d. The formula method

3. Apply critical thinking skills to determine whether the amount you have calculated is reasonable. Recheck your calculation, if necessary.

Using Conversion Factors

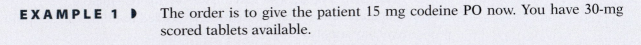

Fraction Proportion Method

EXAMPLE 1 ▶ The order is to give the patient 15 mg codeine PO now. You have 30-mg scored tablets available.

SOLUTION ▶ The dosage ordered *O* is 15 mg. The dose on hand *H* is 30 mg, and the dosage unit *Q* is 1 tablet.

Because the dosage ordered and the dose on hand have the same units, no conversion is needed to find the desired dose *D*, which is 15 mg.

1. Fill in the proportion.

$$\frac{Q \text{ (dosage unit)}}{H \text{ (dose on hand)}} = \frac{A \text{ (amount to dispense)}}{D \text{ (desired dose)}}$$

$$\frac{1 \text{ tablet}}{30 \text{ mg}} = \frac{A}{15 \text{ mg}}$$

2. Cancel units.

$$\frac{1 \text{ tablet}}{30 \text{ mg}} = \frac{A}{15 \text{ mg}}$$

3. Cross-multiply and solve for the unknown.

$$30 \times A = 1 \text{ tablet} \times 15$$

$$A = 1 \text{ tablet} \times \frac{15}{30}$$

$$A = 0.5 \text{ tablet}$$

Think critically about the result. Because 15 mg is one-half of 30 mg, tablet is an appropriate answer since the tablets are scored.

EXAMPLE 2 ▶ The order is Inderal® 80 mg PO qid. You have 40-mg tablets available.

SOLUTION ▶ The dosage ordered *O* is 80 mg. The dose on hand *H* is 40 mg, and the dosage unit *Q* is 1 tablet.

Because the dosage ordered and the dose on hand have the same units, no conversion is needed to find the desired dose *D*, which is 80 mg.

1. Fill in the proportion.

$$\frac{1 \text{ tablet}}{40 \text{ mg}} = \frac{A}{80 \text{ mg}}$$

2. Cancel units.

$$\frac{1 \text{ tablet}}{40 \text{ mg}} = \frac{A}{80 \text{ mg}}$$

3. Cross-multiply and solve for the unknown.

$$40 \times A = 1 \text{ tablet} \times 80$$

$$A = 1 \text{ tablet} \times \frac{80}{40}$$

$$A = 2 \text{ tablets}$$

Thinking critically about this result, you realize 80 is twice 40, so this dose requires twice 1 tablet. The calculated dosage does not call for more than 3 tablets, so this answer seems reasonable.

4. Calculate how much medication is needed to fill the prescription for a 30 day supply.

$$A = 2 \text{ tablets} \times 30 \text{ days} = 60 \text{ tablets}$$

Using Conversion Factors

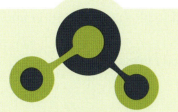

Ratio Proportion Method

EXAMPLE 1 ▶   The order is for 15 mg codeine. You have 30 mg scored tablets available.

SOLUTION ▶   The dosage ordered O is 15 mg. The dose on hand H is 30 mg, and the dosage unit Q is 1 tablet.

Because the dosage ordered and the dose on hand already have the same units, no conversion is needed to find the desired dose D, which is 15 mg.

1. Fill in the proportion.

$$Q:H::A:D$$
$$1 \text{ tablet}:30 \text{ mg}::A:15 \text{ mg}$$

2. Cancel units.

$$1 \text{ tablet}:30 \text{ m\!g}::A:15 \text{ m\!g}$$

3. Multiply means and extremes, then solve for the missing value.

$$30 \times A = 1 \text{ tablet} \times 15$$
$$A = 1 \text{ tablet} \times \frac{15}{30}$$
$$A = 0.5 \text{ tablet}$$

Think critically about the result. Because 15 mg is one-half of 30 mg, $\frac{1}{2}$ tablet is an appropriate answer since the tablets are scored.

EXAMPLE 2 ▶   The order is Inderal 80 mg PO qid. You have 40 mg tablets available.

SOLUTION ▶   The dosage ordered O is 80 mg. The dose on hand H is 40 mg, and the dosage unit Q is 1 tablet.

Because the dosage ordered and the dose on hand already have the same units, no conversion is needed to find the desired dose D, which is 80 mg.

1. Fill in the proportion.

$$1 \text{ tablet}:40 \text{ mg}::A:80 \text{ mg}$$

2. Cancel units.

$$1 \text{ tablet}:40 \text{ m\!g}::A:80 \text{ m\!g}$$

3. Cross-multiply the means and extremes, then solve for the missing value.

$$40 \times A = 1 \text{ tablet} \times 80$$
$$A = 1 \text{ tablet} \times \frac{80}{40}$$
$$A = 2 \text{ tablets}$$

Thinking critically about this result, you realize 80 is 40 × 2, so this dose requires twice 1 tablet. The calculated dosage does not call for more than 3 tablets, so this answer is correct.

4. Calculate how much medication is needed to fill the prescription for a 30 day supply.

$$A = 2 \text{ tablets} \times 30 \text{ days} = 60 \text{ tablets}$$

Using Conversion Factors

Dimensional Analysis

EXAMPLE 1 ▶ The order is 15 mg codeine. You have 30-mg scored tablets available.

SOLUTION ▶

1. The unit of measure for the amount to administer will be tablets.

$$A \text{ tablets} =$$

2. Since the unit of measure for the dosage ordered is the same as that for the dose on hand, this step is unnecessary.

3. The dosage unit is 1 tablet. The dosage on hand is 30 mg.

$$\frac{1 \text{ tablet}}{30 \text{ mg}}$$

4. The dosage ordered is 15 mg.

$$A \text{ tablets} = \frac{1 \text{ tablet}}{30 \text{ mg}} \times \frac{15 \text{ mg}}{1}$$

5. Cancel units.

$$A \text{ tablets} = \frac{1 \text{ tablet}}{30 \text{ mg}} \times \frac{15 \text{ mg}}{1}$$

6. Solve the equation.

$$A \text{ tablets} = \frac{1 \text{ tablet}}{30} \times \frac{15}{1}$$

$$A = 0.5 \text{ tablet} = \frac{1}{2} \text{ tablet}$$

Think critically about the result. Because 15 mg is one-half of 30 mg, tablet is an appropriate answer since the tablets are scored.

EXAMPLE 2 ▶ The order is Inderal 80 mg PO qid. You have 40-mg tablets available.

SOLUTION ▶

1. The unit of measure for the amount to administer will be tablets.

$$A \text{ tablets} =$$

2. Since the unit of measurement for the dosage ordered is the same as that for the dose on hand, this step is unnecessary.
3. The dosage unit is 1 tablet. The dose on hand is 40 mg.

$$\frac{1 \text{ tablet}}{40 \text{ mg}}$$

4. The dosage ordered is 80 mg.

$$A \text{ tablets} = \frac{1 \text{ tablet}}{40 \text{ mg}} \times \frac{80 \text{ mg}}{1}$$

5. Cancel units.

$$A \text{ tablets} = \frac{1 \text{ tablet}}{40 \text{ m\!g}} \times \frac{80 \text{ m\!g}}{1}$$

6. Solve the equation.

$$A \text{ tablets} = \frac{1 \text{ tablet}}{40} \times \frac{80}{1}$$

$$A = 2 \text{ tablets}$$

Thinking critically about this result, you realize 80 is 40 × 2, so this dose requires twice 1 tablet. The calculated dosage does not call for more than 3 tablets so this answer is correct.

7. Calculate how much medication is needed to fill the prescription for a 30-day supply.

$$A = 2 \text{ } tablets \times 30 \text{ days} = 60 \text{ tablets}$$

Using Conversion Factors

Formula Method

EXAMPLE 1 ▶ The order is for 15 mg codeine. You have 30-mg scored tablets available.

SOLUTION ▶ 1. The drug is ordered in milligrams, which is the same unit of measure as that for the dose on hand. Therefore,

$$D = 15 \text{ mg}$$
$$Q = 1 \text{ tablet}$$
$$H = 30 \text{ mg}$$

2. Fill in the formula.

$$\frac{D \times Q}{H} = A$$

or $\dfrac{\text{Desired dose}}{\text{Dose on hand}} \times$ dosage unit = amount to administer

$$\frac{15 \text{ mg} \times 1 \text{ tablet}}{30 \text{ mg}} = A$$

3. Cancel units.

$$\frac{15 \cancel{\text{ mg}} \times 1 \text{ tablet}}{30 \cancel{\text{ mg}}} = A$$

4. Solve for the unknown.

$$\frac{15 \times 1 \text{ tablet}}{30} = A$$

$$A = 0.5 \text{ tablet} = \frac{1}{2} \text{ tablet}$$

Think critically about the result. Because 15 mg is one-half of 30 mg, $\frac{1}{2}$ tablet is an appropriate answer since the tablets are scored.

EXAMPLE 2 ▶ The order is Inderal 80 mg PO qid. You have 40-mg tablets available.

SOLUTION ▶ 1. The drug is ordered in milligrams, which is the same unit of measure as the dose on hand. Therefore,

$$H = 40 \text{ mg}$$
$$D = 80 \text{ mg}$$
$$Q = 1 \text{ tablet}$$

2. Fill in the formula.

$$\frac{80 \text{ mg} \times 1 \text{ tablet}}{40 \text{ mg}} = A$$

3. Cancel units.

$$\frac{80 \cancel{\text{ mg}} \times 1 \text{ tablet}}{40 \cancel{\text{ mg}}} = A$$

4. Solve for the unknown.

$$\frac{80 \times 1 \text{ tablet}}{40} = A$$

$$A = 2 \text{ tablets}$$

Thinking critically about this result, you realize 80 is 40 × 2, so this dose requires twice 1 tablet. The calculated dosage does not call for more than 3 tablets so there is no need to question the order.

5. Calculate how much medication is needed to fill the prescription for a 30-day supply.

$$A = 2 \text{ tablets} \times 30 \text{ days} = 60 \text{ tablets}$$

Super Tech . . .

Open the CD-ROM that accompanies your textbook and select Chapter 7, Exercise 7-2. Review the animation and example problems, and then complete the practice problems. Continue to the next section of the book once you have mastered the information presented.

Crushing Tablets or Opening Capsules

For patients who have difficulty swallowing pills, certain tablets may be crushed (Figure 7-3) and certain capsules may be opened.

Sometimes you can mix a crushed tablet or an opened capsule with soft food or liquid. First check for interactions between the medication and the food or fluid being mixed with it or other medications that are being administered. For example, tetracycline is inactivated by milk. It must not be dissolved in foods that contain milk. In addition, it should not be given with either antacids or vitamin and mineral supplements.

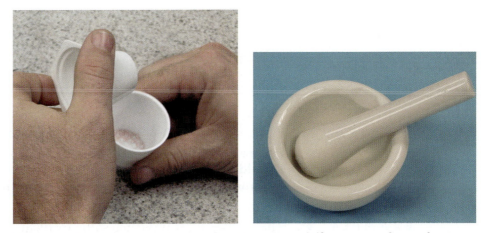

Figure 7-3 Tablets can be crushed by using different crushing devices.

Oral forms of medication are also ordered for patients with nasogastric, gastrostomy, or jejunostomy tubes. Before administering medication through the tube, the contents from a crushed tablet or opened capsule first must be dissolved in a small amount of warm water.

Some medications cannot be crushed. If these medications are ordered for a patient with a feeding tube or one who cannot swallow pills, determine whether an alternative form of the medication exists. Consult a drug reference or pharmacist for information, then ask the physician if the medication could be ordered in one of these forms. Always follow the policy of the facility where you are employed regarding substituting forms of medications.

Enteric-coated: Medications that dissolve only in the alkaline environment of the small intestines.

Enteric-coated tablets have a coating that dissolves only in an alkaline environment, such as the small intestine. These tablets deliver medication that would be destroyed by stomach acid or that could injure the stomach lining. Enteric-coated tablets often look like candies that have a soft center and a hard shell. Some aspirins are enteric-coated, as are certain

Sustained-release: Medications that releases slowly into the blood-stream over several hours.

Spansules: Special capsule that contains coated granules to delay the release of the medication.

iron tablets such as ferrous gluconate. Enteric-coated tablets must *never* be crushed, broken, or chewed. A patient must swallow them with their coating intact (see Figure 7-4).

Some medications are available in a **sustained-release** form that allows the drug to be released slowly into the bloodstream over a period of several hours. If the medication is scored, you may break it at the scored line. Otherwise you must not break it. Crushing or dissolving sustained-release tablets would allow more than the intended amount of medication to be absorbed at one time, causing overdose or toxicity of the drug.

Special capsules, often called **spansules,** contain granules of medication with different coatings to delay the release of the medication. You may open spansules and gently mix the granules in soft food, but you must not crush or dissolve the granules. (See Figure 7-5.)

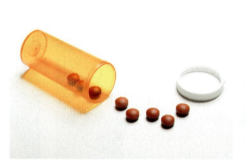

Figure 7-4 Enteric-coated tablets should never be split when given to patients.

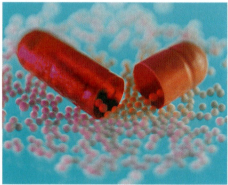

Figure 7-5 Sustained-release capsules are often called spansules.

E X A M P L E ▶ The following list indicates some medications that should not be crushed or altered. Crushing or altering these medications could cause an inaccurate dose of the medication to be administered.

To prevent an incorrect dose of medication do not crush or otherwise alter any of the following:

- Enteric-coated tablets
- Sustained-release forms of medication
- Any tablet with a hard shell or coating
- Any tablet with layers or speckles of different colors
- Tablets for sublingual or buccal use
- Capsules with seals that prevent separating the two parts

Super Tech . . .

Open the CD-ROM that accompanies your textbook and select Chapter 7, Exercise 7-3. Review the animation and example problems, and then complete the practice problems. Continue to the next section of the book once you have mastered the information presented.

Estimated days supply: How long the medication will last the patient if taken correctly.

Calculating estimated days supply for tablets and capsules

To determine **estimated days supply** you will multiply amount of medication to dispense by days needed over the number of dosage units per day.

$$\frac{\text{Amount to dispense}}{\text{Dosage units per day}} = \text{Estimated days supply}$$

EXAMPLE 1 ▶   The physician orders Motrin® 600 mg tablets #20 ipo bid

$$\frac{20 \text{ tablets}}{2} = 10 \text{ days}$$

The prescription should last the patient 10 days.

EXAMPLE 2 ▶   The physician orders Robitussin® AC 240 mL ii tsp tid

Since the order is for 2 tsp (10 mL) three times per day, the number of dosage units per day is 30 mL.

$$\frac{240 \text{ mL}}{30 \text{ mL}} = 8 \text{ days}$$

The prescription should last the patient 8 days.

✓ Review and Practice 7-1 Tablets and Capsules

In Exercises 1–10, calculate the amount to administer and estimated days supply where indicated. Unless otherwise noted, all scored tablets are scored in half.

1. Ordered: Tegretol® 200 mg PO bid, #180
   On hand: Tegretol® 200-mg unscored tablets

   Administer: _____
   Estimated Days Supply: _____

2. Ordered: Seroquel® 75 mg PO tid, # 90
   On hand: Seroquel® 75-mg unscored tablets

   Administer: _____
   Estimated Days Supply: _____

3. Ordered: Tolectin® 300 mg PO tid, # 30
   On hand: Tolectin® 300 mg scored tablets

   Administer: _____
   Estimated Days Supply: _____

4. Ordered: Isordil® Titradose® 15 mg PO now
   On hand: Isordil® Titradose® 10-mg deep-scored tablets

   Administer: _____

5. Ordered: Felbatol® 600 mg PO qid
   On hand: Felbatol® 400-mg scored tablets

   Administer: _____

6. Ordered: Decadron® 1.5 mg PO daily
   On hand: Decadron® 0.75-mg unscored tablets

   Administer: _____

7. Ordered: Coumadin® 5 mg PO daily
   On hand: Coumadin® 2-mg scored tablets

   Administer: _____

8. Ordered: Cardizem® 90 mg PO tid
   On hand: Cardizem® 60-mg scored tablets

   Administer: _____

9. Ordered: Tambocor® 150 mg PO q12h   Administer: _____
   On hand: Tambocor® 100-mg scored tablets

10. Ordered: Clozaril® 75 mg PO daily   Administer: _____
    On hand: Clozaril® 25-mg unscored tablets

Liquid Medications

Many medications are available in liquid form. Liquids can be measured in small units of volume; thus, a greater range of dosages can be ordered and administered. Because they are easier to swallow than tablets and capsules, they are often used for children and elderly patients. Liquids can also be administered easily through feeding tubes.

Liquids may be less stable than solid forms of drugs. Many medications that are intended to be administered as liquids are provided as powders, which must be reconstituted. Many liquids, especially antibiotics, require refrigeration.

When reconstituting liquid medications:

- Use only the liquid specified on the drug label.
- Use the exact amount of liquid specified on the drug label.
- Check the label to determine whether the medication should be shaken before administering.
- Check the label to determine whether the reconstituted medication must be refrigerated.
- Write on the label the date and time you reconstitute the medication. Also, write your initials. Check the label to determine how long the reconstituted medication may be stored. Discard any medication left after this time period has passed.
- When medication can be reconstituted in different strengths, write on the label the strength that you choose.
- When medication can be reconstituted in different strengths, select the strength that will allow the desired dose to be administered in the smallest volume.

Read the order carefully when you calculate the amount to dispense. The physician usually orders the dose in units of drug, not volume of liquid. The person dispensing the medication calculates the volume needed to administer the desired doses.

Review with patients who are taking medications in a home environment the rules for reconstituted liquid medications. If necessary, copy the rules for them, then discuss. If you are dispensing medications, give the patients the same information that the pharmacist would, if you are allowed to do so. Give patients the following information about handling liquid medication:

1. Read the label to learn how to store the medication.
2. Use the measuring device provided or a device purchased specifically to measure medications. Household teaspoons and tablespoons do not measure liquid accurately.

3. Do not store medication longer than the label indicates. Medication used after its expiration date may have lost potency, or its chemical composition may have changed.
4. Wash the measuring device with hot water and a dishwashing detergent after each use. Dry it thoroughly. Store it in a clean container such as a plastic sandwich bag.
5. Keep liquid medication in its original container. Do not transfer it to other containers.

EXAMPLE ▶ How would you reconstitute the following medication? Find the amount to administer.

Ordered: E.E.S. susp 400 mg PO q6h
On hand: E.E.S. susp 200 mg per 5 mL when reconstituted
Label reads: "Add 154 mL water and shake vigorously. This makes 200 mL of suspension."

According to the label, you add 154 mL of water to the bottle of granules and shake vigorously. You then have a total of 200 mL of oral suspension that must be stored in the refrigerator for up to 10 days.

Calculate the amount to administer. The dosage ordered is 400 mg. The dosage strength is 200 mg/5 mL, which makes the dose on hand 200 mg and the dosage unit 5 mL.

Using Conversion Factors

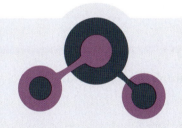

Fraction Proportion Method

1. Fill in the proportion.

$$\frac{Q}{H} = \frac{A}{D} \quad \text{or} \quad \frac{\text{dosage unit}}{\text{dose on hand}} = \frac{\text{amount to administer}}{\text{desired dose}}$$

$$\frac{5\ mL}{200\ mg} = \frac{A}{400\ mg}$$

2. Cancel units.

$$\frac{5\ mL}{200\ \cancel{mg}} = \frac{A}{400\ \cancel{mg}}$$

3. Cross-multiply and solve for the unknown.

$$200 \times A = 5\ mL \times 400$$

$$A = \frac{5\ mL \times 400}{200}$$

$$A = \frac{10\ mL}{1}$$

$$A = 10\ mL$$

Using Conversion Factors

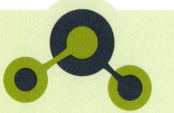

Ratio Proportion Method

1. Fill in the proportion.

$$Q:H::A:D$$

or dosage unit : dose on hand :: amount to administer : desired dose.

$$5 \text{ mL} : 2 \text{ mg} :: A : 5 \text{ mg}$$

2. Cancel units.

$$5 \text{ mL} : 2 \text{ mg} :: A : 5 \text{ mg}$$

3. Multiply the means and extremes, then solve for the missing value.

$$200 \times A = 5 \text{ mL} \times 400$$

$$A = \frac{5 \text{ mL} \times 400}{200}$$

$$A = \frac{10 \text{ mL}}{1}$$

$$A = 10 \text{ mL}$$

Using Conversion Factors

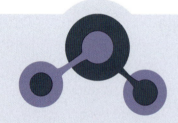

Dimensional Analysis

1. The unit of measure for the amount to administer will be milliliters.

$$A \text{ mL} =$$

2. Since the unit of measure for the dosage ordered is the same as that for the dose on hand, this step is unnecessary.

3. The dosage unit is 5 mL. The dose on hand is 2 mg. This is your first factor.

$$\frac{5 \text{ mL}}{2 \text{ mg}}$$

4. The dosage ordered is 5 mg. Place this over 1 for the second factor.

$$A \text{ mL} = \frac{5 \text{ mL}}{200 \text{ mg}} \times \frac{400 \text{ mg}}{1}$$

5. Cancel units.

$$A \text{ mL} = \frac{5 \text{ mL}}{200 \text{ mg}} \times \frac{400 \text{ mg}}{1}$$

6. Solve the equation.

$$A \text{ mL} = \frac{10 \text{ mL}}{1}$$

$$A = 10 \text{ mL}$$

Using Conversion Factors

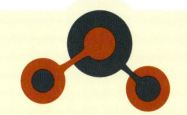

Formula Method

Calculate the amount to administer. The dosage ordered is 400 mg. The dosage strength is 200 mg/5 mL which makes the dose on hand 200 mg and the dosage unit 5 mL.

1. The drug is ordered in milligrams, which is the same unit of measure as that for the dose on hand. Therefore,

$$D = 200 \text{ mg}$$
$$Q = 5 \text{ mL}$$
$$H = 400 \text{ mg}$$

2. Fill in the formula.

$$\frac{D}{H} \times Q = A$$

$$\frac{400 \text{ mg} \times 5 \text{ mL}}{200 \text{ mg}} = A$$

3. Cancel units.

$$\frac{400 \cancel{\text{ mg}} \times 5 \text{ mL}}{200 \cancel{\text{ mg}}} = A$$

4. Solve for the unknown.

$$\frac{10 \text{ mL}}{1} = A$$

$$A = 10 \text{ mL}$$

 Super Tech . . .

Open the CD-ROM that accompanies your textbook and select Chapter 7, Exercise 7-4. Review the animation and example problems, and then complete the practice problems. Continue to the next section of the book once you have mastered the information presented.

Calculating estimated days supply for liquid medications

To determine estimated days supply you will multiply amount of medication to dispense by days needed over the number of dosage units per day.

$$\frac{\text{Amount to dispense}}{\text{Dosage units per day}} = \text{Estimated days supply}$$

Ordered: E.E.S. susp 400 mg PO q6h, dispense 400mL
On hand: E.E.S. susp 200 mg per 5 mL when reconstituted
Label reads: "Add 154 mL water and shake vigorously. This makes 200 mL of suspension."

The patient is to take 10 mL q6h, which is 4 times a day, for a total of 40 mL per day.

$$\frac{400}{40 \text{ mL}} = 10 \text{ days}$$

The prescription should last the patient 10 days.

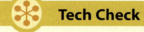

Tech Check

Reconstituting Powders

A pharmacy technician is preparing a bottle of Amoxil® suspension for this order: Amoxil 500 mg PO q8h for 5 days. The pharmacy has available 100-mL bottles and 150-mL bottles containing 250 mg/5 mL.

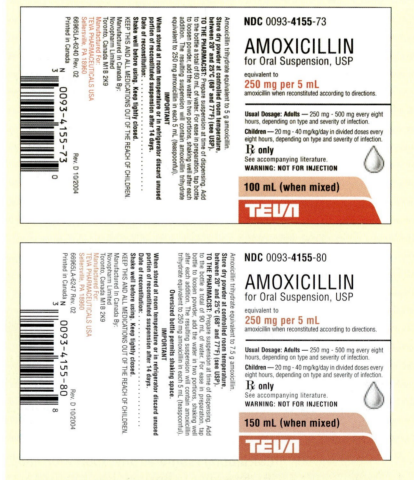

After calculating as follows the technician determines that the patient will receive 10 mL for each dose and 3 doses each day. This will require 30 mL of suspension each day for 5 days, or a total of 150 mL. The reconstituted medication can be refrigerated for 14 days.

The technician selects the 150-mL bottle and adds 150 mL of water to it. However, the liquid overflows from the bottle.

Think Before You Act

Checking the label, the technician realizes that 90 mL of water, *not* 150 mL, should have been used. Furthermore, only $\frac{1}{2}$ of the water, or 45 mL, should have been added at first to wet the powder, followed by the remaining 45 mL.

The powder's volume must be considered when you calculate the final volume of solution. The manufacturer has performed this calculation and listed the correct amount of water to add to the powder. The label calls for 90 mL of water to be added. When the technician added 150 mL of water instead of 90 mL, a volume of 210 mL of suspension was produced, instead of 150 mL.

During the week, the patient will be administered 150 mL of liquid medication, yet 210 mL has been prepared.

The patient will receive $\frac{150}{210}$ of the total solution and, in turn, only 71 percent of the drug itself. Thus, instead of receiving 250 mg/5 mL, the patient will receive only 187.5 mg in each 5 mL.

This lesser amount of medication may be ineffective in treating the patient's infection. If the patient does not improve, the physician may order a different antibiotic. The technician's error, if not corrected, could cause the patient to suffer symptoms for a longer time period, to be exposed to side effects from an unnecessary medication, and to spend additional money to purchase a drug that would not otherwise have been needed.

✔ Review and Practice 7-2 Liquid Medications

In Exercises 1–8, calculate the amount to administer and the estimated days supply where indicated.

1. Ordered: Trilisate® 400 mg PO tid
   On hand: Trilisate® liquid labeled 500 mg/5 mL
   Administer: _____

2. Ordered: MSIR® sol 15 mg PO q4h
   On hand: MSIR® solution labeled 10 mg/5 mL
   Administer: _____

3. Ordered: Megace® 200 mg PO qid
   On hand: Megace® solution labeled 40 mg/mL
   Administer: _____

4. Ordered: Norvir® 60 mg PO bid
   On hand: Norvir® solution labeled 80 mg/mL
   Administer: _____

5. Ordered: Zofran® 8 mg PO q12h, dispense 100 mL
   On hand: Zofran® liquid labeled 4 mg/5 mL
   Administer: _____
   Estimated days supply: _____

6. Ordered: Motrin® 600 mg PO tid, dispense 450 mL
   On hand: Motrin® liquid labeled 100 mg/5 mL
   Administer: _____
   Estimated days supply: _____

7. Ordered: Cefzil® 500 mg PO q24h, dispense 200 mL
   On hand: Cefzil® 125 mg/5 mL oral suspension
   Administer: _____
   Estimated days supply: _____

8. Ordered: Griseofulvin 500 mg PO daily, dispense 140 mL
   On hand: Griseofulvin 125 mg/5 mL suspension
   Administer: _____
   Estimated days supply: _____

Parenteral Dosages

Injections are mixtures that contain the drug dissolved in an appropriate liquid. The dosage or solution strength on an injectable medication's label indicates the amount of drug contained within a volume of solution. Dosage strength may be expressed in milligrams per milliliter, as a percent, or as a ratio. Once you have determined the amount to be administered to the patient, you must select the appropriate syringe.

Selecting a Syringe

1. If the amount of injection to administer is 1 mL or more, use a standard 3-mL syringe.
2. If the amount of injection to administer is less than 1 mL but greater than or equal to 0.5 mL, use a 1-mL tuberculin syringe.
3. If the amount of injection to administer is less than 0.5 mL, use a 0.5-mL tuberculin syringe.

EXAMPLE 1 ▶ The amount to administer is calculated at 2.4 mL. Since this is greater than 1 mL a standard syringe should be used. See Figure 7-6.

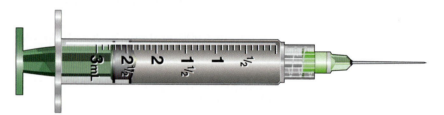

Figure 7-6 Standard syringe with 2.4 mL.

EXAMPLE 2 ▶ The amount to administer is calculated at 0.6 mL. Since this is less than 1 mL and greater than 0.5 mL, a 1-mL tuberculin syringe should be used. See Figure 7-7.

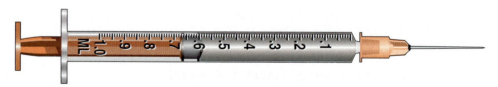

Figure 7-7 A 1-mL tuberculin syringe with 0.6 mL.

The amount to administer will not always be in whole milliliters, and it will sometimes be necessary to round your answer.

Correctly round the amount to administer of an injection.

1. Round volumes greater than 1 mL to the nearest tenth (one decimal) because the 3-mL syringe is calibrated in tenths.
2. Round volumes less than 1 mL to the nearest hundredth (two decimals) because tuberculin syringes are calibrated in hundredths.

EXAMPLE 1 ▶ The amount to administer is calculated at 1.66 mL. Since the volume is greater than 1 mL, you round 1.66 mL to the nearest tenth, which is 1.7 mL (Figure 7-8).

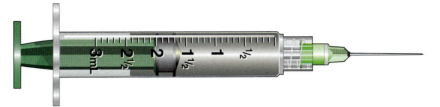

Figure 7-8 Standard Syringe with 1.7 mL.

EXAMPLE 2 ▶ The amount to administer is calculated at 0.532 mL. Since the volume is less than 1 mL, you round 0.532 mL to the nearest hundredth, which is 0.53 mL (Figure 7-9).

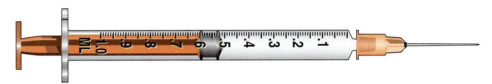

Figure 7-9 A 1-mL tuberculin syringe with 0.53 mL.

EXAMPLE 3 ▶ The amount to administer is calculated at 0.34 mL. Since this is less than 1 mL, a 0.5-mL tuberculin syringe should be used when available (Figure 7-10).

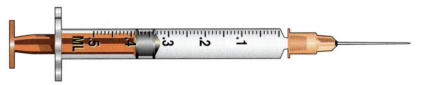

Figure 7-10 A 0.5 mL tuberculin syringe with 0.34 mL.

Using Conversion Factors

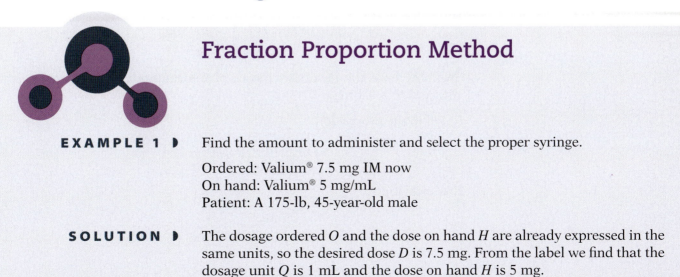

Fraction Proportion Method

EXAMPLE 1 ▶ Find the amount to administer and select the proper syringe.

Ordered: Valium® 7.5 mg IM now
On hand: Valium® 5 mg/mL
Patient: A 175-lb, 45-year-old male

SOLUTION ▶ The dosage ordered O and the dose on hand H are already expressed in the same units, so the desired dose D is 7.5 mg. From the label we find that the dosage unit Q is 1 mL and the dose on hand H is 5 mg.

1. Fill in the proportion.

$$\frac{Q}{H} = \frac{A}{D}$$

$$\frac{1\ \text{mL}}{5\ \text{mg}} = \frac{A}{7.5\ \text{mg}}$$

2. Cancel units.

$$\frac{1\ \text{mL}}{5\ \cancel{\text{mg}}} = \frac{A}{7.5\ \cancel{\text{mg}}}$$

3. Cross-multiply and solve for the unknown.

$$5 \times A = \text{mL} \times 7.5$$
$$A = 1\ \text{mL} \times \frac{7.5}{5}$$
$$A = 1.5\ \text{mL}$$

The amount to administer is 1.5 mL.
A standard syringe would be used.
It is not necessary to round in this example.

EXAMPLE 2 ▶ Find the amount to administer and select the proper syringe.

Ordered: 200 mcg atropine sulfate IM now
On hand: 0.4 mg/mL
Patient: An 80-lb, 10-year-old female

SOLUTION ▶ The dosage ordered O is in micrograms, and the dose on hand H is in milligrams, so the desired dose D, in milligrams, must be calculated.

1. Fill in the proportion, recalling that 1 mg = 1000 mcg.

$$\frac{1\ \text{mg}}{1000\ \text{mcg}} = \frac{D}{200\ \text{mcg}}$$

2. Cancel units.

$$\frac{1\ \text{mg}}{1000\ \cancel{\text{mcg}}} = \frac{D}{200\ \cancel{\text{mcg}}}$$

3. Cross-multiply and solve for the unknown.

$$1000 \times D = 1 \times 200\ \text{mg}$$
$$D = 0.2\ \text{mg}$$

We now have the necessary pieces of information: $D = 0.2$ mg, $Q = 1$ mL, and $H = 0.4$ mg.

1. Fill in the proportion.

$$\frac{1\ \text{mL}}{0.4\ \text{mg}} = \frac{A}{0.2\ \text{mg}}$$

2. Cancel units.

$$\frac{1\ \text{mL}}{0.4\ \cancel{\text{mg}}} = \frac{A}{0.2\ \cancel{\text{mg}}}$$

3. Cross-multiply and solve for the unknown.

$$0.4 \times A = 1 \text{ mL} \times 0.2$$

$$A = 1 \text{ mL} \times \frac{0.2}{0.4}$$

$$A = 0.5 \text{ mL}$$

The amount to administer is 0.5 mL
A 1-mL tuberculin syringe would be used.
It is not necessary to round in this example.

Using Conversion Factors

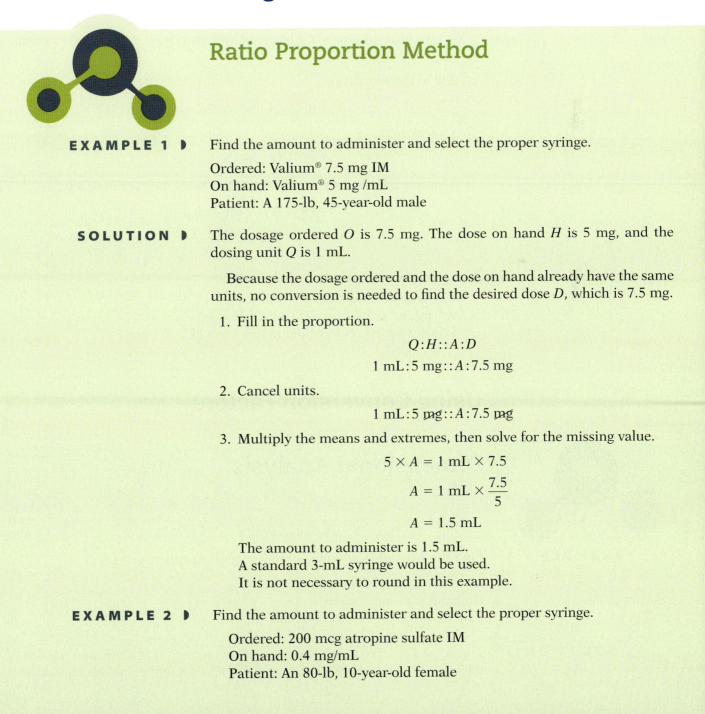

Ratio Proportion Method

EXAMPLE 1 ▶ Find the amount to administer and select the proper syringe.

Ordered: Valium® 7.5 mg IM
On hand: Valium® 5 mg /mL
Patient: A 175-lb, 45-year-old male

SOLUTION ▶ The dosage ordered O is 7.5 mg. The dose on hand H is 5 mg, and the dosing unit Q is 1 mL.

Because the dosage ordered and the dose on hand already have the same units, no conversion is needed to find the desired dose D, which is 7.5 mg.

1. Fill in the proportion.

$$Q:H::A:D$$
$$1 \text{ mL}:5 \text{ mg}::A:7.5 \text{ mg}$$

2. Cancel units.

$$1 \text{ mL}:5 \text{ mg}::A:7.5 \text{ mg}$$

3. Multiply the means and extremes, then solve for the missing value.

$$5 \times A = 1 \text{ mL} \times 7.5$$

$$A = 1 \text{ mL} \times \frac{7.5}{5}$$

$$A = 1.5 \text{ mL}$$

The amount to administer is 1.5 mL.
A standard 3-mL syringe would be used.
It is not necessary to round in this example.

EXAMPLE 2 ▶ Find the amount to administer and select the proper syringe.

Ordered: 200 mcg atropine sulfate IM
On hand: 0.4 mg/mL
Patient: An 80-lb, 10-year-old female

SOLUTION ▶ The dosage ordered O is in micrograms, and the dose on hand H is in milligrams, so the desired dose D, in milligrams, must be calculated.

1. Fill in the proportion, recalling that 1 mg = 1000 mcg.

$$1 \text{ mg} : 1000 \text{ mcg} :: D : 200 \text{ mcg}$$

2. Cancel units.

$$1 \text{ mg} : 1000 \text{ mcg} :: D : 200 \text{ mcg}$$

3. Multiply the means and extremes, then solve for the missing value.

$$1000 \times D = 1 \text{ mg} \times 200$$

$$D = \frac{1 \text{ mg} \times 200}{1000}$$

$$D = 0.2 \text{ mg}$$

We now have the necessary pieces of information: $D = 0.2$ mg, $Q = 1$ mL, and $H = 0.4$ mg.

1. Fill in the proportion.

$$1 \text{ mL} : 0.4 \text{ mg} :: A : 0.2 \text{ mg}$$

2. Cancel units.

$$1 \text{ mL} : 0.4 \text{ mg} :: A : 0.2 \text{ mg}$$

3. Multiply the means and extremes, then solve for the missing value.

$$0.4 \times A = 1 \text{ mL} \times 0.2$$

$$A = \frac{1 \text{ mL} \times 0.2}{0.4}$$

$$A = 0.5 \text{ mL}$$

The amount to administer is 0.5 mL.
A 1-mL tuberculin syringe would be used.
It is not necessary to round in this example.

Using Conversion Factors

Dimensional Analysis

EXAMPLE 1 ▶ Find the amount to administer and select the proper syringe.

Ordered: Valium® 7.5 mg IM
On hand: Valium® 5mg/mL
Patient: A 175-lb, 45-year-old male

SOLUTION ▶ The dosage ordered O is 7.5 mg. The dose on hand H is 5 mg, and the dosing unit Q is 1 mL. Because the dosage ordered and the dose on hand have the same units, no conversion is needed to find the desired dose D, which is 7.5 mg.

1. The unit of measure for the amount to administer will be milliliters.

$$A \text{ mL} =$$

2. Since the unit of measure for the dosage ordered is the same as that for the dose on hand, this step is unnecessary.

3. The dosage unit is 1 mL. The dose on hand is 5 mg. This is your first factor.

$$\frac{1 \text{ mL}}{5 \text{ mg}}$$

4. The dosage ordered is 7.5 mg. Set up the equation.

$$A \text{ mL} = \frac{1 \text{ mL}}{5 \text{ mg}} \times \frac{7.5 \text{ mg}}{1}$$

5. Cancel units.

$$A \text{ mL} = \frac{1 \text{ mL}}{5 \text{ mg}} \times \frac{7.5 \text{ mg}}{1}$$

6. Solve the equation.

$$A \text{ mL} = \frac{1 \text{ mL}}{5} \times \frac{7.5}{1}$$

$$A = 1.5 \text{ mL}$$

The amount to administer is 1.5 mL.
A standard syringe would be used.
It is not necessary to round in this example.

EXAMPLE 2 ▶ Find the amount to administer and select the proper syringe.

Ordered: 200 mcg atropine sulfate IM
On hand: 0.4 mg/mL
Patient: An 80-lb, 10-year-old female

SOLUTION ▶ 1. The unit of measure for the amount to administer will be milliliters.

$$A \text{ mL} =$$

2. The unit of measure for the dosage ordered is micrograms. The unit of measure for the dose on hand is milligrams. Recall that 1 mg = 1000 mcg. Because we wish to convert to milligrams (the units of the dose on hand), our first factor must have milligrams on top.

$$\frac{1 \text{ mg}}{1000 \text{ mcg}}$$

3. The dosage unit is 1 mL. The dose on hand is 0.4 mg. This is our second factor.

$$\frac{1 \text{ mg}}{1000 \text{ mcg}} \times \frac{1 \text{ mL}}{0.4 \text{ mg}}$$

4. The dosage ordered is 200 mcg. Set up the equation.

$$\frac{1 \text{ mg}}{1000 \text{ mcg}} \times \frac{1 \text{ mL}}{0.4 \text{ mg}} \times \frac{200 \text{ mcg}}{1}$$

5. Cancel units.

$$\frac{1 \text{ mg}}{1000 \text{ meg}} \times \frac{1 \text{ mL}}{0.4 \text{ mg}} \times \frac{200 \text{ meg}}{1}$$

6. Solve the equation.

$$A \text{ mL} = \frac{1}{1000} \times \frac{1 \text{ mL}}{0.4} \times \frac{200}{1}$$

$$A = 0.5 \text{ mL}$$

The amount to administer is 0.5 mL.
A 1-mL tuberculin syringe would be used.
It is not necessary to round in this example.

Using Conversion Factors

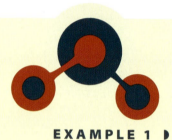

Formula Method

EXAMPLE 1 ▶ Find the amount to administer and select the proper syringe.

Ordered: Valium® 7.5 mg IM
On hand: Valium® 5 mg/mL
Patient: A 175-lb, 45-year-old male

SOLUTION ▶
1. The drug is ordered in milligrams, which is the same unit of measure as that of the dose on hand. Therefore,

Desired dose D = 7.5 mg
Dose on hand H = 5 mg
Quantity to be administered Q = 1 mL

2. Fill in the formula.

$$\frac{D}{H} \times Q = A$$

$$\frac{7.5 \text{ mg} \times 1 \text{ mL}}{5 \text{ mg}} = A$$

3. Cancel units.

$$\frac{7.5 \text{ mg} \times 1 \text{ mL}}{5 \text{ mg}} = A$$

4. Solve for the unknown.

$$\frac{7.5 \times 1 \text{ mL}}{5} = A$$

$$1.5 \text{ mL} = A$$

The amount to administer is 1.5 mL.
A standard syringe would be used.
It is not necessary to round in this example.

EXAMPLE 2 ▶   Find the amount to administer and select the proper syringe.

Ordered: 200 mcg atropine sulfate IM
On hand: 0.4 mg/mL
Patient: An 80-lb, 10-year-old female

SOLUTION ▶   The dosage ordered Q is in micrograms, and the dose on hand H is in milligrams, so the desired dose D in milligrams must be calculated.
   In this example, the fraction proportion method is used.

1. Fill in the proportion, recalling that 1 mg = 1000 mcg.

$$\frac{1 \text{ mg}}{1000 \text{ mcg}} = \frac{D}{200 \text{ mcg}}$$

2. Cancel units.

$$\frac{1 \text{ mg}}{1000 \text{ mcg}} = \frac{D}{200 \text{ mcg}}$$

3. Cross-multiply and solve for the unknown.

$$1000 \times D = 1 \times 200 \text{ mg}$$
$$D = 0.2 \text{ mg}$$

We now have the necessary pieces of information: $D = 0.2$ mg, $Q = 1$ mL, and $H = 0.4$ mg.

1. Fill in the formula.

$$\frac{0.2 \text{ mg} \times 1 \text{ mL}}{0.4 \text{ mg}} = A$$

2. Cancel units.

$$\frac{0.2 \text{ mg} \times 1 \text{ mL}}{0.4 \text{ mg}} = A$$

3. Solve for the unknown.

$$\frac{0.2 \times 1 \text{ mL}}{0.4} = A$$

$$0.5 \text{ mL} = A$$

The amount to administer is 0.5 mL.
A 1-mL tuberculin syringe would be used.
It is not necessary to round in this example.

Super Tech . . .

Open the CD-ROM that accompanies your textbook and select Chapter 7, Exercise 7-5. Review the animation and example problems, and then complete the practice problems. Continue to the next section of the book once you have mastered the information presented.

Medications Expressed in Percent or Ratio Format

When the dosage strength is expressed as a percent or a ratio, you must convert it before calculating the amount to administer. For example, to administer 1 percent lidocaine, you need to rewrite the strength as 1 g (dose on hand) per 100 mL (dosage unit) before beginning your calculations. If the labeled strength were 1:2000, you would rewrite it as 1 g (dose on hand) per 2000 mL (dosage unit). Some drugs, such as heparin, are measured in units and may have their solution strength expressed in ratio format. The ratio indicates the number of units contained in 1 mL. For example, heparin sodium 1:10,000 contains 10,000 units in 1 mL.

When a solution strength is expressed as a percent or ratio:

1. Convert the percent or ratio to the dosage strength, such as grams per milliliter, milligrams per milliliter, or units per milliliter.
2. Calculate the amount to administer, and select the proper syringe.

Using Conversion Factors

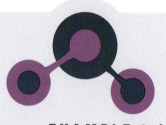

Fraction Proportion Method

EXAMPLE 1 ▶ Find the amount to administer and select the proper syringe.

Ordered: Magnesium sulfate 300 mg IM
On hand: Magnesium sulfate 10 percent solution
Patient: A 75-lb, 8-year-old female

SOLUTION ▶ Convert the dosage strength of a 10 percent solution to 10 g (H) per 100 mL (Q).

The dose on hand H is now in grams, and the dosage ordered O is in milligrams. To calculate the desired dose D, we must first convert the dosage ordered, 300 mg, to the same unit of measure as that of the dose on hand, grams.

1. Fill in the proportion, recalling that 1 g = 1000 mg.

$$\frac{1 \text{ g}}{1000 \text{ mg}} = \frac{D}{300 \text{ mg}}$$

2. Cancel units.

$$\frac{1 \text{ g}}{1000 \text{ mg}} = \frac{D}{300 \text{ mg}}$$

3. Cross-multiply and solve for the unknown.

$$1000 \times D = 300 \times 1 \text{ g}$$

$$D = \frac{300 \times 1 \text{ g}}{1000}$$

$$D = 0.3 \text{ g}$$

We now have the necessary pieces of information: $D = 0.3$ g, $Q = 100$ mL, and $H = 10$ g.

1. Fill in the proportion.

$$\frac{100 \text{ mL}}{10 \text{ g}} = \frac{A}{0.3 \text{ g}}$$

2. Cancel units.

$$\frac{100 \text{ mL}}{10 \text{ g}} = \frac{A}{0.3 \text{ g}}$$

3. Cross-multiply and solve for the unknown.

$$10 \times A = 100 \text{ mL} \times 0.3$$

$$A = \frac{100 \text{ mL} \times 0.3}{10}$$

$$A = 3 \text{ mL}$$

The amount to administer is 3 mL.
A standard syringe would be used.
It is not necessary to round in this example.

EXAMPLE 2 ▶ Find the amount to administer and select the proper syringe.

Ordered: Epinephrine 0.2 mg sub-Q stat
On hand: Vial of epinephrine 1 : 2000 solution for injection
Patient: A 150-lb, 35-year-old adult

SOLUTION ▶ Convert the dosage strength of a 1 : 2000 solution to 1 g (H) per 2000 mL (Q).

The dose on hand H is now in grams, and the dosage ordered O is in milligrams. To calculate the desired dose D, we must first convert the dosage ordered, 0.2 mg, to the same unit of measure as that of the dose on hand, grams.

1. Fill in the proportion, recalling that 1 g = 1000 mg.

$$\frac{1 \text{ g}}{1000 \text{ mg}} = \frac{D}{0.2 \text{ mg}}$$

2. Cancel units.

$$\frac{1 \text{ g}}{1000 \text{ mg}} = \frac{D}{0.2 \text{ mg}}$$

3. Cross-multiply and solve for the unknown.

$$1000 \times D = 0.2 \times 1 \text{ g}$$

$$D = \frac{0.2 \times 1 \text{ g}}{1000}$$

$$D = 0.0002 \text{ g}$$

We now have the necessary pieces of information: $D = 0.0002$ g, $Q = 2000$ mL, and $H = 1$ g.

1. Fill in the proportion.

$$\frac{2000 \text{ mL}}{1 \text{ g}} = \frac{A}{0.0002 \text{ g}}$$

2. Cancel units.

$$\frac{2000 \text{ mL}}{1 \, \cancel{g}} = \frac{A}{0.0002 \, \cancel{g}}$$

3. Cross-multiply and solve for the unknown.

$$1 \times A = 2000 \text{ mL} \times 0.0002$$

$$A = \frac{2000 \text{ mL} \times 0.0002}{1}$$

$$A = 0.4 \text{ mL}$$

The amount to administer is 0.4 mL.
A 0.5-mL tuberculin syringe would be used.
It is not necessary to round in this example.

Using Conversion Factors

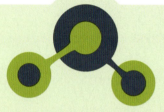

Ratio Proportion Method

EXAMPLE 1 ▶ Find the amount to administer and select the proper syringe.

Ordered: Magnesium sulfate 300 mg IM
On hand: Magnesium sulfate 10 percent solution
Patient: A 75-lb, 8-year-old female

SOLUTION ▶ Convert the dosage strength of a 10 percent solution to 10 g (H) per 100 mL (Q).

The dose on hand H is now in grams, and the dosage ordered O is in milligrams. To calculate the desired dose D, we must first convert the dosage ordered 300 mg to the same unit of measure as that of the dose on hand, grams.

1. Fill in the proportion, recalling that 1 g = 1000 mg.

$$1 \text{ g} : 1000 \text{ mg} :: D : 300 \text{ mg}$$

2. Cancel units.

$$1 \text{ g} : 1000 \, \cancel{\text{mg}} :: D : 300 \, \cancel{\text{mg}}$$

3. Multiply the means and extremes, then solve for the missing value.

$$1 \text{ g} : 1000 \text{ mg} :: D : 300 \text{ mg}$$

$$D = \frac{1 \text{ g} \times 300}{1000}$$

$$D = 0.3 \text{ g}$$

We now have the necessary pieces of information: $D = 0.3$ g, $Q = 100$ mL, and $H = 10$ g.

1. Fill in the proportion.

$$100 \text{ mL} : 10 \text{ g} :: A : 0.3 \text{ g}$$

2. Cancel units.

$$100 \text{ mL} : 10 \cancel{\text{ g}} :: A : 0.3 \cancel{\text{ g}}$$

3. Multiply the means and extremes, then solve for the missing value.

$$10 \times A = 100 \text{ mL} \times 0.3$$

$$A = \frac{100 \text{ mL} \times 0.3}{10}$$

$$A = 3 \text{ mL}$$

The amount to administer is 3 mL.
A standard syringe would be used.
It is not necessary to round in this example.

EXAMPLE 2 ▶   Find the amount to administer and select the proper syringe.

Ordered: Epinephrine 0.2 mg sub-Q stat
On hand: Vial of epinephrine 1 : 2000 solution for injection
Patient: A 150-lb, 35-year-old adult

SOLUTION ▶   Convert the dosage strength of a 1 : 2000 solution to 1 g (H) per 2000 mL (Q).

The dose on hand H is now in grams, and the dosage ordered O is in milligrams. To calculate the desired dose D, we must first convert the dosage ordered, 0.2 mg, to the same unit of measure as that of the dose on hand, grams.

1. Fill in the proportion, recalling that 1 g = 1000 mg.

$$1 \text{ g} : 1000 \text{ mg} :: D : 0.2 \text{ mg}$$

2. Cancel units.

$$1 \text{ g} : 1000 \cancel{\text{ mg}} :: D : 0.2 \cancel{\text{ mg}}$$

3. Multiply the means and extremes, then solve for the missing value.

$$1000 \times D = 1 \text{ g} \times 0.2$$

$$D = \frac{1 \text{ g} \times 0.2}{1000}$$

$$D = 0.0002 \text{ g}$$

We now have the necessary pieces of information: $D = 0.0002$ g, $Q = 2000$ mL, $H = 1$g.

1. Fill in the proportion.

$$2000 \text{ mL} : 1 \text{ g} :: A : 0.0002 \text{ g}$$

2. Cancel units.

$$2000 \text{ mL} : 1 \cancel{\text{ g}} :: A : 0.0002 \cancel{\text{ g}}$$

3. Multiply the means and extremes, then solve for the missing value.

$$1 \times A = 2000 \text{ mL} \times 0.0002 \text{ g}$$

$$A = \frac{2000 \text{ mL} \times 0.0002}{1}$$

$$A = 0.4 \text{ mL}$$

The amount to administer is 0.4 mL.
A 0.5-mL tuberculin syringe would be used.
It is not necessary to round in this example.

Using Conversion Factors

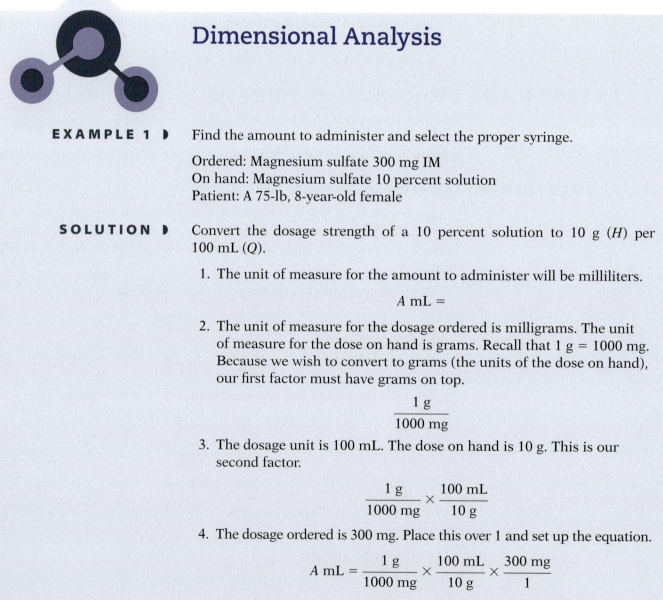

Dimensional Analysis

EXAMPLE 1 ▶   Find the amount to administer and select the proper syringe.

Ordered: Magnesium sulfate 300 mg IM
On hand: Magnesium sulfate 10 percent solution
Patient: A 75-lb, 8-year-old female

SOLUTION ▶   Convert the dosage strength of a 10 percent solution to 10 g (H) per 100 mL (Q).

1. The unit of measure for the amount to administer will be milliliters.

$$A \text{ mL} =$$

2. The unit of measure for the dosage ordered is milligrams. The unit of measure for the dose on hand is grams. Recall that 1 g = 1000 mg. Because we wish to convert to grams (the units of the dose on hand), our first factor must have grams on top.

$$\frac{1 \text{ g}}{1000 \text{ mg}}$$

3. The dosage unit is 100 mL. The dose on hand is 10 g. This is our second factor.

$$\frac{1 \text{ g}}{1000 \text{ mg}} \times \frac{100 \text{ mL}}{10 \text{ g}}$$

4. The dosage ordered is 300 mg. Place this over 1 and set up the equation.

$$A \text{ mL} = \frac{1 \text{ g}}{1000 \text{ mg}} \times \frac{100 \text{ mL}}{10 \text{ g}} \times \frac{300 \text{ mg}}{1}$$

5. Cancel units.

$$A \text{ mL} = \frac{1 \cancel{g}}{1000 \cancel{mg}} \times \frac{100 \text{ mL}}{10 \cancel{g}} \times \frac{300 \cancel{mg}}{1}$$

6. Solve the equation.

$$A \text{ mL} = \frac{1}{1000} \times \frac{100 \text{ mL}}{10} \times \frac{300}{1}$$

$$A = 3 \text{ mL}$$

The amount to administer is 3 mL.
A standard syringe would be used.
It is not necessary to round in this example.

EXAMPLE 2 ▶ Find the amount to administer and select the proper syringe.

Ordered: Epinephrine 0.2 mg sub-Q stat
On hand: Vial of epinephrine 1 : 2000 solution for injection
Patient: A 150-lb, 35-year-old adult

SOLUTION ▶ Convert the dosage strength of a 1 : 2000 solution to 1 g (H) per 2000 mL (Q).

The dose on hand H is now in grams, and the dosage ordered O is in milligrams. To calculate the desired dose D, we must first change the dosage ordered 0.2 mg to the same unit of measure as that of the dose on hand, grams.

1. The unit of measure for the amount to administer will be milliliters.

$$A \text{ mL} =$$

2. The unit of measure for the dosage ordered is milligrams. The unit of measure for the dose on hand is grams. Recall that 1 g = 1000 mg. Because we wish to convert to grams (the units of the dose on hand), our first factor must have grams on top.
3. The dosage unit is 2000 mL. The dose on hand is 1 g. This is our next factor.

$$\frac{1 \text{ g}}{1000 \text{ mg}} \times \frac{2000 \text{ mL}}{1 \text{ g}}$$

4. The dosage ordered is 0.2 mg. Place this over 1 and set up the equation.

$$A \text{ mL} = \frac{1}{1000 \text{ mg}} \times \frac{2000 \text{ mL}}{1} \times \frac{0.2 \text{ mg}}{1}$$

5. Cancel units.

$$A \text{ mL} = \frac{1 \cancel{g}}{1000 \cancel{mg}} \times \frac{2000 \text{ mL}}{1 \cancel{g}} \times \frac{0.2 \cancel{mg}}{1}$$

6. Solve the equation.

$$A \text{ mL} = \frac{2000 \text{ mL} \times 0.2 \text{ mg}}{1000 \text{ mg}}$$

$$A = 0.4 \text{ mL}$$

The amount to administer is 0.4 mL.
A 0.5-mL tuberculin syringe would be used.
It is not necessary to round in this example.

Using Conversion Factors

Formula Method

EXAMPLE 1 ▶ Find the amount to administer and select the proper syringe.

Ordered: Magnesium sulfate 300 mg IM
On hand: Magnesium sulfate 10 percent solution
Patient: A 75-lb, 8-year-old female

SOLUTION ▶ Convert the dosage strength of a 10 percent solution to 10 g (H) per 100 mL (Q).

The dosage ordered O is in milligrams, and the dose on hand H is in grams, so the desired dose D, in grams, must be calculated.
In this example, the fraction proportion method is used.

1. Fill in the proportion, recalling that 1 g = 1000 mg.

$$\frac{1 \text{ g}}{1000 \text{ mg}} = \frac{D}{300 \text{ mg}}$$

2. Cancel units.

$$\frac{1 \text{ g}}{1000 \text{ \cancel{mg}}} = \frac{D}{300 \text{ \cancel{mg}}}$$

3. Cross-multiply and solve for the unknown.

$$1000 \times D = 300 \times 1 \text{ g}$$

$$D = \frac{300 \times 1 \text{ g}}{1000}$$

$$D = 0.3 \text{ g}$$

We now have the necessary pieces of information: $D = 0.3$ g, $Q = 100$ mL, and $H = 10$ g.

1. Fill in the formula.

$$\frac{0.3 \text{ g} \times 100 \text{ mL}}{10 \text{ g}} = A$$

2. Cancel units.

$$\frac{0.3 \text{ \cancel{g}} \times 100 \text{ mL}}{10 \text{ \cancel{g}}} = A$$

3. Solve for the unknown.

$$\frac{0.3 \times 100 \text{ mL}}{10} = A$$

$$3 \text{ mL} = A$$

The amount to administer is 3 mL.
A standard syringe would be used.
It is not necessary to round in this example.

EXAMPLE 1 ▶ Find the amount to administer and select the proper syringe.

Ordered: Epinephrine 0.2 mg sub-Q stat
On hand: Vial of epinephrine 1:2000 solution for injection
Patient: A 150-lb, 35-year-old adult

SOLUTION ▶ Convert the dosage strength of a 1:2000 solution to 1 g (*H*) per 2000 mL (*Q*).

The dose on hand *H* is now in grams, and the dosage ordered *O* is in milligrams. To calculate the desired dose *D*, we must first convert the dosage ordered 0.2 mg to the same unit of measure as that of the dose on hand, grams.

1. Fill in the proportion, recalling that 1 g = 1000 mg.

$$\frac{1 \text{ g}}{1000 \text{ mg}} = \frac{D}{300 \text{ mg}}$$

2. Cancel units.

$$\frac{1 \text{ g}}{1000 \text{ m\!g}} = \frac{D}{0.2 \text{ m\!g}}$$

3. Cross-multiply and solve for the unknown.

$$1000 \times D = 0.2 \times 1 \text{ g}$$

$$D = \frac{0.2 \times 1 \text{ g}}{1000}$$

$$D = 0.0002 \text{ g}$$

We now have the necessary pieces of information: *D* = 0.0002 g, *Q* = 2000 mL, and *H* = 1 g.

1. Fill in the formula.

$$\frac{0.0002 \text{ g} \times 2000 \text{ mL}}{1 \text{ g}} = A$$

2. Cancel units.

$$\frac{0.0002 \text{ g\!\!\!/} \times 2000 \text{ mL}}{1 \text{ g\!\!\!/}} = A$$

3. Solve for the unknown.

$$\frac{0.0002 \times 2000 \text{ mL}}{1} = A$$

$$0.4 \text{ mL} = A$$

The amount to administer is 0.4 mL.
A 0.5-mL tuberculin syringe would be used.
It is not necessary to round in this example.

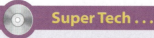

Super Tech . . .

Open the CD-ROM that accompanies your textbook and select Chapter 7, Exercise 7-6. Review the animation and example problems, and then complete the practice problems. Continue to the next section of the book once you have mastered the information presented.

✔ Review and Practice 7-3 Parenteral Dosages

Find the amount to administer for each of the following orders. Then mark the syringe with the correct amount to administer.

1. Ordered: Magnesium sulfate 500 mg IM stat
   On hand: Magnesium sulfate 20 percent solution

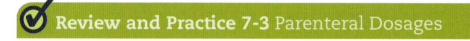

2. Ordered: Lidocaine 80 mg IM stat
   On hand: Lidocaine 4 percent solution

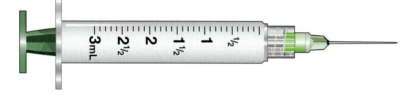

3. Ordered: Epinephrine 0.3 mg sub-Q stat
   On hand: Epinephrine 1 : 1000 solution

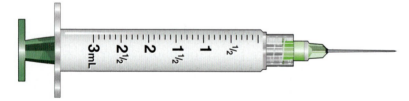

4. Ordered: Adrenalin 0.5 mg sub-Q stat
   On hand: Adrenalin 1 : 1000 solution

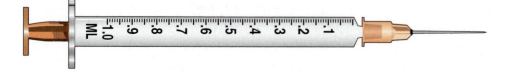

5. Ordered: Prostigmin 0.2 mg IM post-op q6h
   On hand: Prostigmin 1:4000 solution

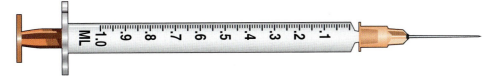

6. Ordered: Prostigmin 0.5 mg IM stat
   On hand: Prostigmin 1:2000 solution

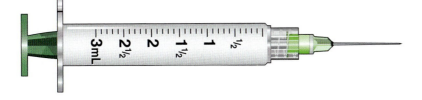

7. Ordered: Heparin sodium 8000 units deep sub-Q q8h
   On hand: Heparin sodium 1:10,000 solution

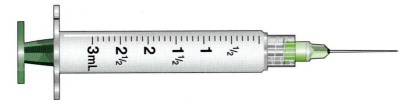

8. Ordered: Heparin sodium 5000 units sub-Q q12h
   On hand: Heparin sodium 1:10,000 solution

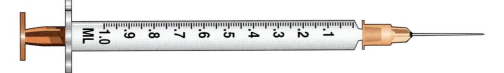

For Exercises 9 to 15, find the amount to administer, and then determine the proper syringe and write it in the space provided.

9. Ordered: Depo-Provera 1000 mg IM
   On hand: Depo-Provera 400 mg/mL

   Administer: _____ Syringe: _____

10. Ordered: Zantac® 50 mg IM q6h
    On hand: Zantac® 25 mg/mL

    Administer: _____ Syringe: _____

11. Ordered: Tigan® 200 mg IM TID
    On hand: Tigan® 100 mg/mL

    Administer: _____ Syringe: _____

12. Ordered: Sandostatin® 200 mcg sub-Q q12h
    On hand: Sandostatin® 500 mcg/mL

    Administer: _____ Syringe: _____

13. Ordered: Neupogen® 180 mcg sub-Q qd
    On hand: Neupogen® 300 mcg/0.5 mL

    Administer: _____ Syringe: _____

14. Ordered: Neupogen® 240 mcg sub-Q qd
    On hand: Neupogen® 480 mcg/1.6 mL

    Administer: _____ Syringe: _____

15. Ordered: Epogen® 3500 units sub-Q tiw
    On hand: 4000 units/mL

    Administer: _____ Syringe: _____

Reconstituting Medications

Medications that lose potency quickly in solution may be supplied in powdered form. When needed, they are reconstituted by dissolving them in an appropriate solvent (or diluent). The drug label, package insert, and PDR provide instructions for reconstituting a medication. Be sure to use the directions specific to the medication you plan to administer.

First, determine what solvent should be used to dilute the medication. Common solvents include sterile water, saline, or a bacteriostatic solution containing a preservative that prevents the growth of microorganisms. Some medications are packaged with a separate container of the appropriate solvent.

Many medications, especially antibiotics, cause severe pain when injected. They may be mixed with lidocaine, a local anesthetic, to reduce this pain. The label or package insert indicates when lidocaine can be used. *Because lidocaine is itself a medication, you need a physician's order to use it.* Therefore, check whether the physician has ordered lidocaine. Do not confuse it with the combination of lidocaine and epinephrine, because epinephrine causes vasoconstriction, a tightening of the blood vessels, which delays medication absorption.

The label or package insert lists how much solvent to combine with the medication. Read the directions carefully. Sometimes different amounts of solvent are used, depending on whether the medication is for IM or IV use.

To reconstitute a powdered medication:

1. Find the directions on the medication label or package insert.
2. Use a sterile syringe and aseptic (germ-free) technique to draw up the correct amount of the appropriate diluent.
3. Inject the diluent into the medication vial.
4. Agitate the mixture by rolling, inverting, or shaking the vial. Check the directions on the label or package insert for which of these methods to use.
5. Make sure that the powdered medication is completely dissolved and that the solution is free of visible particles before you use it.

You must use the exact amount of solvent indicated in the directions to produce a solution with the correct dosage strength. Powder takes up volume even when dissolved. The volume of the reconstituted medication includes the volume of the solvent and the volume of the powder.

If less than the recommended amount of solvent is used, the powder may not dissolve completely, making the solution unsafe to administer. If too much solvent is used, then the patient will not receive the desired dose. When you prepare a suspension, remember that the particles will not dissolve completely. Your goal is to distribute them evenly.

Some vials contain a single dose of medication. Many must be reconstituted immediately before administering them, because they quickly lose potency. Other such medications can be stored for a short time after reconstitution. In some facilities, medications are reconstituted in the pharmacy and delivered ready to use.

When you store a medication after reconstituting it:

1. You must record the date, the time of expiration, and your name or initials.
2. For multiple-dose medications, also record the solution strength.
3. Check the drug label or package insert for the length of time a reconstituted medication may be stored. Storage time may depend on whether the medication is refrigerated.

Super Tech . . .

Open the CD-ROM that accompanies your textbook and select Chapter 7, Exercise 7-7. Review the animation and example problems, and then complete the practice problems. Continue to the next section of the book once you have mastered the information presented.

✓ Review and Practice 7-4 Reconstituting Medications

In Exercises 1–4, refer to the label instructions below.

On hand: Leucovorin 350 mg, single use vial.

Each vial contains 350 mg when reconstituted with 17.5 mL of sterile water for injection, or Bacteriostatic water for injection. Each contains 20 mg of Leucovorin.

1. How much diluent should you add to the 350-mg vial?

2. What solution strength should you print on the label?

3. What can be used to reconstitute the leucovorin?

4. If the dose ordered is 15 mg IM, what would be the amount to administer?

Other Medication Routes

Medications may be given by a variety of routes besides oral and common parenteral routes. These routes are used for inhalants; ophthalmic and otic drops; and topical and transdermal, rectal. and vaginal medications.

Inhalants

Inhalant: Medication administered directly to the lungs, usually through a metered-dose inhaler or nebulizer.

Inhaled medications, or **inhalants,** are administered directly to the lungs usually through a metered-dose inhaler (MDI) or by nebulizer. Metered-dose inhalers provide a measured dose of medication in each puff. The physician orders the number of puffs to be given. No calculation is necessary; see Figure 7-11.

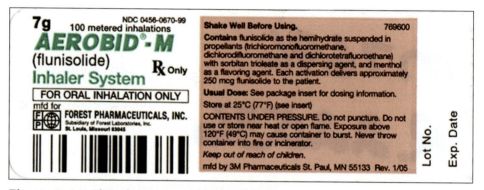

Figure 7-11 This drug is used by inhalation.

Medications given by nebulizer are supplied as liquids that are mixed with sterile saline solution. Single doses premixed with saline are available for most medications. A few are measured in the receptacle of the nebulizer, after which the correct amount of saline is added. Sterile saline is usually provided in 3-mL or 5-mL single-dose ampules.

Inhalant medications in multiple-dose containers are usually packaged with special droppers calibrated for the standard doses. If the dropper is not available or becomes contaminated, a sterile syringe may be used.

The physician usually specifies the solution strength and the amount of inhalant to administer. For example, the order "Mucomyst® 20 percent 3 mL via nebulizer QID" is a complete order. In some cases, the physician will also order an amount of normal saline to be added to the medication. When calculations are necessary, the same methods—fraction proportion, ratio proportion, dimensional analysis, and formula—are used for inhalants as are used for parenteral medications.

Calculating estimated days supply for inhalants
To determine estimated days supply you will multiply amount of medication to dispense by days needed over the number of dosage units per day.

$$\frac{\text{Amount to dispense}}{\text{Dosage units per day}} = \text{Estimated days supply}$$

Ordered: Mucomyst 20 percent 3 mL via nebulizer QID, dispense 60 mL

3 mL taken 4 times a day = 12 mL per day

$$\frac{60 \text{ mL}}{12} = 5 \text{ days}$$

The prescription should last the patient 5 days.

Topical and Transdermal

Topical: Medication applied to the skin.

Transdermal: Medication administered through the skin, typically via a patch.

Topical medications are applied to the skin and include ointments, creams, and lotions. **Transdermal** medications are administered through the skin, typically via a patch. Patches usually consist of a special membrane that releases liquid medication at a constant rate. The patch has adhesive edges to hold it in place so that the membrane rests against the skin. The dosage rate of a transdermal patch is usually expressed in milligrams or micrograms per hour. Patches cannot be divided. If a dose is larger than the amount provided by a single patch, you can use multiple patches. Before you administer a patch, be certain to remove any patches that are already in place and wipe off any residual medication; see Figure 7-12.

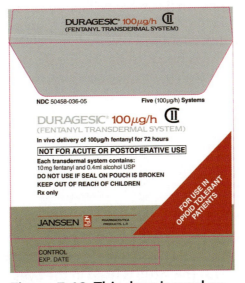

Figure 7-12 **This drug is used on the skin, or for dermatologic use only.**

EXAMPLE ▶ Find the amount to be administered.

Ordered: Vivelle® 0.125 mg/day
On hand: Vivelle® in four dosage strengths: 0.0375 mg/day, 0.05 mg/day, 0.075 mg/day, and 0.1 mg/day.

Start with the patch that has the greatest dosage strength (0.1 mg/day). Because all the patches deliver more than 0.025 mg/day, none will work in combination with this patch. Next, try combinations with the 0.075 mg/day patch. Note that 0.075 + 0.05 = 0.125 Dispense a combination of one 0.075 mg/day patch and one 0.05 mg/day patch.

Calculating estimated days supply for topical and transdermal medications
To determine estimated days supply, you will multiply amount of medication to dispense by days needed over the number of dosage units per day.

$$\frac{\text{Amount to dispense}}{\text{Dosage units per day}} = \text{Estimated days supply}$$

Ordered: Vivelle® 0.1 mg # 30, apply one patch daily
On hand: Vivelle® 0.1-mg patches.

$$\frac{30 \text{ patches}}{1} = 30 \text{ days}$$

The prescription should last the patient 30 days.

Ophthalmic and Otic Drops

Ophthalmic medications are used for the eyes and otic medications are used for ears. Both are usually given in liquid/drop form. Some ophthalmic medications are supplied in ointment form. In certain cases ophthalmic medications can be prescribed for otic use, but otic medications can not be prescribed for ophthalmic use. There are approximately 20 drops in 1 mL. When a prescription is received in the pharmacy, the amount to dispense almost always needs to be calculated. Some ophthalmic and otic drops come in more than one package size, for example 2.5- or 5-mL bottles; see Figure 7.13.

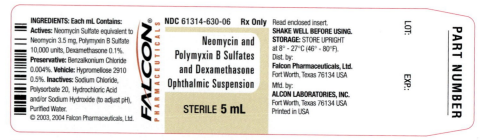

Figure 7-13 **This drug is used in the eyes.**

EXAMPLE 1 ▶

Find the amount to dispense.

Ordered: Alrex® ophthalmic solution, 2 gtts OD qid prn for 8 days.
On hand: Alrex® ophthalmic solution 2.5-mL bottle and 5-mL bottle

SOLUTION ▶

1. Determine how many drops are needed.

$$2 \text{ gtts} \times 4 = 8 \text{ gtts/day}$$
$$8 \text{ gtts/day} \times 8 \text{ days} = \text{gtt dispense}$$

2. Cancel

$$8 \text{ gtts/day} \times 8 \text{ days} = \text{gtt dispense}$$

3. Solve, using the rule that 20 gtts = 1 mL:

$$8 \text{ gtts} \times 8 = 64 \text{ gtts}$$
$$64 \div 20 = 3.2 \text{ mL}$$

3.2 mL is needed to fill the medication order; you dispense the 5-mL bottle.

Calculating estimated days supply for ophthalmic and otic drops

To determine estimated days supply, you will multiply amount of medication to dispense by days needed over the number of dosage units per day.

$$\frac{\text{Amount to dispense}}{\text{Dosage units per day}} = \text{Estimated days supply}$$

Ordered: Alrex® ophthalmic solution 5 mL, 1 gtts OD qid prn
On hand: Alrex® ophthalmic solution 5-mL bottle

SOLUTION ▶

2 drops 4 times a day = 8 drops per day

There are approximately 20 drops per 1 mL

$$20 \text{ drops} \times 5 \text{ mL} = 100 \text{ drops per 5 mL}$$
$$\frac{100 \text{ drops}}{8} = 12.5 \text{ days}$$

The prescription should last the patient 12.5 days.

Rectal and Vaginal Medications

Rectal: Medication administered through the rectum, usually a suppository

Rectal medications are usually given in suppository form. Generally, suppositories cannot be accurately divided. Therefore, in most cases, only doses that are multiples of the available suppository strength may be administered. In some cases, according to their manufacturers, suppositories can be safely divided in half. However, they are not scored. Thus, the physician's order should specify that a divided suppository is to be given. For example, if the order reads "Tigan® 50 mg p.r. t.i.d.," ask the pharmacist to clarify if $\frac{1}{2}$ of a 100-mg suppository is acceptable. The order should then be rewritten: "Tigan® 100 mg supp. Give $\frac{1}{2}$ supp rectally." Note that when suppositories are divided, they must be cut in half lengthwise because of the shape design for insertion rectally. **Vaginal** medications are administered through the vagina and are supplied in suppository, cream, and tablet form. It is extremely important the directions clearly indicated if a medication is to be taken rectally or vaginally.

Vaginal: Medication administered through the vagina, in suppository, cream, or tablet form.

Calculating estimated days supply for rectal and vaginal medications

To determine estimated days supply you will multiply amount of medication to dispense by days needed over the number of dosage units per day.

$$\frac{\text{Amount to dispense}}{\text{Dosage units per day}} = \text{Estimated days supply}$$

Ordered: Tigan® 100 mg supp. # 1 Give $\frac{1}{2}$ supp rectally q12h.
On hand: Tigan® 100-mg suppositories

Write your fraction as a decimal in your equation.

$$\frac{1}{0.5 \times 2} = 1 \ days$$

The prescription should last the patient 1 day.

Super Tech . . .

Open the CD-ROM that accompanies your textbook and select Chapter 7, Exercise 7-8. Review the animation and example problems, and then complete the practice problems. Continue to the next section of the book once you have mastered the information presented.

✓ Review and Practice 7-5 Other Medication Routes

In Exercises 1–10, find the amount to be administered or dispensed.

1. Ordered: Acetylcysteine 1 g via nebulizer
   On hand: Acetylcysteine 20 percent solution 10 mL vial

2. Ordered: Albuterol 2.5 mg via nebulizer
   On hand: Albuterol 5 mg/mL

3. Ordered: Atrovent® 250 mcg via nebulizer
   On hand: Atrovent® 0.02 percent inhalation solution 500 mcg/2.5 mL vial

4. Ordered: Numorphan® 10 mg p.r. PRN (as needed)
   On hand: Numorphan® 5 mg suppositories

5. Ordered: RMS morphine supp 15 mg p.r. PRN (as needed)
   On hand: RMS 5 mg, 10 mg, and 30 mg suppositories

6. Ordered: Phenergan® 12.5 mg pr PRN (as needed)
   On hand: Phenergan® 25 mg suppositories

7. Ordered: Alrex® ophthalmic solution 1 gtt in OU bid for 12 days qsad
   On hand: Alrex® ophthalmic solution, 2.5 mL and 5 mL bottles

8. Ordered: Catapres® 0.5 mg/day top
   On hand: Catapres® TTS-1 (0.1 mg/day), TTS-2 (0.2 mg/day), TTS-3 (0.3 mg/day)

9. Ordered: Alora® 0.15 mg/day
   On hand: Alora® 0.05 mg/day, 0.075 mg/day, and 0.1 mg/day

10. Ordered: Transderm nitro 0.3 mg/h top
    On hand: Transderm nitro 0.1 mg/h, 0.2 mg/h, and 0.6 mg/h patches

In Exercises 11–14, calculate the estimated days supply.

11. Ordered: Alrex® ophthalmic solution, 5 mL 1 gtt in OU q4h.
    On hand: Alrex® ophthalmic solution, 5 mL bottles   Estimated days supply: _____

12. Ordered: Albuterol 2.5 mg, via nebulizer qid, dispense 30 mL
    On hand: Albuterol 5 mg/mL   Estimated days supply: _____

13. Ordered: Alora® 0.1 mg/day #30
    On hand: 0.1 mg/day   Estimated days supply: _____

14. Ordered: RMS morphine supp 5 mg, # 4, p.r. q12h PRN
    (as needed) for pain
    On hand: RMS 5 mg suppositories   Estimated days supply: _____

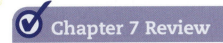

Chapter 7 Review

Test Your Knowledge

Multiple Choice

Select the best answer and write the letter on the line.

_____ 1. Medication, usually liquid, in gela-
tin shells that is not designed to be
opened.
A. Tablet
B. Capsule
C. Gelcap
D. Caplet

_____ 2. Solid oral medication, drug combined
with an inactive ingredient to form a
solid disk or cylinder.
A. Tablet
B. Capsule
C. Gelcap
D. Caplet

_____ 3. Medication, powder or granules, in a
gelatin shell that has two pieces that
fit together.
A. Tablet
B. Capsule
C. Gelcap
D. Caplet

_____ 4. Oval-shaped, has a special coating that
makes it easy to swallow.
A. Tablet
B. Capsule
C. Gelcap
D. Caplet

Practice Your Knowledge

In Exercises 5–21, calculate the amount to administer and estimated days supply where indicated.

NOTE: *Unless otherwise noted, tablets are scored in half.*

5. Ordered: Dilaudid® 4 mg PO q6h   Administer: _____
   On hand: Dilaudid® 8 mg scored tablets

6. Ordered: DiaBeta® 1.25 mg #30 PO qam ac   Administer: _____
   On hand: DiaBeta® 1.25 mg scored tablets   Estimated days supply: _____

7. Ordered: Biltricide® 450 mg PO q8h   Administer: _____
   On hand: Biltricide® 600 mg tablets scored in quarters

8. Ordered: Amoxicillin 300 mg PO q12h dispense 120 mL   Administer: _____
   On hand: Amoxicillin suspension labeled 50 mg/mL Estimated days supply: _____

9. Ordered: Artane® 3 mg PO daily   Administer: _____
   On hand: Artane® solution labeled 2 mg/5 mL

10. Ordered: Fosamax® 10 mg PO qam 30 min ac with water   Administer: _____
    On hand: Fosamax® 5 mg unscored tablets

11. Ordered: Biaxin® liquid 62.5 mg PO q12h dispense 25 mL
    On hand: Biaxin® liquid labeled 125 mg/5 mL

    Administer: _____
    Estimated days supply: _____

12. Ordered: Isoptin® 270 mg PO qam
    On hand: Isoptin® 180 mg scored tablets

    Administer: _____

13. Ordered: Duricef® 0.5 g PO bid, dispense 100 mL
    On hand: Duricef® suspension labeled 250 mg/5 mL

    Administer: _____
    Estimated days supply: _____

14. Ordered: Levoxyl® 0.45 mg PO daily
    On hand: Levoxyl® 300 mcg scored tablets

    Administer: _____

15. Ordered: Hivid® 750 mcg PO q8h
    On hand: Hivid® 0.375 mg unscored tablets

    Administer: _____

16. Ordered: Duricef® 500 mg PO bid
    On hand: Duricef® 1 g scored tablets

    Administer: _____

17. Ordered: MSIR® gr 1/8 PO q4h
    On hand: MSIR® 15 mg scored tablets

    Administer: _____

18. Ordered: Felbatol® 400 mg PO tid
    On hand: Felbatol® liquid labeled 600 mg/5 mL

    Administer: _____

19. What combination will provide the desired dose with the fewest tablets?

    Ordered: Hytrin® 5 mg PO qpm
    On hand: Hytrin® 1-mg unscored tablets and Hytrin 2 mg unscored tablets

20. A patient receives 15 mL of Lortab elixir every 6 h. Lortab® elixir contains 7.5 mg hydrocodone and 500 mg acetaminophen in each 15 mL.

    How much acetaminophen will this patient receive in 24 h?

21. How would you reconstitute the following medication? Find the amount to administer.

    Ordered: Ceftin® 375 mg PO bid
    On hand: Ceftin® 125 mg per 5 mL

In Exercises 22–31, find the amount to administer, then mark the syringe.

22. Ordered: INFeD® (iron dextran) 100 mg deep IM qd
    On hand: INFeD® 50 mg/mL

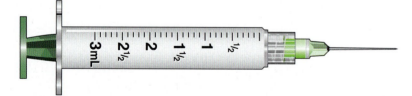

23. Ordered: Haloperidol decanoate 60 mg deep IM stat
    On hand: Haloperidol decanoate 50 mg/mL

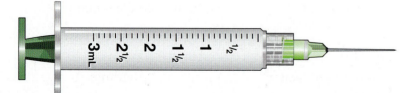

24. Ordered: Loxitane® 30 mg IM bid
    On hand: Loxitane® 50 mg/mL

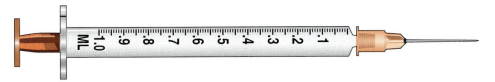

25. Ordered: Epogen® 1400 U sub-Q tiw
    On hand: Epogen® 2000 U/mL

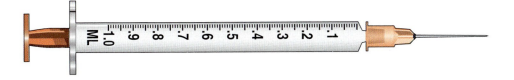

26. Ordered: Lidocaine 300 mg IM stat
    On hand: Lidocaine 20 percent solution

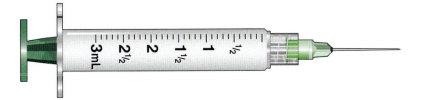

27. Ordered: Magnesium sulfate 250 mg IM qd
    On hand: Magnesium sulfate 10 percent solution

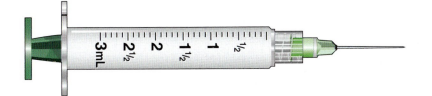

28. Ordered: Levsin® 0.4 mg IM bid
    On hand: Levsin® 0.5 mg/mL

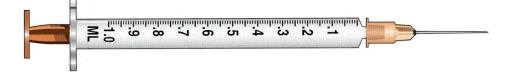

29. Ordered: Robinul® 0.15 mg IM stat
    On hand: Robinul® 0.2 mg/mL

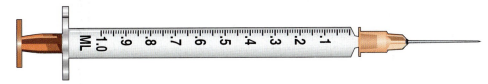

30. Order: Prostigmin 0.75 mg IM q4h
    On hand: Prostigmin 1:1000 solution

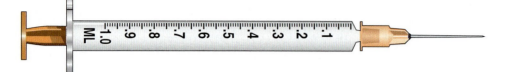

31. Ordered: Epinephrine 0.5 mg sub-Q stat
    On hand: Epinephrine 1:200 solution

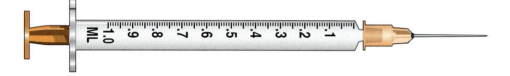

For Exercises 32–36, find the amount to administer, select the proper syringe, and write in the space provided.

32. Ordered: Adrenalin 0.2 mg sub-Q stat
    On hand: Adrenalin 1:2000 solution

    Administer: _____ Syringe: _____

33. Ordered: Calciferol 24,000 IU IM qd
    On hand: Calciferol 500,000 IU/5 mL

    Administer: _____ Syringe: _____

34. Ordered: Heparin sodium 7500 U Sub-Q q8h
    On hand: Heparin 1:20,000 solution

    Administer: _____ Syringe: _____

35. Ordered: Heparin calcium 7500 units Sub-Q q8h
    On hand: Heparin calcium 5000 units/0.2 mL

    Administer: _____ Syringe: _____

36. Ordered: Levsin® 1 mg IM qid
    On hand: Levsin® 0.5 mg per mL.

    Administer: _____ Syringe: _____

In Exercises 37–40, find the amount to administer and the estimated days supply.

37. Ordered: Acetylcysteine 800 mg via nebulizer q6h, dispense 240 mL
    On hand: Acetylcysteine 10 percent solution

38. Ordered: Albuterol 1.25 mg via nebulizer q8h, dispense 15 mL
    On hand: Albuterol 5 mg/mL

39. Ordered: Thorazine® 25mg #12 q8h p.r. as needed
    On hand: Thorazine® 25 mg

40. Ordered: Androderm® 2.5 mg/day top, dispense 21 patches
    On hand: Androderm® 2.5 mg/day patches

Apply Your Knowledge

How much medication needs to be dispensed?

You are the pharmacy technician working in a retail pharmacy. You are working in the pharmacy when the following prescription comes in: "Biaxin® 187.5 mg PO qid for 5 days, qsad." On hand: Biaxin® 125 mg per 5 mL, 100 mL when mixed with 55 mL of water.

Answer the following questions:

1. How many milliliters need to be dispensed to fill the prescription?

   _____

2. How many milliliters will the patient take per dose?

   _____

3. How many milliliters will the patient take in 24 hours?

   _____

Internet Activity

The pharmacist discovers that a patient who has trouble swallowing has been crushing Glucotrol® XL tablets. Because this sustained-release medication should not be crushed, the patient has been receiving too much medication at one time. You realize that this problem could occur with any patient who is taking a sustained-release medication.

Assignment: Search the Internet for patient education materials warning patients about crushing medications.

Suggested key words: medication + crushing; medication + swallowing; pills + swallowing

Super Tech...

Open the CD-ROM that accompanies your textbook and a final review of Chapter 7. For a final evaluation, take the chapter test and email or print your results for your instructor. A score of 95 percent or above indicates mastery of the chapter concepts.

8

Intravenous Calculations

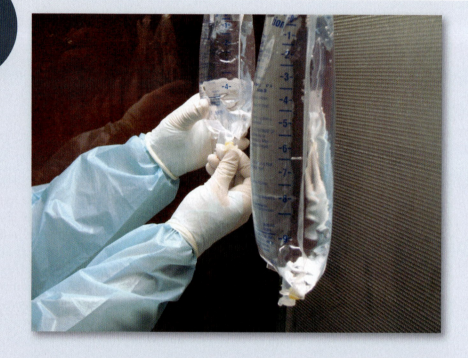

Learning Outcomes

When you have successfully completed Chapter 8, you will have mastered skills to be able to:

▶ Identify the components and concentrations of IV solutions.

▶ Calculate IV flow rates.

▶ Calculate infusion time based on volume and flow rate.

▶ Calculate infusion completion time based on flow rate.

▶ Calculate volume based on infusion time and flow rate.

▶ Calculate medications for intermittent IV infusions.

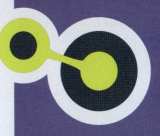

Introduction

This chapter teaches intravenous (IV) calculations and theory. As a pharmacy technician you will need to know how to perform accurate IV calculations. Pharmacy technicians who prepare IV solutions should know the principles discussed in this chapter.

Intravenous (IV) fluids are solutions that include medications that are delivered directly into the bloodstream through a vein. Blood, a suspension, is also delivered intravenously. Fluids delivered directly into the bloodstream have a rapid effect, which is necessary during emergencies or other critical care situations when medications are needed. However, the results can be fatal if the wrong medication or dosage is given. Many IV drugs are available. Each has its own guidelines regarding its use, based on specifications developed by the manufacturers.

The guidelines typically outline recommended dosages, infusion rates, compatibility, and patient monitoring. For example, some medications cannot be combined with others, or must be administered over a specific length of time.

Furthermore, most states regulate who may administer IV medications and what training is required.

PTCB Correlations

When you have completed this chapter you will have the building block of knowledge needed to perform IV drip rate calculations and prepare IV mixtures.

▶ Knowledge of pharmacy calculations (Statement I-50).

▶ Knowledge of procedures to prepare IV admixtures (Statement I-55).

Intravenous (IV) fluids: Solutions that include medication delivered directly to the bloodstream through a vein.

Critical Thinking in the Pharmacy
How Long Will That IV Last?

You are the pharmacy technician working in a hospital pharmacy. You are working in the pharmacy when the following order comes in: "D5W 3000 mL at 120 mL per hour." The IV solution comes in 1000-mL bags.

When you have completed Chapter 8 you will be able to determine how many hours a 1000-mL bag will last and how many bags are needed to complete the order.

IV Solutions

IV solutions fall into four functional categories: **replacement fluids, maintenance fluids, KVO fluids,** and **therapeutic fluids.**

- *Replacement fluids* replace electrolytes and fluids lost or depleted due to hemorrhage, vomiting, or diarrhea. Examples include whole blood, nutrient solutions, or fluids administered to treat dehydration.
- *Maintenance fluids* help patients maintain normal electrolyte and fluid balance. They include IV fluids such as normal saline given during and after surgery.
- *KVO fluids* are prescribed to keep the veins open (KVO or TKO) to provide access to the vascular system for emergency situations; these include 5 percent dextrose in water.
- *Therapeutic fluids* are IV fluids that deliver medication to the patient.

Replacement fluids: Fluids that replace electrolytes or fluids lost from dehydration, hemorrhage, vomiting, or diarrhea.

Maintenance fluids: Fluids that maintain the fluid and electrolyte balance for patients.

KVO fluids: Fluids prescribed to keep the veins open that provide access to the vascular system for emergency situations.

Therapeutic fluids: IV fluids that deliver medication to patients.

Electrolytes

A patient's fluid and electrolyte balance helps determine the solution's concentration. Calcium, potassium, chloride, phosphorus, and magnesium are electrolytes that can be added to an IV solution to help correct a fluid or chemical imbalance.

IV solutions are classified as **isotonic, hypotonic,** or **hypertonic,** depending on their effect on the fluid content of cells.

- Isotonic IV solutions, such as D5W, NS, and lactated Ringer's, do not affect the fluid balance of the surrounding cells or tissues. These solutions help patient maintain normal electrolyte and fluid balance.
- Hypotonic IV solutions such as 0.45 percent sodium chloride (NaCl) and 0.3 percent sodium chloride move across the cell membrane into surrounding cells and tissues. This movement restores the proper fluid level in cells and tissues of patients who are dehydrated.
- Hypertonic IV solutions such as 3 percent saline draw fluids from cells and tissues across the cell membrane into the bloodstream. They are helpful for patients with severe fluid shifts, such as those caused by burns.

Isotonic: Fluids that do not affect the fluid balance of the surrounding cells or tissues, such as D5W, NS, and lactated Ringer's.

Hypotonic: Fluids that move across the cell membrane into surrounding cells and tissues, such as ½ NS or 0.45% sodium chloride (NaCL) and 0.3% NaCL.

Hypertonic: Fluids that draw fluids from cells and tissues across the cell membrane into the bloodstream, such as 3 percent saline.

Patients with normal electrolyte levels are likely to receive isotonic solutions, which helps maintain normal electrolyte and fluid balance. Those with high electrolyte levels will receive hypotonic solutions. Those with low electrolyte levels will receive hypertonic solutions.

EXAMPLE 1 ▶

Patient A is a 35-year-old healthy female who will have an IV infusion during a diagnostic test.

She will require an isotonic solution such as D5W, NS, or lactated Ringer's.

EXAMPLE 2 ▶

Patient B is an 8-year-old female who has been vomiting and has had diarrhea for 24 h and is dehydrated. She may require a hypotonic solution like 0.45 or 0.3 percent saline to restore the proper fluid level in her cells and tissues.

EXAMPLE 3 ▶   Patient C is a 50-year-old male with burns over 35 percent of his body. He may require hypertonic solution such as 3 percent NaCl to help draw fluids from cells and tissues.

IV Labels

IV solutions are labeled with the name and exact amount of components in the solution. The label in Figure 8-1 is clearly marked as 5 percent dextrose and lactated Ringer's injection. Table 8-1 summarizes abbreviations often used for IV solutions.

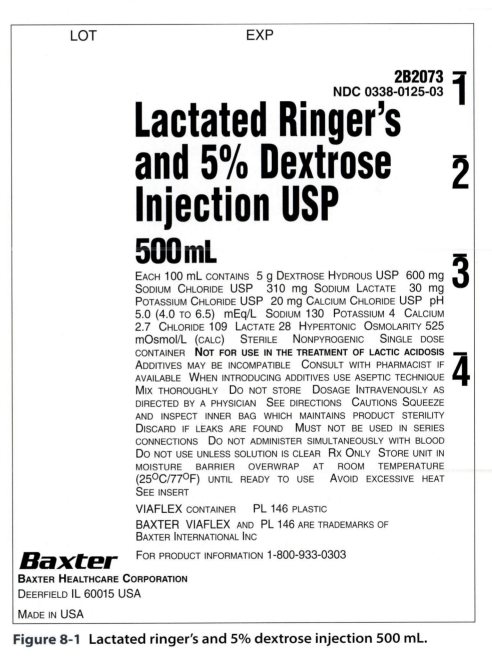

LOT   EXP

2B2073
NDC 0338-0125-03   **1**

Lactated Ringer's and 5% Dextrose Injection USP   **2**

500 mL   **3**

EACH 100 mL CONTAINS 5 g DEXTROSE HYDROUS USP 600 mg SODIUM CHLORIDE USP 310 mg SODIUM LACTATE 30 mg POTASSIUM CHLORIDE USP 20 mg CALCIUM CHLORIDE USP pH 5.0 (4.0 TO 6.5) mEq/L SODIUM 130 POTASSIUM 4 CALCIUM 2.7 CHLORIDE 109 LACTATE 28 HYPERTONIC OSMOLARITY 525 mOsmol/L (CALC) STERILE NONPYROGENIC SINGLE DOSE CONTAINER **NOT FOR USE IN THE TREATMENT OF LACTIC ACIDOSIS** ADDITIVES MAY BE INCOMPATIBLE CONSULT WITH PHARMACIST IF AVAILABLE WHEN INTRODUCING ADDITIVES USE ASEPTIC TECHNIQUE MIX THOROUGHLY DO NOT STORE DOSAGE INTRAVENOUSLY AS DIRECTED BY A PHYSICIAN SEE DIRECTIONS CAUTIONS SQUEEZE AND INSPECT INNER BAG WHICH MAINTAINS PRODUCT STERILITY DISCARD IF LEAKS ARE FOUND MUST NOT BE USED IN SERIES CONNECTIONS DO NOT ADMINISTER SIMULTANEOUSLY WITH BLOOD DO NOT USE UNLESS SOLUTION IS CLEAR RX ONLY STORE UNIT IN MOISTURE BARRIER OVERWRAP AT ROOM TEMPERATURE (25°C/77°F) UNTIL READY TO USE AVOID EXCESSIVE HEAT SEE INSERT   **4**

VIAFLEX CONTAINER   PL 146 PLASTIC

BAXTER VIAFLEX AND PL 146 ARE TRADEMARKS OF BAXTER INTERNATIONAL INC

FOR PRODUCT INFORMATION 1-800-933-0303

Baxter
BAXTER HEALTHCARE CORPORATION
DEERFIELD IL 60015 USA

MADE IN USA

Figure 8-1 Lactated ringer's and 5% dextrose injection 500 mL.

Table 8-1   Commonly Used Abbreviations

D10W	10% dextrose in water
D5W	5% dextrose in water
W, H$_2$O	Water
NS, NSS	Normal saline (0.9% NaCl)
LR	Lactated Ringer's
RL	Ringer's lactate
$\frac{1}{2}$ NS, $\frac{1}{2}$ NSS	One-half normal saline solution (0.45% NaCl)
$\frac{1}{3}$ NS, $\frac{1}{3}$ NSS	One-third normal saline solution (0.3% NaCl)
$\frac{1}{4}$ NS, $\frac{1}{4}$ NSS	One-fourth normal saline solution (0.225% NaCl)

In abbreviations for IV solutions, letters identify the component and numbers identify the concentration.

EXAMPLE ▶ An order for 5 percent dextrose in lactated Ringer's solution might be abbreviated in any of the following ways:

D5LR   D$_5$LR   5%D/LR   D5%LR

IV Concentrations

IV solutions may have different concentrations of dextrose (glucose) or saline (sodium chloride, or NaCl). For example, 5 percent dextrose contains 5 g of dextrose per 100 mL (Figure 8-2).

Normal saline is 0.9 percent saline; it contains 900 mg, or 0.9 g, of sodium chloride per 100 mL (Figure 8-3). In turn, 0.45 percent saline, or $\frac{1}{2}$ NS, has 450 mg of sodium chloride per 100 mL—one-half the amount of normal saline. Other saline concentrations include 0.3 percent saline, or $\frac{1}{3}$ NS, and 0.225% saline, or $\frac{1}{4}$ NS.

EXAMPLE ▶ How much dextrose is contained in 500 mL D5W?

D5W represents 5 percent dextrose in water; it has 5 g of dextrose per 100 mL of water. Using ratio proportion (refer to Procedure Checklist 6-2, Chapter 6) gives:

$$500 \text{ mL} : ? \text{ g} :: 100 \text{ mL} : 5 \text{ g}$$
$$? \text{ g} \times 100 \text{ mL} = 500 \text{ mL} \times 5 \text{ g}$$
$$? = 25$$

So 25 g of dextrose is contained in 500 mL D5W.

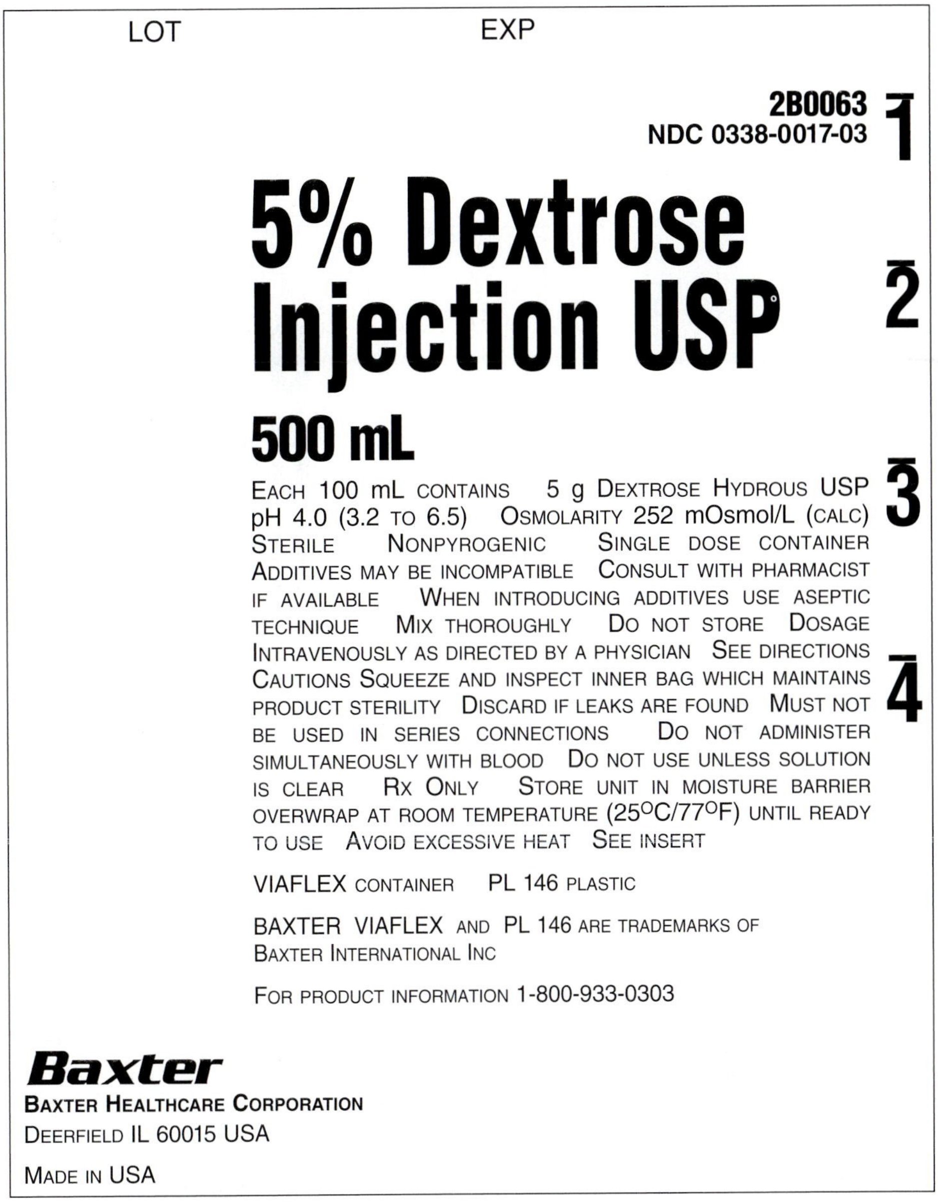

LOT   EXP

2B0063
NDC 0338-0017-03   **1**

5% Dextrose Injection USP

2

500 mL

EACH 100 mL CONTAINS   5 g DEXTROSE HYDROUS USP
pH 4.0 (3.2 TO 6.5)   OSMOLARITY 252 mOsmol/L (CALC)   **3**
STERILE   NONPYROGENIC   SINGLE DOSE CONTAINER
ADDITIVES MAY BE INCOMPATIBLE   CONSULT WITH PHARMACIST
IF AVAILABLE   WHEN INTRODUCING ADDITIVES USE ASEPTIC
TECHNIQUE   MIX THOROUGHLY   DO NOT STORE   DOSAGE
INTRAVENOUSLY AS DIRECTED BY A PHYSICIAN   SEE DIRECTIONS
CAUTIONS SQUEEZE AND INSPECT INNER BAG WHICH MAINTAINS   **4**
PRODUCT STERILITY   DISCARD IF LEAKS ARE FOUND   MUST NOT
BE USED IN SERIES CONNECTIONS   DO NOT ADMINISTER
SIMULTANEOUSLY WITH BLOOD   DO NOT USE UNLESS SOLUTION
IS CLEAR   RX ONLY   STORE UNIT IN MOISTURE BARRIER
OVERWRAP AT ROOM TEMPERATURE (25°C/77°F) UNTIL READY
TO USE   AVOID EXCESSIVE HEAT   SEE INSERT

VIAFLEX CONTAINER   PL 146 PLASTIC

BAXTER VIAFLEX AND PL 146 ARE TRADEMARKS OF
BAXTER INTERNATIONAL INC

FOR PRODUCT INFORMATION 1-800-933-0303

Baxter
BAXTER HEALTHCARE CORPORATION
DEERFIELD IL 60015 USA
MADE IN USA

Figure 8-2 500 mL of D5W.

Compatibility

Medications, electrolytes, and nutrients are additives that can be combined with IV solutions. Potassium chloride, vitamins B and C, and antibiotics are common additives. While additives are often prepackaged in the solution, as a pharmacy technician you may need to mix the additive and IV solution. The physician's order will tell you how much additive to administer, the amount and type of basic IV solution to use, and the length of time over which the additive/IV mixture should infuse. For example, an order may call for 20 milliequivalents (mEq) of potassium chloride in 1000 mL of 5 percent dextrose and normal saline over 8 h, or 1000 mL D5NS c̄ 20 mEq KCl IV over 8 h.

Before you combine any medications, electrolytes, or nutrients with an IV solution, you must be sure the components are compatible.

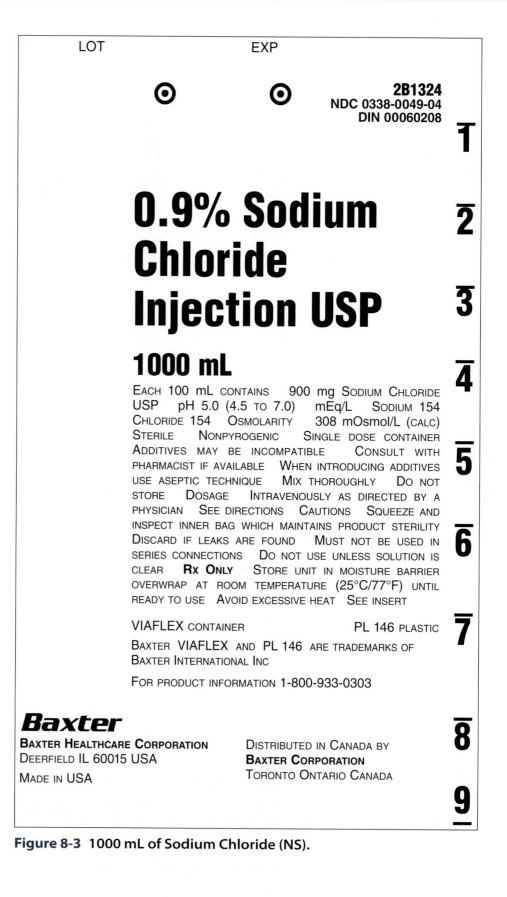

Figure 8-3 1000 mL of Sodium Chloride (NS).

EXAMPLE ▶ Incompatible additives may cause the resulting solution to turn cloudy or crystallize (harden to crystals). If you mix an IV base solution with an additive that is incompatible (see Table 8-2), you place the patient's health at serious risk. Verify compatibility by checking with the pharmacist, a compatibility chart, a drug reference book, the Internet, or a package insert.

Table 8-2 Incompatible Solutions*

Ampicillin	5% dextrose in water
Cefotaxime sodium	Sodium bicarbonate
Diazepam	Potassium chloride
Dopamine HCl	Sodium bicarbonate
Penicillin	Heparin
Penicillin	Vitamin B complex
Sodium bicarbonate	Lactated Ringer's
Tetracycline HCl	Calcium chloride

* These are a few examples of incompatible combinations. Always check the compatibility of IV solutions and additives.

Tech Check

Checking Compatibility

A patient in respiratory distress with congestive heart failure is started on D5/0.45% NaCl. The next day she is diagnosed with an upper respiratory infection. The physician orders 500 mg ampicillin IVPB q6h. The pharmacy technician pulls the medication from the shelf and does not check the patient's medication record or a compatibility chart.

Think Before You Act

The pharmacist suspects that the additive is not compatible with the IV solution. She uses a compatibility chart to verify her suspicions. After which she calls the physician to obtain a new order. This error could have been avoided by the pharmacy technician by checking the patient's medication record and a compatibility chart.

In this case, the pharmacist caught the error. However, in many cases, failing to verify compatibility **before** introducing an additive can have severe consequences for the patient, including death.

Super Tech . . .

Open the CD-ROM that accompanies your textbook and select Chapter 8, Exercise 8-1. Review the animation and example problems, and then complete the practice problems. Continue to the next section of the book once you have mastered the information presented.

✓ Review and Practice 8-1 IV Solutions

Fill in the blanks using the following word bank.

Maintenance fluids   KVO fluids   Hypertonic
Isotonic   Replacement fluids   Therapeutic fluids
Hypotonic

_____ 1. Type of fluid given to a patient with a severe burn.

_____ 2. Type of fluid given to a patient who is dehydrated.

_____ 3. Helps patient maintain normal electrolyte and fluid balance.

_____ 4. Provides access to the vascular system for emergency situation.

_____ 5. Replaces electrolytes and fluid lost because of hemorrhage, vomiting, or diarrhea.

_____ 6. Type of fluid given to a patient having an IV infusion during a diagnostic test.

_____ 7. Delivers medication to the patient.

Calculating Flow Rates

Milliliters per Hour

An order for IV fluids indicates the *amount of an IV fluid* to be administered and the *length of time* over which it is to be given. Before the IV can be administered, you must calculate a *flow rate* for the intravenous solution from these two values.

To calculate flow rates in milliliters per hour, you need to identify the following:

- V (volume) expressed in milliliters.
- T (time) expressed in hours. (Convert the units when necessary by using fraction proportion, ratio proportion, or dimensional analysis.)
- F (flow rate) rounded to the nearest whole number.

Use the formula method with $F = \frac{V}{T}$ or dimensional analysis to determine the flow rate in milliliters per hour.

Using Conversion Factors

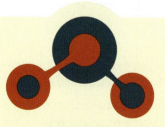

Formula Method

EXAMPLE 1 ▶   Find the flow rate.

Ordered: 500 mg ampicillin in 100 mL NS to infuse over 30 minutes

In this case the volume is expressed in milliliters, and $V = 100$ mL.

SOLUTION ▶ Since time is expressed in minutes, you must first convert 30 minutes (min) to hours to find T.

(In this example we will use the fraction proportion Procedure Checklist 6-1 in Chapter 6 to convert. You may prefer to use the ratio proportion Procedure Checklist 6-2 or the dimensional analysis Procedure Checklist 6-3.)

$$\frac{1h}{60 \text{ min}} = \frac{?}{30 \text{ min}}$$

$$\frac{1h}{60 \text{ min}} = \frac{?}{30 \text{ min}}$$

$$60 \times ? = 1\text{ h} \times 30$$

$$? = \frac{1\text{ h} \times 30}{60}$$

$$? = 0.5\text{ h}$$

We now have the information needed in the proper units.

$$V = 100 \text{ mL} \quad \text{and} \quad T = 0.5 \text{ h}$$

Using the formula $F = \frac{V}{T}$, we find that

$$F = \frac{100 \text{ mL}}{0.5 \text{ h}}$$

$$F = 200 \text{ mL/h}$$

EXAMPLE 2 ▶ Find the flow rate.

Ordered: 500 mL 5% D 0.45%S over 3 hours

SOLUTION ▶ In this case the units are already expressed in milliliters and hours.

$$V = 500 \text{ mL} \quad \text{and} \quad T = 3 \text{ h}$$

Using the formula $F = \frac{V}{T}$, we have

$$F = \frac{500 \text{ mL}}{3 \text{ h}}$$

$$F = 166.666 \text{ mL/h}$$

$$F = 167 \text{ mL/h rounded to the nearest whole number}$$

Using Conversion Factors

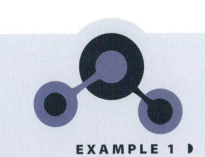

Dimensional Analysis

EXAMPLE 1 ▶ Find the flow rate.

Ordered: 500 mg ampicillin in 100 mL NS to infuse over 30 min

SOLUTION ▶

1. Determine the units of measure for the answer (*F*), and place it as the unknown on one side of the equation.

$$F \text{ mL/h} =$$

2. Write a factor with the number of milliliters to be administered on top (*V*) and the length of time to be administered (*T*) on the bottom.

$$\frac{100 \text{ mL}}{30 \text{ min}}$$

3. Multiply by a second factor to convert the minutes to hours, and place minutes in the numerator. Set up the equation.

$$F \text{ mL/h} = \frac{100 \text{ mL}}{30 \text{ min}} \times \frac{60 \text{ min}}{1 \text{ h}}$$

4. Cancel units on the right side of the equation. The remaining unit of measure on the right side of the equation should match the unknown unit of measure on the left side of the equation.

$$F \text{ mL/h} = \frac{100 \text{ mL}}{30 \text{ \cancel{min}}} \times \frac{60 \text{ \cancel{min}}}{1 \text{ h}}$$

5. Solve the equation.

$$F \text{ mL/h} = \frac{100 \times 60}{30}$$

$$F = 200 \text{ mL/h}$$

EXAMPLE 2 ▶ Find the flow rate.

Ordered: 500 mL 5% D 0.45%S over 3 hours

SOLUTION ▶

1. Determine the units of measure for the answer (*F*), and place it as the unknown on one side of the equation.

$$F \text{ mL/h} =$$

2. On the right side of the equation, write a factor with the number of milliliters to be administered on top (*V*) and the length of time to be administered (*T*) on the bottom.

$$F \text{ mL/h} = \frac{500 \text{ mL}}{3 \text{ h}}$$

3. Since the units of measure on the left side of the equation match the units of measure on the right side of the equation, no additional conversion factors are necessary. Solve the equation.

$$F \text{ mL/h} = \frac{500 \text{ mL}}{3 \text{ h}}$$

$$F = 166.666 \text{ mL/h}$$

$$F = 167 \text{ mL/h}$$

Number of Drops per Minute

When using a manual set, IV flow rates need to be calculated by the number of drops per minute (gtt/min). Before this can be calculated, you must first know how many drops are in a milliliter. IV tubing packages are labeled with a drop factor, which tells you how many drops of IV solution are equal to 1 mL when you are using that tubing. *Macrodrip* tubing has larger drops and one of three typical drop factors: 10 gtt/mL, 15 gtt/mL, or 20 gtt/mL. *Microdrip* tubing has a drop factor of 60 gtt/mL.

To determine the flow rate f in drops per minute:

Change the flow rate in milliliters per hour (F) to drops per minute (f), using the formula

$$f = \frac{F \times C}{60}$$

where F = flow rate, mL/h
  C = calibration factor of tubing, gtt/mL
  60 = number of minutes in 1 h (hour)

Round your answer to the nearest whole number.

Using Conversion Factors

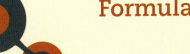

Formula Method

EXAMPLE 1 ▶ Find the flow rate in drops per minute that is equal to 75 mL/h when you are using 20 gtt/mL macrodrip tubing.

SOLUTION ▶
$$F = 75 \text{ mL/h}$$
$$C = 20 \text{ gtt/mL}$$

Substituting into the formula gives:

$$f = \frac{F \times C}{60 \text{ min/h}}$$

$$f = \frac{75 \text{ mL/h} \times 20 \text{ gtt/mL}}{60 \text{ min/h}}$$

Cancel the units.

$$f = \frac{75 \text{ mL/h} \times 20 \text{ mL/gtt}}{60 \text{ min/h}}$$

Solve the equation.

$$f = \frac{75 \times 20 \text{ gtts}}{60 \text{ min}}$$

$$f = 25 \text{ gtt/min}$$

EXAMPLE 2 ▶ Find the flow rate in drops per minute that is equal to 35 mL/h when you are using 60 gtt/mL microdrip tubing.

SOLUTION ▶

$$F = 35 \text{ mL/h}$$
$$C = 60 \text{ gtt/mL}$$

Substituting into the formula gives:

$$f = \frac{F \times C}{60}$$

$$f = \frac{35 \text{ mL/h} \times 60 \text{ gtt/mL}}{60 \text{ min/h}}$$

Cancel the units.

$$f = \frac{35 \text{ m\cancel{L}/\cancel{h}} \times 60 \text{ gtt/m\cancel{L}}}{60 \text{ min/\cancel{h}}}$$

$$f = 35 \text{ gtt/min}$$

Note: The value of the flow rate is the same in drops per minute or milliliters per hour when 60 gtt/mL microdrip tubing is used. In other words, for microdrip tubing, $F = f$.

Using Conversion Factors

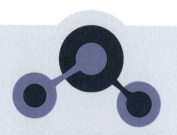

Dimensional Analysis

EXAMPLE 1 ▶ Find the flow rate in drops per minute that is equal to 75 mL/h when you are using 20-gtt/mL macrodrip tubing.

SOLUTION ▶

1. Determine the unit of measure for the answer f, and place it with f as the unknown on one side of the equation.

$$f \text{ gtt/min} =$$

2. Determine the first factor. The number of milliliters to be administered on top (V) and the length of time to be administered (T) on the bottom.

$$\frac{75 \text{ mL}}{1 \text{ h}}$$

3. Multiply by a second factor to convert the hours to minutes, placing hours in the numerator.

$$75 \text{ mL/h} \times \frac{1 \text{ h}}{60 \text{ min}}$$

4. Multiply by the drop factor of the tubing being used. This is the third factor. Set up the equation.

$$f \text{ gtt/min} = \frac{75 \text{ mL}}{1 \text{ h}} \times \frac{1 \text{ h}}{60 \text{ min}} \times \frac{20 \text{ gtt}}{1 \text{ mL}}$$

5. Cancel units on the right side of the equation. The remaining unit of measure on the right side of the equation should match the unknown unit of measure on the left side of the equation.

$$f \text{ gtt/min} = \frac{75 \text{ m\cancel{L}}}{1 \text{ \cancel{h}}} \times \frac{1 \text{ \cancel{h}}}{60 \text{ min}} \times \frac{20 \text{ gtt}}{1 \text{ m\cancel{L}}}$$

6. Solve the equation.

$$f = \frac{75 \times 20 \text{ gtt}}{60 \text{ min}}$$

$$f = 25 \text{ gtt/min}$$

EXAMPLE 2 ❯   Find the flow rate in drops per minute that is equal to 35 mL/h when you are using 60 gtt/mL microdrip tubing.

SOLUTION ❯   1. Determine the unit of measure for the answer (f), and place it as the unknown on the left side of the equation.

$$f \text{ gtt/min} =$$

2. Determine the first factor. Place the number of milliliters to be administered on top (V) and the length of time to be administered (T) on the bottom.

$$\frac{35 \text{ mL}}{\text{h}}$$

3. Multiply by a second factor to convert the hours to minutes, place hours in the numerator.

$$35 \text{ mL/h} \times \frac{1 \text{ h}}{60 \text{ min}}$$

4. Multiply by the drop factor of the tubing being used. Set up the equation.

$$f \text{ gtt/min} = \frac{35 \text{ mL}}{1 \text{ h}} \times \frac{1 \text{ h}}{60 \text{ min}} \times \frac{60 \text{ gtt}}{1 \text{ mL}}$$

5. Cancel units on the right side of the equation. The remaining unit of measure on the right side of the equation should match the unknown unit of measure on the left side of the equation.

$$f \text{ gtt/min} = \frac{35 \text{ m\cancel{L}}}{1 \text{ \cancel{h}}} \times \frac{1 \text{ \cancel{h}}}{60 \text{ min}} \times \frac{60 \text{ gtt}}{1 \text{ m\cancel{L}}}$$

6. Solve the equation.

$$f \text{ gtt/min} = 35 \times \frac{1}{\cancel{60} \text{ min}} \times \frac{\cancel{60} \text{ gtt}}{1}$$

$$f = 35 \text{ gtt/min}$$

Note: The value of the flow rate is the same in drops per minute or milliliters per hour when 60 gtt/mL microdrip tubing is used. In other words, for microdrip tubing, $F = f$.

Tech Check

Calculate with Care!

Always use critical thinking skills to evaluate your answer before you distribute a drug. For example, in Example 1 the tubing used is 20 gtts/mL. If you set up the problem incorrectly and forget to include the tubing drop factor, you would get the answer 1.25 drops per minute; this would deliver 75 drops per hour, not 75 mL per hour, and the patient would not receive enough of the prescribed IV solution.

Think Before You Act

With critical thinking you would determine that the answer appears incorrect and should recalculate. *Never distribute a medication if you are uncertain or uncomfortable with the answer you obtain.*

Super Tech . . .

Open the CD-ROM that accompanies your textbook and select Chapter 8, Exercise 8-2 and 8-3. Review the animation and example problems, and then complete the practice problems. Continue to the next section of the book once you have mastered the information presented.

 Review and Practice 8-2 Calculating Flow Rates

In Exercises 1–10, calculate the flow rate in milliliters per hour.

1. Ordered: 1000 mL LR over 6 h

2. Ordered: 300 mL NS over 2 h

3. Ordered: 3000 mL 0.45% NS q 24 h

4. Ordered: 20 mEq KCl in 500 mL NS over 5 hours

5. Ordered: 1500 mL RL over 12 h

6. Ordered: 1000 mL NS over 12 h

7. Ordered: 750 mL NS over 8 h

8. Ordered: 20 mEq KCl in 50 mL NS over 30 min

9. Ordered: 1800 mL 0.45% S per day

10. Ordered: 250 mL D5W over 3 h

In Exercises 11–22, calculate the flow rate in number of drops per minute.

11. Ordered: 1000 mL NS over 24 h, tubing is 20 gtt/mL

12. Ordered: 400 mL RL over 8 h, tubing is 10 gtt/mL

13. Ordered: 1500 mL 0.45% S over 12 h, tubing is 15 gtt/mL

14. Ordered: 250 mL D5W over 3 h, tubing is 10 gtt/mL

15. Ordered: 40 meq KCl in 100 mL NS over 40 min, tubing is 20 gtt/mL

16. Ordered: 500 mL NS over 8 h, tubing is 15 gtt/mL

17. Ordered: 3000 mL NS over 24 h, tubing is 10 gtt/mL

18. Ordered: 50 mL penicillin IV over 1 h, tubing is 60 gtt/mL

19. Ordered: 750 mL 5%D NS over 5 h, tubing is 20 gtt/mL

20. Ordered: 100 mL gentamicin over 30 min, tubing is 15 gtt/mL

21. Ordered: 1000 mL D5W over 9 h, tubing is 15 gtt/mL

22. Ordered: 750 mL RL over 8 h, tubing 15 gtt/mL

Infusion Time and Volume

An IV order may call for a certain amount of fluid to infuse at a specific rate, without specifying the duration. In this case you will need to calculate the duration or amount of time the IV will take to infuse, so that the IV can be monitored properly. In other cases, you may know the duration and the flow rate, and you will need to calculate the fluid volume.

Calculating Infusion Time

In the previous section, you calculated the rate of infusion when given the volume and time. Sometimes the infusion rate and volume are given in the order, and you will need to calculate the duration or amount of time the infusion will take to be administered.

To calculate infusion time in hours T, you need to identify to following:

- V (volume) expressed in milliliters
- F (flow rate) expressed in milliliters per hour
- Fractional hours expressed in minutes by multiplying by 60

Use the formula $T = \frac{V}{F}$ or dimensional analysis to find T, the infusion time in hours.

Using Conversion Factors

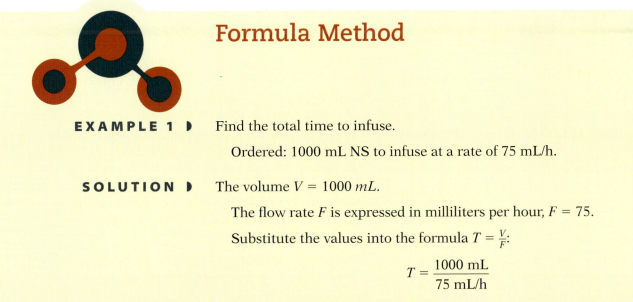

Formula Method

EXAMPLE 1 ▶   Find the total time to infuse.

Ordered: 1000 mL NS to infuse at a rate of 75 mL/h.

SOLUTION ▶   The volume $V = 1000 \ mL$.

The flow rate F is expressed in milliliters per hour, $F = 75$.

Substitute the values into the formula $T = \frac{V}{F}$:

$$T = \frac{1000 \ \text{mL}}{75 \ \text{mL/h}}$$

Cancel the units.

$$T = \frac{1000 \ \cancel{mL}}{75 \ \cancel{mL}/h}$$

$T = 13.33 \ h = $ total time to infuse 1000 mL

Note that 0.33 h does not represent 33 minutes. Because there is 60 min in 1 h, you **must** multiply the fractional hours by 60 to convert to minutes.

$$0.33 \ h \times 60 \ min/h = 20 \ min$$

The total time to infuse the solution is 13 h 20 min.

EXAMPLE 2 ▶   Find the total time to infuse.

Ordered: 750 mL **LR** to infuse at a rate of 125 mL/h started at 11 p.m.

SOLUTION ▶   The volume $V = 750$ mL

The flow rate F is expressed in milliliters per hour, $F = 125$ mL/h

Substitute the values into the formula $T = \frac{V}{F}$:

$$T = \frac{750 \ mL}{125 \ mL/h}$$

Cancel the units.

$$T = \frac{750 \ \cancel{mL}}{125 \ \cancel{mL}/h}$$

$T = 6 \ h = $ total time to infuse 750 mL

Using Conversion Factors

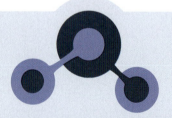

Dimensional Analysis

EXAMPLE 1 ▶   Find the total time to infuse.

Ordered: 1000 mL **NS** to infuse at a rate of 75 mL/h.

SOLUTION ▶   1. Determine the unit of measure for the answer T, and place it with T as the unknown on the left side of the equation.

$$T \ h =$$

2. The first factor is the number of milliliters to be administered on over 1. The second factor is the inverted flow rate. The flow rate is inverted in order to solve for hours (h).

$$T \ h = \frac{1000 \ mL}{1} \times \frac{1 \ h}{75 \ mL}$$

3. Cancel units on the right side of the equation. The remaining unit of measure on the right side of the equation should match the unknown unit of measure on the left side of the equation.

$$T\,\text{h} = \frac{1000\ \cancel{\text{mL}}}{1} \times \frac{1\ \text{h}}{75\ \cancel{\text{mL}}}$$

4. Solve the equation.

$$T\,\text{h} = \frac{1000\ \text{h}}{75}$$

$$T = 13.33\ \text{h} = \text{total time to infuse } 1000\ \text{mL}$$

Note that 0.33 h does not represent 33 minutes. Because there is 60 min in 1 h, you **must** multiply the fractional hours by 60 to convert to minutes.

$$0.33\ \text{h} \times 60\ \text{min/h} = 20\ \text{min}$$

The total time to infuse the solution is 13 h 20 min.

EXAMPLE 2 ▶   Find the total time to infuse.

Ordered: 750 mL LR to infuse at a rate of 125 mL/h, started at 11 p.m.

SOLUTION ▶

1. Determine the unit of measure for the answer T, and place it with T as the unknown on the left side of the equation.

$$T\,\text{h} =$$

2. The first factor is the number of milliliters to be administered, V over 1. The second factor is the inverted flow in order to solve for hours.

$$T\,\text{h} = \frac{750\ \text{mL}}{1} \times \frac{1\ \text{h}}{125\ \text{mL}}$$

3. Cancel units on the right side of the equation. The remaining unit of measure on the right side of the equation should match the unknown unit of measure on the left side of the equation.

$$T\,\text{h} = \frac{750\ \cancel{\text{mL}}}{1} \times \frac{1\ \text{h}}{125\ \cancel{\text{mL}}}$$

4. Solve the equation.

$$T\,\text{h} = \frac{750\ \text{h}}{125}$$

$$T = 6\ \text{h} = \text{total time to infuse } 750\ \text{mL}$$

Calculating Infusion Completion Time

In some cases, you will need to determine the time an infusion will take to complete. To calculate the time when an infusion will be completed, you must first know the time the infusion started in military time and the total time in hours and minutes to infuse the solution ordered. Since each day is only 24 h long, when the sum is greater than 2400 (midnight), you must start a new day by subtracting 2400. This will determine the time of completion, which will be the next calendar day.

EXAMPLE 1 ▶ Determine when the following infusion will be completed.

Ordered: 1000 mL NS to infuse at a rate of 75 mL/h.
You start the infusion at 7 a.m. on 6/06/09. First determine the start time in military time: 7 a.m. = 0700. Add the total amount of time to infuse, which was determined as 13 h 20 min, or 1320:

$$
\begin{array}{r}
0700 \\
+\ 1320 \\
\hline
2020
\end{array}
$$

The infusion will be completed at 2020, which is 8:20 p.m.

EXAMPLE 2 ▶ Determine when the infusion will be completed.

Ordered: 750 mL LR to infuse at a rate of 125 mL/h, started at 11 p.m. on 8/04/09.
First determine the start time in military time: 11 p.m. = 2300.
Add the total amount of time to infuse, which was determined as 6 h:

$$
\begin{array}{r}
2300 \\
+\ \ 600 \\
\hline
2900 \\
-\ 2400 \\
\hline
500
\end{array}
$$

The infusion will be complete at 0500, or 5:00 a.m., on 8/05/09.

Calculating Infusion Volume

When infusion rate and infusion time are given in the order, the volume infused over a given period of time can be calculated so that the IV can be monitored properly.

To calculate infusion volume, use the formula $V = T \times F$ or dimensional analysis to find the infusion volume V in milliliters, where:

- T (time) must be expressed in hours.
- F (flow rate) must be expressed in milliliters per hour.

Using Conversion Factors

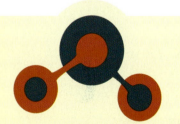

Formula Method

EXAMPLE 1 ▶ Find the total volume infused in 5 h if the infusion rate is 35 mL/h.

SOLUTION ▶
$$T = 5\ \text{h}$$
$$F = 35\ \text{mL/h}$$

Substitute the values into the formula $V = T \times F$.

$$V = 5\ \text{h} \times 35\ \text{mL/h}$$
$$V = 175\ \text{mL} = \text{volume that will be infused over 5 h}$$

EXAMPLE 2 ▶ Find the total volume infused in 12 h if the infusion rate is 200 mL/h.

SOLUTION ▶ Substitute the values into the formula.

$$V = 12 \text{ h} \times 200 \text{ mL/h}$$

$$V = 2400 \text{ mL} = \text{volume that will be infused over 12 h}$$

Using Conversion Factors

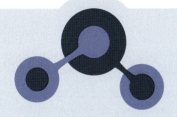

Dimensional Analysis

EXAMPLE 1 ▶ Find the total volume infused in 5 h if the infusion rate is 35 mL/h.

SOLUTION ▶ 1. Determine the unit of measure for the answer T, and place it as the unknown on the left side of the equation.

$$V \text{ mL} =$$

2. The first factor is the length of time of the infusion over 1.

$$\frac{5}{1}$$

3. Multiply by the flow rate of the infusion, the second factor.

$$V \text{ mL} = \frac{5 \text{ h}}{1} \times \frac{35 \text{ mL}}{1 \text{ h}}$$

4. Cancel units on the right side of the equation. The remaining unit of measure on the right side of the equation should match the unknown unit of measure on the left side of the equation.

$$V \text{ mL} = \frac{5 \cancel{h}}{1} \times \frac{35 \text{ mL}}{1 \cancel{h}}$$

5. Solve the equation.

$$V \text{ mL} = 175 \text{ mL to be infused in 5 h}$$

EXAMPLE 2 ▶ Find the total volume infused in 12 h if the infusion rate is 200 mL/h.

SOLUTION ▶ 1. Determine the unit of measure for the answer V, and place it with V as the unknown on the left side of the equation.

$$V \text{ mL} =$$

2. The first factor is the length of time of the infusion over 1.

$$\frac{12 \text{ h}}{1}$$

3. Multiply by the flow rate of the infusion, the second factor.

$$V \text{ mL} = \frac{12 \text{ h}}{1} \times \frac{200 \text{ mL}}{\text{h}}$$

4. Cancel units on the right side of the equation. The remaining unit of measure on the right side of the equation should match the unknown unit of measure on the left side of the equation.

$$V \text{ mL} = \frac{12 \cancel{\text{h}}}{1} \times \frac{200 \text{ mL}}{\cancel{\text{h}}}$$

5. Solve the equation.

$$V \text{ mL} = 2400 \text{ mL to be infused in } 12 \text{ h}$$

Super Tech . . .

Open the CD-ROM that accompanies your textbook and select Chapter 8, Exercise 8-4. Review the animation and example problems, and then complete the practice problems. Continue to the next section of the book once you have mastered the information presented.

Review and Practice 8-3 Infusion Time and Volume

In Exercises 1–5, find the total time to infuse.

1. Ordered: 1000 mL NS at 83 mL/h

2. Ordered: 500 mL LR at 125 mL/h using microdrip tubing

3. Ordered: 750 mL 0.45% NS at 31 mL/h

4. Ordered: 1000 mL NS at 200 mL/h

5. Ordered: 250 mL D5W at 100 mL/h

In Exercises 6–10, find when the infusion will be completed.

6. Ordered: 1500 mL D5W with 30 meq KCl/L at a rate of 75 mL/h. The infusion started at noon.

7. Ordered: 2000 mL NS at 100 mL/h. The infusion started at 3:30 p.m.

8. Ordered: 750 mL RL at 50 mL/h. The IV was started at 1000.

9. Ordered: 250 mL via a microdrip set at 40 mL/h. The infusion started at 9:45 p.m.

10. Ordered: 500 mL at 75 mL/h. The infusion started at 1615.

In Exercises 11–15; find the total volume to administer.

11. 75 mL/h 0.45% NS for 2 h 30 min

12. D5RL set at 100 mL/h for 8 h

13. D5W at 125 mL/h for 12 h

14. An antibiotic solution infused over 2 h at 75 mL/h

Intermittent IV Infusions

IV medications are sometimes delivered on an intermittent basis. Intermittent medications can be delivered through an IV secondary line or a saline or heparin lock. Intermittent IV infusions are usually delivered through an IV secondary line when the patient is receiving continuous IV therapy. Intermittent IV infusions or IV push medications can also be delivered through a saline or heparin lock when the patient does not require continuous or replacement fluids.

Secondary Lines (Piggyback)

Secondary line: Also known as piggyback; line used to add medications or other additives to an existing IV or infusion port.

A secondary line, also known as a piggyback or IVPB, is an IV line used to add medications or other additives to an existing IV or infusion port.

It can be used to infuse medication or other compatible fluids on an intermittent basis, such as q6h. Although shorter than primary tubing, secondary tubing has the same basic components. IVPB bags are usually smaller, often holding 50, 100, or 150 mL of fluid. Some medications require a larger amount fluid as a diluent, such as 250 mL.

Intermittent Peripheral Infusion Devices

Heparin lock: An infusion port attached to an already inserted catheter for IV access; flushed with heparin.

Saline lock: An infusion port attached to an already inserted catheter for IV access; flushed with saline.

Medication can be administered to a patient on a regular schedule, though not continuous, by using an *intermittent peripheral infusion device*. These devices are commonly known as a **heparin lock** or a **saline lock.** A heparin lock is an infusion port attached to an already inserted catheter for IV access, flushed with heparin. A saline lock, is an infusion port attached to an already inserted catheter for IV access, flushed with saline. These locks allow medication to be directly injected into the vein by using a syringe or to be infused intermittently. Physicians' orders will list IV push or bolus for medication that is injected into an IV line or through a saline or heparin lock. Fluids do not flow continuously through the IV needle or catheter when a lock is used. To prevent blockage of the line, the device must be flushed 2 or 3 times a day or after administering medication. When a device is flushed, either saline or heparin fills the infusion port and IV catheter, preventing blood from entering and becoming trapped. If blood were trapped, a clot would form, blocking the catheter.

A saline lock is flushed or irrigated with saline. A heparin lock is flushed or irrigated with heparin, an anticoagulant that retards clot formation. The policy of the facility and the device used will dictate the amount and concentration of solution to use.

Preparing and Calculating Intermittent Infusions

Frequently intermittent medications are already reconstituted and prepared for administration by way of a piggyback or through a heparin or saline lock. The flow rate for prepared medications is calculated in the same manner as regular IV infusions. The amount of fluid may be less and the amount of time to infuse may be less than an hour, so to calculate the flow rate you may need to change the number of minutes into hours.

In some cases, you will be required to reconstitute and prepare a medication for IV infusion or calculate the amount to administer for an IV push medication.

When you prepare medication for an intermittent IV infusion:

- Reconstitute the medication, using the information on the label and package insert.
- Calculate the amount to administer and the flow rate.

Using Conversion Factors

Fraction Proportion Method

EXAMPLE ▶   Ordered: Eloxatin® 75 mg in 250 mL D5W IV piggyback over 90 min
On hand: Eloxatin® 100 mg

Eloxatin® should be reconstituted with 20 mL of water for injection or 5 percent dextrose for injection. The dosage strength of the medication will be 100 mg/20 mL.

SOLUTION ▶   Since the dosage ordered is 75 mg, you will calculate the amount to administer using the following information:

D (desired dose) = 75 mg
H (dose on hand) = 100 mg
Q (dosage unit) = 20 mL

Follow Procedure Checklist 6-4 in Chapter 6.

1. Fill in the proportion.

$$\frac{Q}{H} = \frac{A}{D}$$

$$\frac{20\ mL}{100\ mg} = \frac{A}{75\ mg}$$

2. Cancel units.

$$\frac{20\ mL}{100\ \cancel{mg}} = \frac{A}{75\ \cancel{mg}}$$

3. Cross-multiply and solve for the unknown.

$$100 \times A = 20\ mL \times 75$$

$$A = 20\ mL \times \frac{75}{100}$$

$$A = 15\ mL$$

Using Conversion Factors

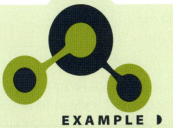

Ratio Proportion Method

EXAMPLE ▶ Ordered: Eloxatin® 75 mg in 250 mL D5W IV piggyback over 90 min
On hand: Eloxatin® 100 mg

Eloxatin® should be reconstituted with 20 mL of water for injection or 5 percent dextrose for injection. The dosage strength of the medication will be 100 mg/20 mL.

SOLUTION ▶ Since the dosage ordered is 75 mg, you will calculate the amount to administer using the following information:

D (desired dose) = 75 mg
H (dose on hand) = 100 mg
Q (dosage unit) = 20 mL

Follow Procedure Checklist 6-5 in Chapter 6.

1. Fill in the proportion.

$$Q : H : : A : D$$
$$20\ \text{mL} : 100\ \text{mg} : : A : 75\ \text{mg}$$

2. Cancel units.

$$20\ \text{mL} : 100\ \cancel{\text{mg}} : : A : 75\ \cancel{\text{mg}}$$

3. Multiply the means and extremes, then solve for the missing value.

$$100 \times A = 20\ \text{mL} \times 75$$
$$A = 20\ \text{mL} \times \frac{75}{100}$$
$$A = 15\ \text{mL}$$

Using Conversion Factors

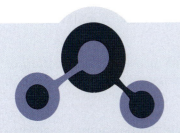

Dimensional Analysis

EXAMPLE ▶ Ordered: Eloxatin® 75 mg in 250 mL D5W IV piggyback over 90 min
On hand: Eloxatin® 100 mg

Eloxatin® should be reconstituted with 20 mL of water for injection or 5 percent dextrose for injection. The dosage strength of the medication will be 100 mg/20 mL.

SOLUTION ▶ Since the dosage ordered is 75 mg, you will calculate the amount to administer using the following information:

$$D \text{ (desired dose)} = 75 \text{ mg}$$

$$H \text{ (dose on hand)} = 100 \text{ mg}$$

$$Q \text{ (dosage unit)} = 20 \text{ mL}$$

Follow Procedure Checklist 6-6 in Chapter 6.

1. The unit of measure for the amount to administer will be milliliters.
2. Since the unit of measurement for the dosage ordered is the same as that for the dose on hand, this step in Procedure Checklist 6-6 is unnecessary.
3. The dosage unit is 20 mL. The dose on hand is 100 mg. This is the first factor.

$$\frac{20 \text{ mL}}{100 \text{ mg}}$$

4. The dosage ordered is 75 mg.

$$A \text{ mL} = \frac{20 \text{ mL}}{100 \text{ mg}} \times \frac{75 \text{ mg}}{1}$$

5. Cancel units.

$$A \text{ mL} = \frac{20 \text{ mL}}{100 \text{ \cancel{mg}}} \times \frac{75 \text{ \cancel{mg}}}{1}$$

6. Solve the equation.

$$A \text{ mL} = \frac{20 \text{ mL}}{100} \times \frac{75}{1}$$

$$A = 15 \text{ mL}$$

Using Conversion Factors

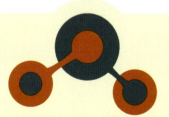

Formula Method

EXAMPLE ▶ Ordered: Eloxatin® 75 mg in 250 mL D5W IV piggyback over 90 min
On hand: Eloxatin® 100 mg

  Eloxatin® should be reconstituted with 20 mL of water for injection or 5 percent dextrose for injection. The dosage strength of the medication will be 100 mg/20 mL.

SOLUTION ▶ Since the dosage ordered is 75 mg, you will calculate the amount to administer using the following information:

$$D \text{ (desired dose)} = 75 \text{ mg}$$

$$H \text{ (dose on hand)} = 100 \text{ mg}$$

$$Q \text{ (dosage unit)} = 20 \text{ mL}$$

Follow Procedure Checklist 6-7 in Chapter 6.

1. The drug is ordered in milligrams, which is the same unit of measure as that for the dose on hand. No conversion is necessary.

2. Fill in the formula.

$$\frac{D \times Q}{H} = A$$

$$\frac{75 \text{ mg} \times 20 \text{ mL}}{100 \text{ mg}} = A$$

3. Cancel units.

$$\frac{75 \cancel{\text{ mg}} \times 20 \text{ mL}}{100 \cancel{\text{ mg}}} = A$$

4. Solve for the unknown.

$$\frac{75 \times 20 \text{ mL}}{100} = A$$

$$15 \text{ mL} = A$$

Super Tech . . .

Open the CD-ROM that accompanies your textbook and select Chapter 8, Exercise 8-5. Review the animation and example problems, and then complete the practice problems. Continue to the next section of the book once you have mastered the information presented.

✓ Review and Practice 8-4 Intermittent IV Infusions

In Exercises 1–4, calculate the flow rate in milliliters per hour and drops per minute.

Ordered: Gemzar® 150 mg in 500 mL NS over 2 h
On hand: 15 gtt per mL IV tubing

1. Flow rate in milliliters per hour: _____

2. Flow rate in drops per minute: _____

Ordered: Fortaz® 1.5 g IVPB over 30 min
On hand: 10 gtt per mL IV tubing and Fortaz® 2% solution

3. Flow rate in milliliters per hour: _____

4. Flow rate in drops per minute: _____

✅ Chapter 8 Review

Test Your Knowledge

Match the following. Write the answer in the space provided.

_____ 1. Maintenance fluids

a. Type of fluid given to a patient with a severe burn

_____ 2. KVO fluids

b. Type of fluid given to a patient who is dehydrated

_____ 3. Hypertonic

c. Helps patient maintain normal electrolyte and fluid balance

_____ 4. Isotonic

d. Provides access to the vascular system for emergency situation

_____ 5. Replacement fluids

e. Replaces electrolytes and fluid lost due to hemorrhage, vomiting, or diarrhea

_____ 6. Therapeutic fluids

f. Type of fluid given to a patient having an IV infusion during a diagnostic test

_____ 7. Hypotonic

g. Delivers medication to the patient

Practice Your Knowledge

In Exercises 8–13, calculate the flow rate for orders in mL per hour.

8. 3000 mL D5W IV q24h

9. 500 mL LR IV q8h

10. 1200 mL $\frac{1}{2}$ NS IV q12h

11. 250 mL NS IV q4h

12. 1 g Claforan® in 100 mL D5W IV over 90 min

13. 500 mg ampicillin in 50 mL D5W IV over 30 min

In Exercises 14–22, find the flow rate for the orders, rounded to the nearest drop.

14. 2200 mL IV RL q24h (15 gtt/mL tubing)

15. 300 mL IV NS q8h (10 gtt/mL tubing)

16. 1000 mL IV D5W q6h (15 gtt/mL tubing)

17. 1800 mL IV D5/$\frac{1}{2}$ NS q12h (20 gtt/mL tubing)

18. 1500 mL IV $\frac{1}{3}$ NS q8h (10 gtt/mL tubing)

19. 300 mL D5/Ringer's IV q6h (microdrip tubing)

20. Ordered: 1000 mL RL over 8 h (15 gtt/mL tubing)

21. Ordered: 2500 mL NS over 24 h (10 gtt/mL tubing)

22. Ordered 500 mL $\frac{1}{2}$ NS over 8 hours (60 gtt/mL tubing)

In Exercises 23–26, find the total time to infuse.

23. Ordered: 1000 mL D5/0.45% NS at 125 mL/h

24. Ordered: 800 mL $\frac{1}{4}$ NS at 50 mL/h

25. Ordered: 600 mL LR IV at 25 mL/h

26. Ordered: 1200 mL D5/NS IV at 70 mL/h

In Exercises 27–30, find when the infusion will be completed.

27. 800 mL via at 90 mL/h, starting at 0820

28. 1000 mL at 125 mL/h, starting at 1 p.m.

29. 500 mL at 175 mL/h, starting at 2230

30. 750 mL at 35 mL/h, starting at 4 p.m.

In Exercises 31–34, find the total volume to administer.

31. $\frac{1}{4}$ NS at 125 mL/h over 5 h 30

32. RL at 25 mL/h over 12 h

33. NS at 125 mL/h over 7 h 30 min

34. D5W at 80 mL/h over 8 h 20 min

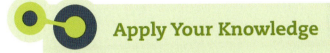

Apply Your Knowledge

How Long Will That IV Last?

You are the pharmacy technician working in a hospital pharmacy. You are working in the pharmacy when the following order comes in: "D5W 3000 mL at 120 mL per hour." The IV solution comes in 1000 mL bags.

Answer the following questions:

1. How many hours will a 1000-mL bag take to infuse?

   _____

2. How many bags will be needed to fill the order?

   _____

3. How many hours will it take to infuse 3000 mL?

   _____

Internet Activity

You are applying for a new job that will require you to work with IV fluids exclusively. To prepare for the position, you want to learn more about the types of fluids and when and how they are used. Additionally you would like to become familiar with IV equipment made by various companies. Research the Internet and learn more about fluids and IV equipment. You may want to make yourself a chart or table with pictures to use as a reference tool.

Super Tech . . .

Open the CD-ROM that accompanies your textbook and complete a final review of Chapter 8. For a final evaluation, take the chapter test and email or print your results for your instructor. A score of 95 percent or above indicates mastery of the chapter concepts.

9

Special Preparations and Calculations

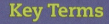

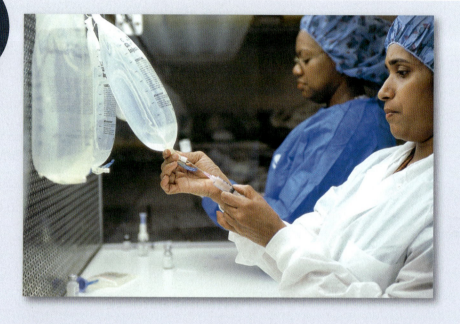

Key Terms

Alligation

Compound

Dilution

Final volume/final strength

Insulin

QSAD

Solute

Solvent

U-100

Learning Outcomes

When you have successfully completed Chapter 9, you will have mastered skills to be able to:

▶ Determine the percentages of solutions, dilutions, and solids.

▶ Prepare solutions from a concentrate.

▶ Prepare a compound.

▶ Calculate and measure insulin doses accurately.

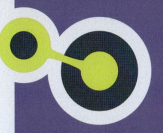

Introduction

As a pharmacy technician you will be required to have additional knowledge related to dosage calculations. This chapter will introduce you to specialized calculations required of pharmacy employees. Information relating to the use of insulin, preparation of solutions, and the alligation method of calculations will be learned in this chapter. These calculations, like all other calculations, require attention to detail and 100 percent accuracy; completing them successfully will help you step into your new career as a pharmacy technician.

Critical Thinking in the Pharmacy
What Is the "Recipe"?

You are the pharmacy technician working in a hospital pharmacy. You are working in the pharmacy when the following order comes in: "10 percent ethanol 100 mL." You have 90 percent ethanol on hand. You will have to make the 10 percent ethanol solution using 90 percent ethanol and water.

When you have completed Chapter 9, you will be able to perform this calculation and determine the "recipe" needed to complete the order.

PTCB Correlations

When you have completed this chapter you will have the building block of knowledge needed to work with compounds.

- Knowledge of pharmacy calculations (Statement I-50).
- Knowledge of procedures to compound sterile non-injectable products (Statement I-62).
- Knowledge of procedures to compound non-sterile products (Statement I-63).

Compounds

Compound: Two or more chemicals mixed together to make a specific mixture or solution.

When two or more chemicals are mixed together to make a specific mixture or solution, it is known as a **compound** in the pharmacy industry. It is occasionally necessary to prepare a solution "from scratch," dilute a solution that is more concentrated than what is needed, or mix two solids together. To do this, you will need to know how concentrations of solutions are expressed.

We will work with percent solutions and solids, and then work with **alligations,** which is one method for calculating dilutions.

Alligation: One method for calculating dilutions.

Preparation of Solutions, Dilutions, and Solids

Solvent: Diluent liquid used to dissolve other chemicals, making a solution.

Solutes: Chemicals dissolved in a solvent, making a solution; a drug or substance being dissolved in a solution.

Solutions are liquid mixtures containing two or more different chemicals. The liquid that is used to dissolve the other chemicals is called the **solvent,** while the chemicals dissolved in the solvent are called **solutes.** The most commonly used solvent is water, which is sometimes referred to as the *universal solvent*. An example of a solution is normal saline, which contains 0.9 grams of sodium chloride (table salt) in every 100 mL of solution. In this example, sodium chloride is the solute, and water is used as the solvent.

Drug manufacturers prepare most of the solutions used in health care. Some common examples are injection medications, eye drops, and cough syrups. When the solute is a solid, the percent concentration tells you how many grams of the solute are contained in every 100 mL of the solution. For example, a 2 percent lidocaine solution contains 2 g of lidocaine in every 100 mL of solution. In other words, 100 mL of 2% lidocaine solution is 2 g of lidocaine mixed with enough solvent to make a total of 100 mL.

When the solute is a liquid, the percent concentration tells you how many milliliters of solute are contained in every 100 mL of the solution. A 70 percent isopropyl alcohol solution has 70 mL of isopropyl alcohol in every 100 mL of solution. In this case, 100 mL of 70% isopropyl solution is 70 mL of isopropyl alcohol mixed with enough solvent (30 mL) to make a total of 100 mL (70 + 30 = 100). When the solute is a solid and the solvent is a solid, the percent concentration tells you how many grams of the solute are contained in 100 g of the product. For example, 2 percent hydrocortisone ointment means that every 100 g of ointment will contain 2 g of hydrocortisone. If the preparation were being compounded in the pharmacy, 2 g of hydrocortisone would be incorporated (mixed) in 98 g of petroleum jelly (2 + 98 = 100).

Final Volume/Final Strength

Final volume/final strength: The amount and strength of a prepared mixture from dilutions or concentrations.

Final volume/final strength is the amount and strength of a prepared mixture from dilutions or concentrations. As a pharmacy technician you may have to find the final volume, initial volume, initial strength, or final strength of a mixture. To find the missing value you can use either the ratio proportion method or the fractional proportion method.

Set up the equation for ratio proportion method as:

initial strength : initial volume :: final strength : final volume

Set up the equation for the fraction proportion method as:

$$\frac{\text{initial strength}}{\text{initial volume}} = \frac{\text{final strength}}{\text{final volume}}$$

As you work through this chapter, both methods are used to solve for final volume/final strength.

Preparing Percent Solutions and Solids

To prepare a liquid solution, you would first measure the solute and then add a *sufficient quantity of solvent to bring the total to the desired volume.*

EXAMPLE 1 ▶ A "recipe" for preparing 100 mL (final volume) of 2 percent lidocaine solution (final strength) would look like this:

2% lidocaine solution	
Lidocaine	2 g
Water	QSAD 100 mL

QSAD: Abbreviation of a Latin phrase meaning "a sufficient quantity to adjust the dimensions to"; used in preparing solutions.

The abbreviation **QSAD** is taken from a Latin phrase meaning "a sufficient quantity to adjust the dimensions to." In this case, you are adding enough water to make the final volume 100 mL. When you are preparing a liquid solution, the diluent should be added to the desired volume.

In this example you were asked how to prepare 100 mL of the solution, and no calculations were needed.

For a percent solution prepared from a solid solute, the percent strength is equal to the number of grams of solute contained in 100 mL of the solution.

EXAMPLE 2 ▶ Write a recipe for preparing 100 g of 10 percent zinc oxide from zinc oxide powder and petroleum jelly.

10% zinc oxide	
Zinc oxide	10 g
Petroleum jelly	90 g

In this example a solid (zinc oxide) is being added to another solid (an ointment base). Once you determine the number of grams for the solute, you must subtract from the total number of grams to create the recipe to compound this ointment. You do not use the expression *QSAD* when preparing solid mixtures.

EXAMPLE 3 ▶ Write out a recipe for preparing 250 mL of 0.9 percent sodium chloride.

Up to this point, you have been asked to make 100 mL of solution. Here you are asked to make a larger volume, which means that you will need more than 0.9 g of NaCl. You can calculate the quantity needed by using the methods introduced earlier in this text—the fraction proportion method, the ratio proportion method, or dimensional analysis.

Using Conversion Factors

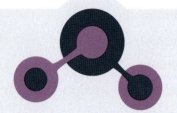

Fraction Proportion Method

1. Write a conversion factor with the units needed in the answer in the numerator and the units you are converting from in the denominator.
2. Write a fraction with the unknown ? as the numerator and the number that you need to convert as the denominator.
3. Set up the two fractions as a proportion.
4. Cancel units.
5. Cross-multiply, then solve for the unknown value.

EXAMPLE 3 ▶

1. The percent concentration tells us that 100 mL (initial volume) solution contains 0.9 g NaCl (initial strength). We need to calculate how many grams of NaCl are needed to prepare 250 mL of solution (final volume). Since we are calculating grams, our conversion factor will be written

$$\frac{0.9 \text{ g NaCl}}{100 \text{ mL solution}}$$

We need to solve for the final strength.

2. The other fraction for our proportion has the unknown ? (final strength) as the numerator and 250 mL solution (final volume) as the denominator:

$$\frac{?}{250 \text{ mL solution}}$$

3. Setting up the two fractions as a proportion gives us the following equation:

$$\frac{0.9 \text{ g NaCl}}{100 \text{ mL solution}} = \frac{?}{250 \text{ mL solution}}$$

4. Cancel units.

$$\frac{0.9 \text{ g NaCl}}{100 \text{ mL solution}} = \frac{?}{250 \text{ mL solution}}$$

5. Cross-multiply to solve for the unknown.

$$100 \times ? = 0.9 \text{ g NaCl} \times 250$$

$$\frac{100 \times ?}{100} = \frac{0.9 \text{ g NaCl} \times 250}{100}$$

$$? \text{ (final strength)} = 2.25 \text{ g NaCl}$$

Using Conversion Factors

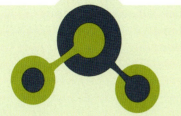

Ratio Proportion Method

1. Write the conversion factor as a ratio $A:B$ so that A has the units needed in the answer.
2. Write a second ratio $C:D$ so that C is the missing value and D is the number that is being converted.
3. Write the proportion in the form $A:B::C:D$.
4. Cancel units.
5. Solve the proportion by multiplying the means and extremes.

EXAMPLE 3

1. Since we are converting to grams, our conversion ratio will have grams as the first part. In a 0.9 percent NaCl solution, 100 mL of solution contains 0.9 g NaCl. Our first ratio is 0.9 g NaCl (initial strength) : 100 mL (initial volume)

2. The second ratio is ? (final strength) : 250 mL (final volume).

$$?:250 \text{ mL}$$

3. Our proportion is

$$0.9 \text{ g NaCl} : 100 \text{ mL} :: ? : 250 \text{ mL}$$

4. Cancel units.

$$0.9 \text{ g NaCl} : 100 \text{ m\cancel{L}} :: ? : 250 \text{ m\cancel{L}}$$

5. Solve for the missing value.

$$100 \times ? = 0.9 \text{ g NaCl} \times 250$$

$$\frac{100 \times ?}{100} = \frac{0.9 \text{ g NaCl} \times 250}{100}$$

$$? \text{ (final strength)} = 2.25 \text{ g NaCl}$$

Using Conversion Factors

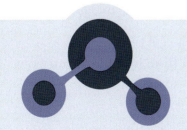

Dimensional Analysis

1. Write the unknown as ? alone on one side of an equation.
2. On the other side of the equation, write a conversion factor with the units of measure for the answer in the numerator and the units you are converting from in the denominator.
3. Multiply the conversion factor by the number that is being converted over 1.
4. Cancel units.
5. Solve the equation.

EXAMPLE 3 ▶

1. ? grams =

2. The percent concentration tells us that in 100 mL of solution there is 0.9 g of NaCl. We need to calculate how many grams of NaCl are needed to prepare 250 mL of solution. Since we are calculating grams, our conversion factor will be written

$$\frac{0.9 \text{ g NaCl}}{100 \text{ mL solution}}$$

$$? = \frac{0.9 \text{ g NaCl}}{100 \text{ mL solution}}$$

3. $? = \dfrac{0.9 \text{ g NaCl}}{100 \text{ mL solution}} \times \dfrac{250 \text{ mL solution}}{1}$

4. $? = \dfrac{0.9 \text{ g NaCl}}{100 \text{ mL solution}} \times \dfrac{250 \text{ mL solution}}{1}$

5. $? = 2.25 \text{ g NaCl}$

Regardless of the method used, we find that 2.25 g of NaCl is needed to prepare 250 mL of a 0.9 percent solution.

Our "recipe" looks like this:

0.9% sodium chloride	
NaCl	2.25 g
Water	QSAD 250 mL

Super Tech . . .

Open the CD-ROM that accompanies your textbook and select Chapter 9, Exercise 9-1. Review the animation and example problems, and then complete the practice problems. Continue to the next section of the book once you have mastered the information presented.

✓ Review and Practice 9-1 Compounds

1. Write a recipe for preparing 500 mL of 0.9 percent sodium chloride.

2. Write a recipe for preparing 50 mL of a 2 percent lidocaine solution.

3. Write a recipe for preparing 100 g of a 3 percent hydrocortisone ointment from hydrocortisone powder and petroleum jelly.

Alligations

One of the most common ways of expressing the concentration of a solution is as a percent. Remember that *percent* means *per hundred*. Alligations are a method of calculation used to determine the amounts of two solutions with different percents of concentration needed to get a desired percent of a concentrated solution. When a concentration is expressed as a percent, it tells you how much of the solute is found in every 100 mL of the solution. In alligations, when you are working with two concentrated solutions, one will have a higher concentration and one will have a lesser concentration.

To perform a calculation using the alligation method you will use a tic-tac-toe grid to set up your equation and you will write the concentration of the higher concentrated solution in the upper left corner, write the concentration of the lesser concentrated solution in lower left corner, and write the concentration needed in the center of the tic-tac-toe grid, and then take the differences diagonally. This means you subtract the concentration needed from the higher concentration solution to determine parts of the higher concentration and then subtract the lesser concentration solution from the concentration needed to determine the parts of the lesser concentration needed.

EXAMPLE ▶

1. Write out a tic-tac-toe grid, and fill in the following values.

The concentration of the **higher** concentrated solution		Parts of the **higher** concentrated solution needed[†]
	The **desired** concentration needed	
The concentration of the **less** concentrated solution*		Parts of the **less** concentrated solution needed[‡]

* When you are diluting with water, the less concentrated solution has a concentration of **_ZERO._**

[†] The difference between the concentration needed and the concentration of the LESSER concentrated solution. (The **diagonal** difference)

[‡] The difference between the concentration needed and the concentration of the HIGHER concentrated solution. (The **diagonal** difference)

2. Find the total number of parts in the solution by adding the two values in the right column, which are your parts-needed values.
3. Find the volume of one part by dividing the total number of parts into the volume of solution needed.
4. Multiply the volume of one part (answer from step 3) by the number in the top right of the grid (parts of higher concentration solution needed). The result is the amount of the higher concentrated solution needed.
5. Add a sufficient quantity of the lesser concentrated solution to bring the final volume up to the desired volume by subtracting the amount of the higher concentration needed (answer from step 4) from the total volume needed.

In the next section we will apply the alligation method of calculation to the process of preparing a dilution from a concentrate.

Super Tech . . .

Open the CD-ROM that accompanies your textbook and select Chapter 9, Exercise 9-2. Review the animation and example problems, and then complete the practice problems. Continue to the next section of the book once you have mastered the information presented.

✓ Review and Practice 9-2 Alligations

1. How much D5W must be mixed with D20W to make 1 L of a D12W solution?

2. How many milliliters of 95 percent ethyl alcohol should be mixed with water to make 1.5 L of 30 percent ethyl alcohol solution?

3. How would you prepare 100 mL of 20 percent iodine from 25 and 10 percent iodine solutions?

Preparing a Dilution from a Concentrate

As a pharmacy technician you may need to prepare a solution by mixing a solution that is more concentrated than needed with one that is less concentrated than needed. (The less concentrated solution often is pure water, which would have a concentration of zero.) For example, you may need a 50 percent ethanol solution but find that you have only a 90 percent solution. In this case, you need to prepare a **dilution,** which is a solution created from an already prepared concentrated solution.

Dilution: A solution created from an already prepared concentrated solution.

Two methods will be presented for calculating how to prepare dilutions: alligation and formula.

Preparing Dilutions from a Concentrate

To prepare a dilution from a concentrate, determine:

- The volume needed
- The concentration needed
- The concentration(s) available

(If water is being used, one of the concentrations is zero.) Then use the alligation method or the formula method to obtain your answer.

EXAMPLE ▶

How would you prepare 500 mL of 50 percent ethanol from 90 percent ethanol? (You will use water as a diluent.)

Before you do the calculation, break down the problem to find the information that is needed.

- The volume needed is 500 mL.
- The concentration needed is 50 percent.
- The concentrations available are 90 and 0 percent.

SOLUTION ▶

The Alligation Method

1. Write the concentration of the higher concentrated solution in the upper left, the concentration of the less concentrated solution in lower left, and the concentration needed in the center of a tic-tac-toe grid, and then take the differences diagonally.

   a. 90 (higher concentration) − 50 (concentration needed) = 40, place 40 in the lower right corner as the parts of the lesser concentration needed.

b. 50 (concentration needed) − 0 (lesser concentration) = 50, place 50 in the upper right corner as the parts of the higher concentration needed.

Alligation grid

90		50
	50	
0		40

2. Add the numbers in the right column to find the total number of parts.

$$50 + 40 = 90 \text{ parts total}$$

3. Determine the volume of 1 part by dividing the volume needed by the total number of parts.

$$\frac{500 \text{ mL}}{90 \text{ parts}} = 5.56 \text{ mL/part}$$

4. Determine how much of the **higher** concentrated solution is needed.

$$5.56 \text{ mL/part} \times 50 \text{ parts of concentration needed} = 278 \text{ mL}$$

So 278 mL of the 90 percent solution is needed to prepare 500 mL of a 50 percent solution.

5. Since the desired volume is 500 mL, you would dilute the 90 percent solution by adding water up to a final volume of 500 mL.

$$500 \text{ mL (final volume)} - 278 \text{ mL (higher concentration solution needed)} = 222 \text{ mL water needed}$$

SOLUTION ▶ **The Formula Method**

1. Identify the following information in the problem.

   a. The volume of solution needed (this is V_n, for volume needed)
   b. The concentration of the solution needed (this is C_n, for concentration needed)
   c. The concentration of the solution that is available (this C_a, for concentration available)

2. Plug the value into the following formula, in which V_a is the volume of the available solution needed to prepare the dilution.

$$V_a = \frac{V_n \times C_n}{C_a}$$

3. Cancel units.
4. Solve the equation for V_a.

Note: The formula method for dilutions can be used only when one of the solutions being mixed has a concentration of zero.

EXAMPLE ▶ How would you prepare 500 mL of 50 percent ethanol from 90 percent ethanol? (You will use water as a diluent.)

Before you do any calculations, you must break down the problem to find the information that is needed and that which is available.

- The volume needed is 500 mL.
- The concentrations available are 90 percent and 0 percent.

SOLUTION ▶ 1. Identify the information in the problem.

  a. The volume of solution needed: $V_n = 500$ mL
  b. The concentration of the solution needed: $C_n = 50\%$
  c. The concentration of the solution that is available: $C_a = 90$

2. Plug the values into the formula.

$$V_a = \frac{500 \text{ mL} \times 50\%}{90\%}$$

3. Cancel units.

$$V_a = \frac{500 \text{ mL} \times 50\%}{90\%}$$

4. Solve the equation.

$$V_a = 278 \text{ mL}$$

Regardless of the method used, we find that 278 mL of the 90 percent ethanol solution is needed to prepare 500 mL of a 50 percent solution. Our "recipe" looks like this:

50% ethanol	
90% ethanol	278 mL
Water	QSAD 500 mL

When preparing a dilution from a concentrate and both solutions being mixed have a concentration of greater than zero, the alligation method must be used.

EXAMPLE ▶ How would you prepare 100 mL of 5 percent iodine from 10 percent and 2 percent iodine solutions?

In this case, because neither of the solutions has a concentration of zero, we must use the alligation method.

SOLUTION ▶ 1. Write the concentration of the more concentrated solution in the upper left, the concentration of the less concentrated solution in the lower left, and the concentration needed in the center of a tic-tac-toe grid, and then take the differences diagonally.

10		3
	5	
2		5

2. Add the numbers in the right column to find the total number of parts.

$$3 + 5 = 8 \text{ parts total}$$

3. Determine the volume of 1 part by dividing the volume needed by the total number of parts.

$$\frac{100 \text{ mL}}{8 \text{ parts}} = 12.5 \text{ mL/part}$$

4. Determine how much of the more concentrated solution is needed.

$$12.5 \text{ mL/part} \times 3 \text{ parts of } 10\% \text{ solution} = 37.5$$

So 37.5 mL of the 10 percent solution is needed to prepare 100 mL of a 10 percent solution.

5. Since the desired volume is 100 mL, you would dilute the 10 percent solution by adding 2 percent iodine up to a final volume of 100 mL.

Our "recipe" looks like this:

5% iodine	
10% iodine	37.5 mL
2% iodine	QSAD 100 mL

Super Tech . . .

Open the CD-ROM that accompanies your textbook and select Chapter 9, Exercise 9-3. Review the animation and example problems, and then complete the practice problems. Continue to the next section of the book once you have mastered the information presented.

✓ Review and Practice 9-3 Preparing a Dilution from a Concentrate

In Exercises 1 and 2, write a recipe for creating a percent solution or solid.

1. 50 g of 1 percent hydrocortisone cream using a 2.5 percent hydrocortisone cream and a cream base?

2. 250 mL of 40 percent dextrose from 80 percent dextrose solution?

In Exercises 3 and 4, write a recipe for preparing a dilution from a concentrate.

3. How many milliliters of 95 percent ethyl alcohol should be mixed with water to make 1.5 L of 30 percent ethyl alcohol solution?

4. How would you prepare 100 mL of 20 percent iodine from 25 percent and 10 percent iodine solutions?

Insulin

Insulin: A pancreatic hormone that stimulates glucose metabolism.

Insulin is a pancreatic hormone that stimulates glucose metabolism. People who have low or no insulin production may have insulin-dependent diabetes. They often need regular injections of insulin to keep their glucose (blood sugar) from rising to levels that could be life-threatening. These regular injections must be rotated to various sites of the body to prevent scarring of the tissue at a single injection site. Insulin is commonly supplied in a 10-mL vial.

Insulin Syringes

U-100: Common concentration of insulin, meaning that 100 units of insulin is contained in 1mL of solution.

Insulin is commonly administered with special U-100 insulin syringes marked in units. **U-100** indicates the common concentration of insulin, meaning that 100 units of insulin are contained in 1 mL of solution. A standard U-100 insulin syringe holds up to 100 units, or 1 mL, of solution. Most of these syringes are calibrated for every 2 units, though some are marked for each unit. Insulin administration is different from the administration of most other injectable medications because the syringe measures the amount of insulin rather than a volume of solution.

Smaller insulin syringes, holding up to 50 units of 100 units/mL of insulin (0.5 mL of solution) or 30 units of 100 units/mL of insulin (0.3 mL), are usually calibrated for each unit. Their larger numbers make them easier to use for visually impaired patients.

For more accurate measurements, use a 50 unit insulin syringe for insulin doses of less than 50 units of 100 units/mL of insulin, and a 30 unit insulin syringe for insulin doses less than 30 units of 100 units/mL of insulin if these syringes are available. As a pharmacy technician you may have to calculate how much insulin is to be dispensed to fill a prescription. Now we will determine the proper dose, syringe to be used, and how much to dispense.

To determine the amount to be dispensed, you will use the fact that there are 100 units of insulin in 1 mL. Therefore a 10-mL vial of insulin contains 1000 units of insulin.

EXAMPLE 1 ▶ Ordered: Novolin® N 66 units sub-Q with breakfast, QSAD for 30 days.

Because this order is for more than 50 units, use a U-100 insulin syringe. Find the mark for 66 units and fill the syringe to that calibration (see Figure 9-1).

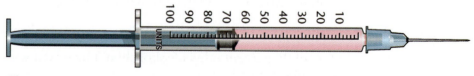

Figure 9-1 U-100 (1 mL) Syringe

Determine the amount to be dispensed:

1. 66 units × 30 (days) = 1980 units
2. 1980 units ÷ 1000 units per vial = 1.98

You will dispense two 10-mL vials.

EXAMPLE 2 ▶   Ordered: Humulin® R 55 units sub-Q daily as directed, QSAD 90 days.

Because this order is for more than 50 units, you will need a 100-unit (U-100) syringe. Your best choice would be a syringe calibrated for each unit (see Figure 9-2). If you use a syringe calibrated for every 2 units, then fill it to the imaginary line between 54 and 56 units.

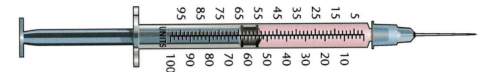
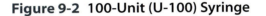

Figure 9-2 100-Unit (U-100) Syringe

Determine the amount to be dispensed:

1. 55 units × 90 (days) = 4950 units
2. 4950 units ÷ 1000 units per vial = 4.95

You will dispense five 10-mL vials.

EXAMPLE 3 ▶   Ordered: Humulin® R 35 units sub-Q before lunch, QSAD 30 days.

Because this order is for less than 50 units, you may use a smaller syringe in which each unit is calibrated (Figure 9-3).

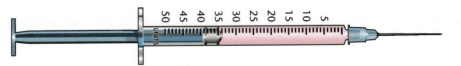

Figure 9-3 50-Unit (0.5 mL) Syringe

Determine the amount to be dispensed:

1. 35 units × 28 (days) = 980 units
2. 980 units ÷ 1000 units per vial = 0.98

You will dispense one 10-mL vial.

EXAMPLE 4 ▶ Ordered: Novolin® R 8 units, sub-Q with breakfast, QSAD 90 days.

Because this order is for less than 30 units, you may use either a 30 unit or 50 unit insulin syringe in which each unit is calibrated (Figure 9-4).

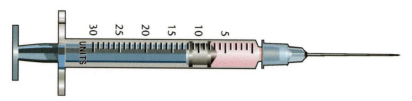

Figure 9-4 **30-Unit (0.3 mL) Syringe**

Determine the amount to be dispensed:

1. 8 units × 90 (days) = 720 units
2. 720 ÷ 1000 units per vial = 0.72

You will dispense one 10-mL vial.

U-500 insulin is used for patients with highly elevated blood sugars. Insulin may also be given intravenously for elevated blood sugars. On the occasion that U-500 is ordered or an insulin dose is over 100 units, a tuberculin or standard syringe may be necessary.

U-500 insulin and U-100 insulin over 100 units will not fit in a U-100 syringe and must be measured in milliliters.

If the order is for U-500 insulin (which contains 500 units in each milliliter), use a tuberculin syringe. Calculate the amount to administer in milliliters.

EXAMPLE 1 ▶ Ordered: Humulin® R U-500 insulin 80 units.

$$80 \text{ units} \times \frac{1 \text{ mL}}{500 \text{ units}} = A \quad \text{(Amount to be administered)}$$

$$\overset{4}{\cancel{80 \text{ units}}} \times \frac{1 \text{ mL}}{\underset{25}{\cancel{500 \text{ units}}}} = 4 \times \frac{1}{25} \text{ mL} = \frac{4}{25} \text{ mL} = 0.16 \text{ mL}$$

Amount to be administered is 0.16 mL drawn up in a tuberculin syringe. (See Figure 9-5.)

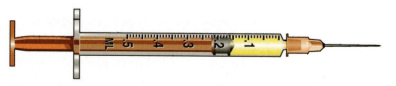

Figure 9-5 **0.5 mL Tuberculin Syringe**

EXAMPLE 2 ▶   Ordered: 150 units Humulin® R IV STAT.

On hand: Humulin® R U-100.

$$150 \text{ units} \times \frac{1 \text{ mL}}{100 \text{ units}} = A$$

$$150 \text{ units} \times \frac{1 \text{ mL}}{100 \text{ units}} = A = 15 \times \frac{1 \text{ mL}}{10} = \frac{15 \text{ mL}}{10} = 1.5 \text{ mL}$$

Administer 1.5 mL in a standard syringe. (See Figure 9-6.)

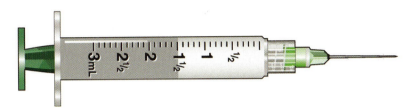

Figure 9-6 3-mL Standard Syringe

Super Tech . . .

Open the CD-ROM that accompanies your textbook and select Chapter 9, Exercise 9-4. Review the animation and example problems, and then complete the practice problems. Continue to the next section of the book once you have mastered the information presented.

Review and Practice 9-4 Insulin

In Exercises 1–10, determine how many 10-mL vials to dispense.

1. Ordered: Novolin® R 15 units sub-Q ac breakfast, QSAD for 60 days.

2. Ordered: Humalog® 5 units sub-Q 15 min before lunch, QSAD for 90 days.

3. Ordered: Novolin® N 33 units sub-Q daily, QSAD for 60 days.

4. Ordered: Humulin® N 66 units sub-Q daily, QSAD for 90 days.

5. Ordered: Humulin® 50/50 42 units sub-Q ac breakfast, QSAD for 30 days.

6. Ordered: Humalog® 75/25 BR 17 units ac breakfast, QSAD for 90 days.

7. Ordered: Novolin® 70/30 53 units sub-Q ac dinner, QSAD for 90 days.

8. Ordered: Novolin® 70/30 R 32 units sub-Q ac breakfast, QSAD for 90 days.

9. Ordered: Novolin® R insulin 48 units sub-Q ac breakfast and dinner, QSAD for 60 days.

10. Ordered: Humalog® 15 units sub-Q ac breakfast, QSAD for 60 days.

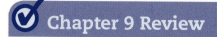

Chapter 9 Review

Test Your Knowledge

Multiple Choice

Select the best answer and write the letter on the line.

_____ 1. What is a combined mixture?
    A. The solution
    B. The solute
    C. The diluent
    D. The solvent

_____ 2. What is the liquid used to dissolve chemicals in?
    A. The solvent
    B. The solute
    C. The diluent
    D. Both A and C

_____ 3. What is the chemical being dissolved in a combined mixture?
    A. The solvent
    B. The solute
    C. The diluent
    D. The solution

Practice Your Knowledge

In Exercises 4 & 5, write a recipe for creating a percent solution or solid.

4. Write a recipe for preparing 250 mL of a $\frac{1}{2}$ NS solution.

5. Write a recipe for preparing 75 g of a 20 percent zinc oxide ointment from zinc oxide powder and petroleum jelly.

In Exercises 6 and 7, write a recipe for preparing a dilution from a concentrate.

6. Using water as a diluent, how would you prepare 2 L of 50 percent ethanol from 90 percent ethanol?

7. How many grams of 10 percent ointment should be mixed with a 2 percent ointment to make a $\frac{1}{2}$ lb of a 5 percent ointment?

In Exercises 8–12 determine how many 10-mL vials to dispense.

8. Ordered: Humulin® R 11 units sub-Q ac breakfast, QSAD for 90 days.

9. Ordered: Humulin® 50/50 48 units sub-Q ac dinner, QSAD for 60 days.

10. Ordered: Novolin® 70/30 57 units sub-Q ac breakfast, QSAD for 30 days.

11. Ordered: Humulin® U 24 units sub-Q Daily, QSAD for 60 days.

12. Ordered: Novolin® N 65 units sub-Q ac dinner, QSAD for 30 days.

Apply Your Knowledge

What Is the "Recipe"?

You are the pharmacy technician working in a hospital pharmacy. You are working in the pharmacy when the following order comes in: "10 percent ethanol 100 mL." You have 90 percent ethanol on hand. You will have to make the 10 percent ethanol solution using 90 percent ethanol and water.

Answer the following questions:

1. Write the "recipe" needed to complete the order.

   _____

2. How much 90 percent ethanol is needed to make the solution?

   _____

3. How much water is needed to make the solution?

   _____

Internet Activity

To get additional reinforcement with alligations, perform an Internet search for: alligations. The Internet will ask you if you meant allegations; do not select allegations and continue your search for alligations. There are some good brain bruisers out there.

Super Tech...

Open the CD-ROM that accompanies your textbook and complete a final review of Chapter 9. For a final evaluation, take the chapter test and email or print your results for your instructor. A score of 95 percent or above indicates mastery of the chapter concepts.

10 Pediatric and Geriatric Considerations

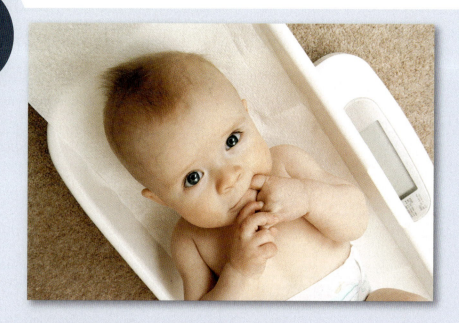

Learning Outcomes

When you have successfully completed Chapter 10, you will have mastered skills to be able to:

▶ Explain why dosage calculations for special populations must be based on the individual patient.

▶ Identify factors that affect the absorption, distribution, biotransformation, and elimination of drugs in special populations.

▶ Determine safe doses for special populations.

▶ Calculate patient dosages based on body weight.

▶ Calculate pediatric dosages using Clark's Rule.

▶ Calculate pediatric dosages using Young's Rule.

▶ Find a patient's body surface area (BSA).

▶ Calculate patient dosages based on a patient's BSA.

Introduction

Working as a pharmacy technician you need to be aware of two special populations that require extra consideration when you are calculating medication dosages. These are **pediatric** patients [under the age of 18 years (children)] and **geriatric** patients, [typically considered anyone over the age of 65 (mature adults)]. The risk of harm to these populations is far greater because of how they break down and absorb medications. You must clarify all confusing drug orders; calculate with absolute accuracy, verifying that the dose is safe; and seek assistance from the pharmacist if you have concerns. No matter how rushed you may feel, you cannot take shortcuts with any medication calculations, especially patients from special populations. This chapter will show you several methods that are used for calculating dosages for pediatric and geriatric patients. Pharmacy technicians must calculate medication dosages with 100 percent accuracy!

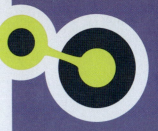

PTCB Correlations

When you have completed this chapter you will have the building block of knowledge needed to work with special populations.

▶ Knowledge of effects of patient's age on drug and nondrug therapy (Statement I-14).

▶ Knowledge of pharmacology (Statement I-16).

Pediatric: Patients under the age of 18 years.

Geriatric: Typically considered anyone over the age of 65.

Critical Thinking in the Pharmacy
What Is the Patient's Weight?

You are the pharmacy technician working in a hospital pharmacy. You are working in the pharmacy when the following order comes in: "8.23mg/kg/day PO TID." The patient weights 187 lb.

When you have completed Chapter 10, you will be able to perform this calculation and determine the total daily medication order and the amount needed per dose.

Pharmacokinetics—How Drugs Are Used by the Body

Pharmacokinetics: The study of what happens to a drug after it is administered to a patient.

Absorption: Movement of a drug from the site where it is given into the bloodstream.

Distribution: Movement of a drug from the bloodstream into other body tissues and fluids.

Biotransformation: Chemical changes of a drug in the body.

Elimination: The process by which a drug leaves the body.

Pharmacokinetics is the study of what happens to a drug after it is administered to a patient. There are four processes that affect a drug after it is administered: absorption, distribution, biotransformation, and elimination. Pharmacokinetics is the study of these four processes. Understanding the processes allows adjustments to be made for patients whose body systems are not fully developed or are not functioning at a certain level.

Absorption is the movement of a drug from the site where it is given into the bloodstream. Intravenous medications bypass the absorption process because they are administered directly into the bloodstream. Oral medications are absorbed through the digestive system, while topical medications are absorbed through the skin.

Distribution is the movement of a drug from the bloodstream into other body tissues and fluids. The blood and each of these other areas are called compartments. Some examples of compartments are blood, fat, cerebrospinal fluid, and the target site. The target site is the site where the drug produces its desired effect. The compartments that a drug will go to are different for different drugs, depending on the chemical nature of the drug.

Biotransformation is the chemical change of a drug in the body. Such changes, which occur primarily in the liver, help to protect the body from foreign chemicals.

Elimination is the process by which a drug leaves the body. The main way of eliminating most drugs is through the urine, although the drug can also be eliminated in the air that we exhale and in sweat, feces, breast milk, or any other body secretion.

The dose of a drug may need to be adjusted if one of these four processes is not functioning within certain limits. Certain conditions affect these four processes, thus affecting the dose. A dose adjustment is based upon the nature and severity of the patient's condition. Thus, the dose ordered might be lower or higher than normal in some circumstances, yet still be the proper dose for the patient. These dosing considerations for various conditions are normally included in the package insert and are considered when the order for the medication is written. You are not expected to make the dosage adjustments; however, understanding these processes will make you aware of the many factors that need to be taken into consideration when determining the appropriate dose for an individual. The functions of the digestive and urinary systems may be affected. Some examples are found in Table 10-1.

Table 10-1   Conditions That May Impact Dosing

Condition	Process Affected	Affect on Dosing
Stomach or intestinal disorders	Absorption	Dose of oral medications may need to be changed.
Liver disorders	Biotransformation	The dose of some drugs needs to be decreased.
Obesity	Distribution	Dose of drugs distributed to fat may need to be increased.
Kidney disease	Elimination	Dose of drugs eliminated in urine may need to be changed.

✔ Review and Practice 10-1 Pharmacokinetics—How Drugs Are Used by the Body

Fill in the blanks using the following word bank.

Absorption   Distribution   Biotransformation   Elimination

_____ 1. The process that chemically changes the drug in the body.

_____ 2. The process that moves a drug from the site where it is given into the bloodstream.

_____ 3. The process in which the drug leaves the body.

_____ 4. The process that moves a drug from the bloodstream into other body tissues and fluids.

Pediatric and Geriatric Dosing

For most drugs, there is a normal recommended dose, based primarily on the patient's weight. This "normal" dose of a medication takes into account a number of assumptions about the patient's body and age. It is assumed that the body systems are fully developed and functioning at a certain level. The function of many body systems changes over the life of a person. In newborns, some systems are not yet fully developed. This is especially true for premature infants. In geriatric patients, those over 65, the function of some body systems begins to deteriorate. Skin and veins become more fragile. The functions of the digestive and urinary systems may be affected. Table 10-2 describes some of the age-related factors that can affect dosing. Pediatric and geriatric doses need to be adjusted and calculated for each individual patient's bodies needs.

Pediatric patients will have a parent or guardian and geriatric patients may have a caretaker who will administer or assist them with medications. These individuals will need education on how much and how often the patient is to have their medication. You may be called upon to teach

Table 10-2   Age-Related Factors That May Affect Dosing

Age Group	Condition	Process Affected	Affect on Dosing
Pediatric	pH of stomach is lower	Absorption	Dose of oral medications may need to be changed.
	Thinner skin	Absorption	Dose of topical medications may need to be decreased.
	Liver still developing	Biotransformation	Dose of some drugs needs to be decreased.
	Less circulation to muscles	Absorption	Dose of IM medications may need to be increased.
Geriatric	Thinner skin	Absorption	Dose of topical medications needs to be decreased.
	Decreased liver function	Biotransformation	Dose of some drugs needs to be decreased.
	Decreased kidney function	Elimination	Dose of some drugs eliminated in the urine needs to be decreased.
	Poor circulation	Absorption and distribution	Dose of some drugs needs to be adjusted.

Table 10-3 **What Should Be Known about Patient Medications**

Name of the medication
Purpose of taking the medication
How to store the medication
How long the patient will need to take the medication
How and when to take the medication
How to know if the medication is effective
Required follow-up (lab tests, doctor appointments)
Possible side effects and what to do about them
Interactions with other drugs and foods
Symptoms to report to the doctor
What to do if a dose is missed
Keeping a list of all medications

the patients or the caregivers about the medications they will be taking. Table 10-3 provides a list of what each patient or caregiver should know about medications.

Ensuring Safe Dosages

When you are working with special populations, always check the package insert, drug label, or product literature to ensure the safety of the dose to be administered. Drug orders may be written in several ways. If you measure the medication, you have the responsibility to check whether the dose is the standard recommended dose. The recommended dose is sometimes written as a range, with a minimum and a maximum recommended dose. In this case, you will need to determine if the dose ordered is not less than the minimum or greater than the maximum recommended dose.

Super Tech . . .

Open the CD-ROM that accompanies your textbook and select Chapter 10, Exercise 10-1. Review the animation and example problems, and then complete the practice problems. Continue to the next section of the book once you have mastered the information presented.

Dosages Based on Body Weight

Many medication orders, especially pediatric and geriatric orders, are based on body weight. This is especially common for small children. An order based on body weight will often state an amount of medication per weight of the patient per unit of time. For example, the order may read "8 mg/kg/day PO q6h." This order says that, over the course of the day, the patient is to be administered 8 mg of medication for every kilogram that he or she weighs. It also says that the total daily dosage is to be divided into 4 doses given at 6-h intervals. You will calculate the amount to be dispensed from the information on the drug order, the patient's weight, and the dose on hand.

Calculating Dosage Based on Body Weight

1. To convert the patient's weight to kilograms you will use the standard conversion factor of 1 kg = 2.2 lb. For accuracy when converting to kilograms, round to the nearest hundredth.
2. Calculate the desired dose *D* by multiplying the dose ordered by the weight in kilograms.

$$\frac{mg}{kg} \times kg = \text{desired dose}$$

3. Confirm whether the desired dose is safe by checking the label, package insert, or product literature. If it is unsafe, consult the pharmacist.
4. Calculate the amount to be dispensed, using the fraction proportion, ratio proportion, dimensional analysis, or formula method.

Using Conversion Factors

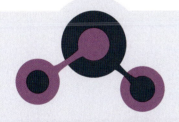

Fraction Proportion Method

EXAMPLE ▶   Calculate the amount to be dispensed to a 3-year-old who weighs 34 lb.

Ordered: Hyoscyamine sulfate 5 mcg/kg sub-Q 1 h preanesthesia
On hand: Hyoscyamine sulfate 0.5 mg/mL

SOLUTION ▶   1. Convert the patient's weight to kilograms.

$$\frac{1\ kg}{2.2\ \cancel{lb}} = \frac{?}{34\ \cancel{lb}}$$

$$2.2 \times ? = 34 \times 1\ kg$$

$$? = \frac{34\ kg}{2.2}$$

$$? = 15.45 = \text{patient's weight in kilograms}$$

2. Calculate the desired dose.

$$\frac{5\ mcg}{kg} \times 15.45\ kg = 77.25\ mcg = \text{Rounded to 77 mcg}$$

3. Confirm that the desired dose is safe.
Checking the *Facts and Comparisons* or other pharmacy resources, you find that 5 mcg/kg is the recommended dose for pediatric patients over 2 years of age.

4. Calculate the amount to be dispensed. Because the unit of measure for the dose on hand is milligrams, the desired dose must also be expressed in milligrams.

Convert the unit of measure.

$$\frac{1 \text{ mg}}{1000 \text{ mcg}} = \frac{?}{77 \text{ mcg}}$$

$$1000 \times ? = 77 \times 1 \text{ mg}$$

$$? = \frac{77 \text{ mg}}{1000}$$

$$? = 0.077 \text{ mg}$$

Fill in the proportion.

$$\frac{Q}{H} = \frac{A}{D}$$

$$\frac{1 \text{ mL}}{0.5 \text{ mg}} = \frac{A}{0.077 \text{ mg}}$$

Cancel units.

$$\frac{1 \text{ mL}}{0.5 \text{ mg}} = \frac{A}{0.077 \text{ mg}}$$

Cross-multiply and solve for the unknown.

$$0.5 \times A = 1 \text{ mL} \times 0.077$$

$$A = 1 \text{ mL} \times \frac{0.077}{0.5}$$

$$A = 0.154 \text{ mL}$$

Since the volume of the injection is less than 1 mL, we round to the nearest hundredth.

$$A = 0.15 \text{ mL}$$

Using Conversion Factors

Ratio Proportion Method

EXAMPLE ▶   Calculate the amount to be dispensed to a 3-year-old who weighs 34 lb.

Ordered: Hyoscyamine sulfate 5 mcg/kg sub-Q 1 h preanesthesia
On hand: Hyoscyamine sulfate 0.5 mg/mL

SOLUTION ▶   1. Convert the patient's weight to kilograms.

$$1 \text{ kg} : 2.2 \text{ lb} :: ? : 34 \text{ lb}$$

$$2.2 \times ? = 1 \text{ kg} \times 34$$

$$? = \frac{1 \text{ kg} \times 34}{2.2}$$

$$? = 15.45 \text{ kg} \quad \text{(Patient's weight in kilograms)}$$

2. Calculate the desired dose.

$$\frac{5 \text{ mcg}}{\text{kg}} \times 15.45 \text{ kg} = 77.25 \text{ mcg} = \text{Rounded to 7 mcg}$$

3. Confirm that the desired dose is safe.
   Checking the *Facts and Comparisons* or other pharmacy resources, you find that 5 mcg/kg is the recommended dose for pediatric patients over 2 years of age.
4. Calculate the amount to be dispensed.
   Because the unit of measure for the dose on hand is milligrams, the desired dose must also be expressed in milligrams.

Convert the unit of measure.

$$1 \text{ mg} : 1000 \text{ mcg} :: ? : 77 \text{ mcg}$$

$$1000 \times ? = 77 \times 1 \text{ mg}$$

$$? = \frac{77}{1000} \text{ mg}$$

$$? = 0.077 \text{ mg}$$

Fill in the proportion.

$$Q : H :: A : D$$

$$1 \text{ mL} : 0.5 \text{ mg} :: A : 0.077 \text{ mg}$$

Cancel units.

$$1 \text{ mL} : 0.5 \text{ mg} :: A : 0.077 \text{ mg}$$

Multiply the means and extremes then solve for the missing value.

$$0.5 \times A = 1 \text{ mL} \times 0.077$$

$$A = 1 \text{ mL} \times \frac{0.077}{0.5}$$

$$A = 0.154 \text{ mL}$$

Since the volume of the injection is less than 1 mL, we round to the nearest hundredth.

$$A = 0.15 \text{ mL}$$

Using Conversion Factors

Dimensional Analysis

EXAMPLE ▶   Calculate the amount to be dispensed to a 3-year-old who weighs 34 lb.

Ordered: Hyoscyamine sulfate 5 mcg/kg sub-Q 1 h preanesthesia
On hand: Hyoscyamine sulfate 0.5 mg/mL

SOLUTION ▶   1. Convert the patient's weight to kilograms.

$$? \text{ kg} = \frac{1 \text{ kg}}{2.2 \text{ lb}} \times 34 \text{ lb}$$

$$? = 15.45 \text{ kg}$$

2. Calculate the desired dose.

$$\frac{5 \text{ mcg}}{\text{kg}} \times 15.45 \text{ kg} = 77.25 \text{ mcg} = \text{Rounded to 77 mcg}$$

3. Confirm that the desired dose is safe.
   Checking the *Facts and Comparisons* or other pharmacy resources, you find that 5 mcg/kg is the recommended dose for pediatric patients over 2 years of age.
4. Calculate the amount to be dispensed.

Convert the unit of measure.

The unit of measure for the dosage ordered is mcg. The unit of measure for the dose on hand is mg. Use the conversion factor 1 mg = 1000 mcg. Since we will be converting the dosage ordered to mg place mg on top. This is the first factor.

$$\frac{1 \text{ mg}}{1000 \text{ mcg}}$$

The dosage unit is 1 mL; the dose on hand is 0.5 mg. This is the second factor.

$$\frac{1 \text{ mg}}{1000 \text{ mcg}} \times \frac{1 \text{ mL}}{0.5 \text{ mg}}$$

The desired dose is 0.077 mg. Place this over 1 and set up your equation.

$$A \text{ mL} = \frac{1 \text{ mg}}{1000 \text{ mcg}} \times \frac{1 \text{ mL}}{0.5 \text{ mg}} \times \frac{77 \text{ mcg}}{1}$$

Since the volume of the injection is less than 1 mL, we round to the nearest hundredth.

$$A = 0.15 \text{ mL}$$

Using Conversion Factors

Formula Method

EXAMPLE ▶ Calculate the amount to be dispensed to a 3-year-old who weighs 34 lb.

Ordered: Hyoscyamine sulfate 5 mcg/kg sub-Q 1 h preanesthesia
On hand: Hyoscyamine sulfate 0.5 mg/mL

SOLUTION ▶

1. Convert the patient's weight to kilograms.

$$? \text{ kg} = \frac{1 \text{ kg}}{2.2 \text{ lb}} \times 34 \text{ lb}$$

$$? = 15.45 \text{ kg}$$

2. Calculate the desired dose.

$$\frac{5 \text{ mcg}}{\text{kg}} \times 15.45 \text{ kg} = 77.25 \text{ mcg} = \text{Rounded to 77 mcg}$$

3. Confirm that the desired dose is safe. Checking the *Facts and Comparisons* or other pharmacy resources, you find that 5 mcg/kg is the recommended dose for pediatric patients over 2 years of age.

4. Calculate the amount to be dispensed.

Because the unit of measure for the dose on hand is milligrams, the desired dose must also be expressed in milligrams.

Convert the unit of measure.

$$\frac{1 \text{ mg}}{1000 \text{ mcg}} = \frac{?}{77 \text{ mcg}}$$

$$1000 \times ? = 77 \times 1 \text{ mg}$$

$$? = \frac{77 \text{ mg}}{1000}$$

$$? = 0.077 \text{ mg}$$

$$D = 0.077 \text{ mg}$$

$$Q = 1 \text{ mL}$$

$$H = 0.5 \text{ mg}$$

Fill in the formula.

$$\frac{0.077 \text{ mg} \times 1 \text{ mL}}{0.5 \text{ mg}} = A$$

Cancel units.

$$\frac{0.077 \; \cancel{mg} \times 1 \; mL}{0.5 \; \cancel{mg}} = A$$

Solve for the unknown.

$$\frac{0.077 \; mg \times 1 \; mL}{0.5 \; mg} = A$$

$$A = 0.154 \; mL$$

Since the volume of the injection is less than 1 mL, we round to the nearest hundredth.

$$A = 0.15 \; mL$$

Super Tech . . .

Open the CD-ROM that accompanies your textbook and select Chapter 10, Exercise 10-2. Review the animation and example problems, and then complete the practice problems. Continue to the next section of the book once you have mastered the information presented.

Tech Check

Converting Ounces Carefully

Infants, especially premature infants, may be weighed in pounds and ounces or grams. On occasion, you will need to convert between these two units to determine if a dose is safe. When you are doing these conversions, remember an ounce is not one-tenth of a pound. A baby whose weight is 8 lb 6 oz does not weigh 8.6 lb.

Convert 6 oz to pounds, using the conversion factor of $\frac{1 \; lb}{16 \; oz}$.

Here, $6 \; oz \times \frac{1 \; lb}{16 \; oz} = 0.375 \; lb$. Thus, 8 lb 6 oz = 8.375 lb.

✓ Review and Practice 10-2 Pediatric and Geriatric Dosing

In Exercises 1–6, convert the following weights to kilograms. Round to the nearest hundredth.

1. 66 lb   3. 54 lb   5. 152 lb

2. 77 lb   4. 37 lb   6. 202 lb

In Exercises 7–10, determine if the order is safe. If it is, then determine the amount to be dispensed.

7. The patient is a 3-day-old newborn who weighs 6 lb 5 oz.

   Ordered: Tobramycin 5 mg IM Q12H

   On hand: Tobramycin multidose vial, 20 mg/2 mL. According to the package insert, a premature or full-term neonate up to 1 week of age may be given up to 4 mg/kg/day in 2 equal doses every 12 h.

8. The patient is a 4-year-old child who weighs 32 lb.

   Ordered: Proventil® 1 tsp syrup PO TID

   On hand: Proventil® syrup, 2 mg/5 mL. According to the package insert, for children 2 to 6 years of age, dosing should be initiated at 0.1 mg/kg of body weight 3 times a day. This starting dose should not exceed 2 mg 3 times per day.

9. The patient is a 5-year-old child who weighs 34 lb and has a severe infection.

   Ordered: Augmentin® 225 mg PO Q8H

   On hand: According to the package insert, the dosing regimen for pediatric patients aged 12 weeks and older, but less than 40 kg, is 40 mg/kg/day Q8H.

10. The patient is a 7-year-old child who weighs 52 lb.

    Ordered: 2.5 g vial of Zantac®. Zantac® 30 mg IV q8h

    On hand: The contents are mixed with diluent to produce 100 mL of solution. According to the package insert, the recommended dose in pediatric patients is for a total daily dose of 2 to 4 mg/kg, to be divided, and may be given every 6 to 8 hours, up to a maximum of 50 mg given every 6 to 8 hours.

Clark's Rule: Calculation that uses the weight of the child to determine the desired dose of medication.

Young's Rule: Calculation that uses the age of the child to determine the desired dose of medication.

***Memory tip** Young = age; the word "young" refers to the age of an individual, and Young's Rule uses the age of the child to determine the desired dose.*

Pediatric Specific Dosage Calculations

There are two other forms of calculations used to calculate pediatric doses, Clark's Rule and Young's Rule. **Clark's Rule** uses the weight of the child to determine the desired dose and **Young's Rule** uses the age of the child to determine the desired dose.

Clark's Rule for children's dosage calculations uses the following formula:

$$\frac{\text{Child's weight in pounds}}{150 \text{ pounds}} \times \text{Average adult dose} = \text{Pediatric patient's dose}$$

EXAMPLE ▶ Using Clark's Rule, find the amount to be dispensed. The patient is a 6-year-old child who weighs 50 lb; the average adult dose is 250 mg.

$$\frac{50 \ lb}{150 \ lb} \times 250 \ mg = 83.3 \ mg$$

Young's Rule for children's dosage calculations uses the following formula. (this formula can be used only if the child is a least 1 year of age):

$$\frac{\text{Child's age in years}}{\text{Child's age in years} + 12 \text{ years}} \times \text{Average adult dose} = \text{Pediatric patient's dose}$$

EXAMPLE ▶ Using Young's Rule, find the amount to be dispensed. The patient is a 6-year-old child who weighs 50 lb; the average adult dose is 250 mg.

$$\frac{6 \ years}{6 \ years + 12 \ years} \times 250 \ mg = 83.3 \ mg$$

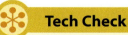

Tech Check

Looking for Warnings

Elena, a pharmacy technician working in a hospital pharmacy, received an order for 1.5 mL of Pediazole® per dose for a 7-week-old infant who weighs 12 lb. The schedule on the package insert has an instruction to adjust the dosage by body weight. She notices that for a 13-lb infant, the recommended dosage is 2.5 mL every 6 or 8 h. Her first instinct tells her that 1.5 mL seems like a safe amount to be dispensed.

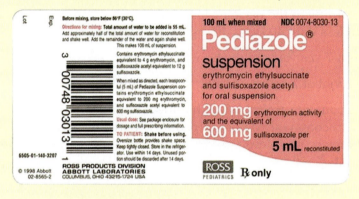

DOSAGE AND ADMINISTRATION

PEDIAZOLE SHOULD NOT BE ADMINISTERED TO INFANTS UNDER 2 MONTHS OF AGE BECAUSE OF CONTRAINDICATIONS OF SYSTEMIC SULFONAMIDES IN THIS AGE GROUP.

For Acute Otitis Media in Children: The dose of Pediazole can be calculated based on the erythromycin component (50 mg/kg/day) or the sulfisoxazole component (150 mg/kg/day to a maximum of 6 g/day). The total daily dose of Pediazole should be administered in equally divided doses three or four times a day for 10 days. Pediazole may be administered without regard to meals.

Think Before You Act

Fortunately, Elena acts on more than instinct. Reading the dosage and administration section of the package insert, she finds a warning that Pediazole® should not be given to patients less than 2 months of age. This patient, 7 weeks old, should not receive Pediazole®. Elena has the pharmacist contact the physician to discuss the order further.

Super Tech . . .

Open the CD-ROM that accompanies your textbook and select Chapter 10, Exercise 10-3. Review the animation and example problems, and then complete the practice problems. Continue to the next section of the book once you have mastered the information presented.

✓ **Review and Practice 10-3** Pediatric Specific Dosage Calculations

In Exercises 1–4, use Young's Rule or Clark's Rule to calculate the pediatric dose.

1. An 8-year-old child needs a dose of medication; the average adult dose is 750 mg.

2. A 3-year-old child needs a dose of medication; the average adult dose is 300 mg.

3. A child who weighs 90 lb needs a dose of medication; the average adult dose is 250 mg.

4. A child who weighs 75 lb needs a dose of medication; the average adult dose is 150 mg.

Dosages Based on Body Surface Area (BSA)

Some medications are prescribed on the basis of a patient's body weight. Others factor in both weight and height to determine a patient's body surface area, or BSA. Many pediatric medications use a patient's BSA to determine the daily dosage. BSA is also important for burn victims and for patients undergoing chemotherapy, radiation treatments, and open heart surgery. BSA calculations are used to provide more accurate dosage calculations specific to the patient's size and severity of the illness.

Calculating a Patient's BSA

Nomogram: A special chart used to determine a patient's body surface area (BSA).

A patient's BSA is stated in square meters (m^2). You can calculate the BSA by using one of the two formulas listed below. Your calculator should have a program or button that will help you find a square root ($\sqrt{}$). You can also use a **nomogram,** which is a special chart used to determine a patient's body surface area. Nomograms provide an estimate of BSA and are easier to use than an equation. Nomograms are available for children and adults. See Figures 10-1 and 10-2.

Calculating the Body Surface Area Using a Formula

To determine a patient's BSA (body surface area):

1. If you know the height in centimeters and weight in kilograms, calculate

$$\text{BSA} = \sqrt{\frac{\text{height (cm)} \times \text{weight (kg)}}{3600}} \; m^2$$

2. If you know the height in inches and weight in pounds, calculate

$$\text{BSA} = \sqrt{\frac{\text{height (in)} \times \text{weight (lb)}}{3131}} \; m^2$$

Note: When using a formula to calculate BSA, if the result is less than one, round to the nearest hundredth. When the result is greater than one, round to the nearest tenth.

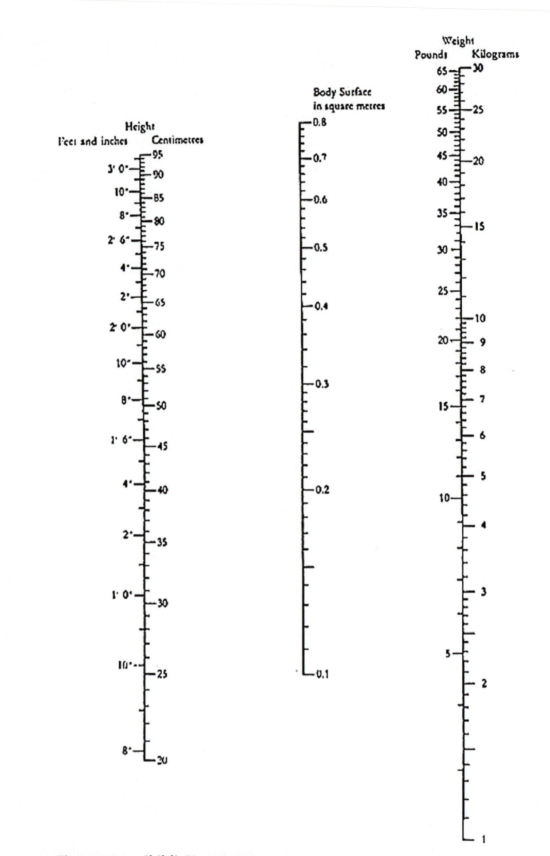

Figure 10-1 Child's Nomogram

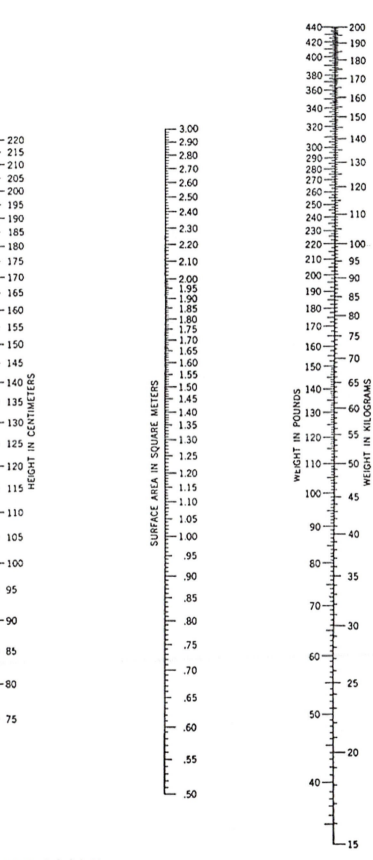

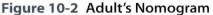

Figure 10-2 Adult's Nomogram

EXAMPLE 1 ▶ Find the body surface area for a child who is 85 cm tall and weighs 13.9 kg.

$$\text{BSA} = \sqrt{\frac{85 \times 13.9}{3600}} \text{ m}^2 = \sqrt{\frac{1181.5}{3600}} \text{ m}^2 \cong 0.572 \text{ m}^2 \cong 0.57 \text{ m}^2$$

EXAMPLE 2 ▶ Find the body surface area for a baby who is 24 in. tall and who weighs 12 lb 3 oz.

First, convert the pounds and ounces to pounds and a fraction of a pound.

$$12 \text{ lb } 3 \text{ oz} = 12.1875 \text{ lb}$$

$$\text{BSA} = \sqrt{\frac{24 \times 12.2}{3131}} \text{ m}^2 = \sqrt{\frac{292.5}{3131}} \text{ m}^2 \cong 0.305 \text{ m}^2 \cong 0.31 \text{ m}^2$$

EXAMPLE 3 ▶ Find the body surface area for an adult who is 5 ft 6 in. tall and who weighs 168 lb.

First, convert the height to inches. Since 1 ft equals 12 in., multiply the number of feet by 12 and then add the inches.

$$5 \times 12 = 60$$

$$60 + 6 = 66 \text{ in}$$

$$\text{BSA} = \sqrt{\frac{66 \times 168}{3131}} \text{ m}^2 = \sqrt{\frac{11,088}{3131}} \text{ m}^2 \cong 1.88 \text{ m}^2 \cong 1.9 \text{ m}^2$$

Calculating the Body Surface Area by Using a Nomogram

Align a straightedge (such as a ruler or piece of paper) so that it intersects at the height and weight. Doing so will create an intersection in the BSA scale. *Note:* Read the calibrations carefully; the spaces and lines vary depending upon where you intersect the line.

EXAMPLE 1 ▶ Find the body surface area for a child who is 85 cm tall and weighs 13.9 kg, using the child's nomogram (Figure 10-3).

$$\text{BSA} = 0.57 \text{ m}^2$$

EXAMPLE 2 ▶ Find the body surface area for a baby who is 24 in. tall and weighs 12 lb 3 oz, using the child's nomogram (Figure 10-4).

$$\text{BSA} = 0.3 \text{ m}^2$$

EXAMPLE 3 ▶ Find the body surface area for an adult who is 5 ft 6 in. tall and who weighs 168 lb, using the adult nomogram (Figure 10-5).

$$\text{BSA} = 1.9 \text{ m}^2$$

$$\text{BSA} = 1.86 \text{ m}^2 \qquad \text{or } 1.9 \text{ m}^2$$

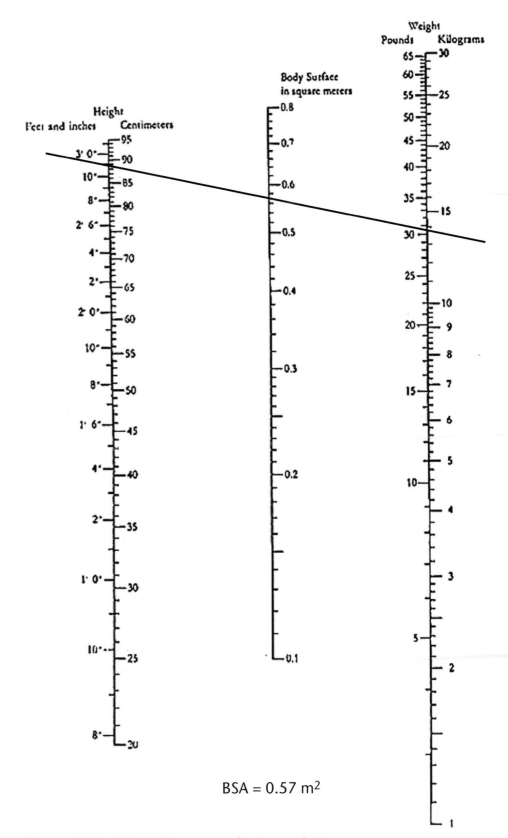

BSA = 0.57 m²

Figure 10-3 Child's Nomogram for Example 1

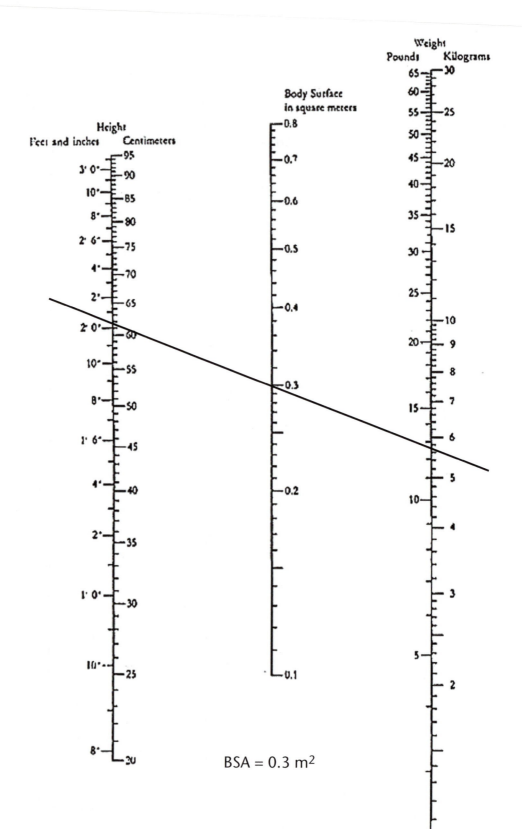

BSA = 0.3 m²

Figure 10-4 Child's Nomogram for Example 2

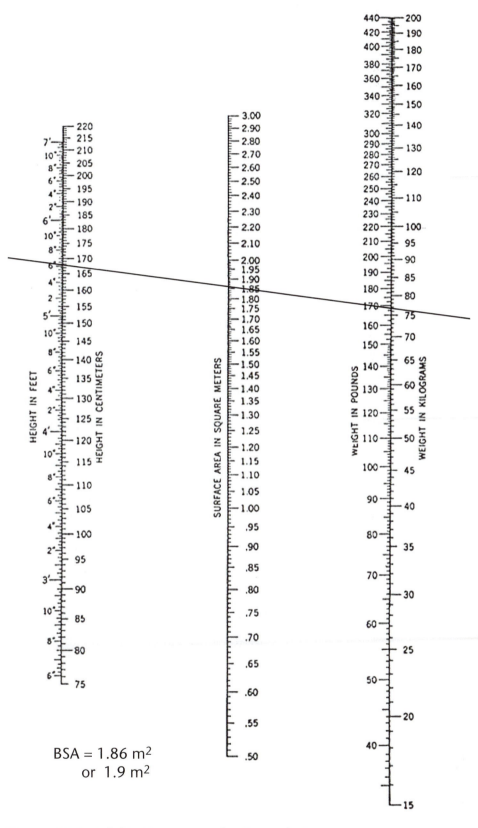

BSA = 1.86 m²
or 1.9 m²

Figure 10-5 Adult's Nomogram for Example 3

Calculating Dosage Based on BSA

1. Calculate the patient's BSA.
2. Calculate the desired dose:

$$\text{Dosage ordered per m}^2 \times \text{BSA} = \text{desired dose}$$

3. Confirm whether the desired dose is safe. If it is unsafe, consult the physician who wrote the order.
4. Calculate the amount to be dispensed, using fraction proportion, ratio proportion, dimensional analysis, or the formula method.

EXAMPLE ▶ Ordered: CeeNU® (first dose) 150 mg now for a patient who is 99 cm tall and weighs 50 kg.

According to the package insert, the first recommended dose of CeeNU® is a single oral dose providing 130 mg/m².

1. The recommended dose is in square meters (m²), so you need to find the BSA. You know the patient's height and weight in centimeters and kilograms. Use the BSA formula for cm and kg.

$$\text{BSA} = \sqrt{\frac{99 \times 50}{3600}} \text{ m}^2 = \sqrt{\frac{4950}{3600}} \text{ m}^2 = 1.2 \text{ m}^2$$

2. Calculate the desired dose.

$$\frac{130 \text{ mg}}{\text{m}^2} \times 1.2 \text{ m}^2 = 156 \text{ mg}$$

3. The dose ordered is safe, since the dose of 150 mg is less than the calculated desired dose of 156 mg.
4. Calculate the amount to be dispensed. CeeNU® is available in 100-mg, 40-mg, and 10-mg capsules. Thinking critically and realizing the capsules cannot be divided, you must provide the dose to the nearest whole number. This would be 150 mg. You determine to dispense 1 capsule of each strength, 100 mg + 40 mg + 10 mg.

Super Tech . . .

Open the CD-ROM that accompanies your textbook and select Chapter 10, Exercise 10-4. Review the animation and example problems, and then complete the practice problems. Continue to the next section of the book once you have mastered the information presented.

✓ Review and Practice 10-4 Dosages Based on Body Surface Area (BSA)

In Exercises 1–8, use the appropriate formula to calculate the BSA for patients with the following heights and weights.

1. 88 cm and 13.2 kg
2. 58 cm and 21 kg
3. 38 cm and 6 kg
4. 48 cm and 10 kg
5. 52 in and 64 lb
6. 43 in and 35 lb
7. 22 in and 18 lb
8. 26 in and 21 lb

In Exercises 9–12, calculate the recommended dosage in the appropriate unit.

9. The child's BSA is 0.82 m². The recommended dosage is 175 mcg/m².

10. The child's BSA is 0.65 m². The recommended dosage is 0.4 mg/m².

11. The child's height is 62 cm and weight is 15 kg. The recommended dosage is 50 mcg/m².

12. The child's height is 41 in. and weight is 63 lb. The recommended dosage is 0.2 mg/m².

In Exercises 13–15, calculate the amount to dispense.

13. The patient is 42 in. tall and weighs 71 lb.

    Ordered: Chemotherapy medication 6 mg/m²/ day IV q12h
    On hand: Chemotherapy medication 200 mcg/mL for IV use

14. The patient is 86 cm tall and weighs 12 kg.

    Ordered: Antibiotic 25 mg/m²/day IM q6h
    On hand: Antibiotic 2 mg/mL for IM use

15. The patient is 34 cm tall and weighs 5 kg.

    Ordered: Cerubidine® IV qw
    On hand: Cerubidine® for injection. When reconstituted, each milliliter contains 5 mg of drug. The recommended pediatric dosage is 25 mg/m² IV the first day every week.

✓ Chapter 10 Review

Test Your Knowledge

Multiple Choice

Select the best answer and write the letter on the line.

_____ 1. The process that chemically changes the drug in the body.
   A. Absorption
   B. Distribution
   C. Biotransformation
   D. Elimination

_____ 2. The process that moves a drug from the site where it is given into the bloodstream.
   A. Absorption
   B. Distribution
   C. Biotransformation
   D. Elimination

_____ 3. The process in which the drug leaves the body.
   A. Absorption
   B. Distribution
   C. Biotransformation
   D. Elimination

_____ 4. The process that moves a drug from the bloodstream into other body tissues and fluids.
   A. Absorption
   B. Distribution
   C. Biotransformation
   D. Elimination

Practice Your Knowledge

In Exercises 5–8, convert the following weights to kilograms.

5. 49 lb   6. 61 lb   7. 6 lb 9 oz   8. 12 lb 13 oz

In Exercises 9–12, calculate the BSA for patients with the following heights and weights.

9. 105 cm and 19 kg   10. 74 cm and 12.1 kg   11. 41 in and 33 lb   12. 30 in and 23 lb

In Exercises 13–18 determine if the dose is safe and the amount to dispense.

13. The child weighs 30 lb.

    Ordered: Depakene® syrup 100 mg po q12h.
    On hand: Depakene® syrup 250 mg/5 mL
    According to the package insert, the initial daily dose for pediatric patients is 15 mg/kg/day.

14. The patient is a 4-year-old child who weighs 16 kg.

    Ordered: Ventolin® syrup 1.6 mg PO TID.
    On hand: Ventolin® syrup 2 mg/5 mL
    According to the package insert, for children from 2 to 6 years of age, dosing should be initiated at
    0.1 mg/kg of body weight 3 times a day. This starting dosage should not exceed 2 mg 3 times a day.

15. The patient is 72 cm tall and weighs 16 kg.

    Ordered: Oncaspar® 1300 IU IM every 14 days
    On hand: Oncaspar® 5 mL/vial, 750 IU/mL
    The recommended pediatric dosage is 2500 IU/m² for children whose BSA is greater than or equal to
    0.6 m² and 82.5 IU/kg for children whose BSA is less than 0.6 m².

16. The patient is a 44-lb child who is $5\frac{1}{2}$ years old.

    Ordered: Tolectin® 100 mg PO QID.
    On hand: Tolectin® 200-mg scored tablets. The package insert indicates that for children 2 years and
    older, the usual dose ranges from 15 to 30 mg/kg/day.

17. The patient weighs 47 lb.

    Ordered: Antibiotic 3 mcg/kg/day IM divided in 2 equal doses.
    On hand: Antibiotic in 50 mcg/mL vials

18. The patient weighs 27 kg.

    Ordered: Muscle relaxant 10 mg/kg/day IM daily.
    On hand: Muscle relaxant in 50 mg/mL suspension

In Exercises 19–22, using Clark's and Young's Rules, determine the desired dose.

19. A 4-year-old child needs a dose of medication; the average adult dose is 375 mg.

20. A 5-year-old child needs a dose of medication; the average adult dose is 500 mg.

21. A child who weights 45 lb needs a dose of medication; the average adult dose is 250 mg.

22. A child who weights 67 lb needs a dose of medication; the average adult dose is 125 mg.

Apply Your Knowledge

What Is the Patient's Weight?

You are the pharmacy technician working in a hospital pharmacy. You are working in the pharmacy when the following order comes in: "8.23 mg/kg/day PO TID." The patient weights 187 lb.

Answer the following questions:

1. How many kilograms does the patient weigh?

   _____

2. What is the total daily medication order?

   _____

3. What is the amount per dose?

   _____

Internet Activity

When you are calculating dosage for special populations, you need to know the patient's actual weight. In some circumstances, it is also important to know the ideal weight for a patient based upon the patient's height. Various charts are available to determine if a patient is of ideal weight. Search the Internet and find a current and reliable height-to-weight ratio chart. Keep this chart handy when you are calculating for special populations.

Super Tech...

Open the CD-ROM that accompanies your textbook and complete a final review of Chapter 10. For a final evaluation, take the chapter test and email or print your results for your instructor. A score of 95 percent or above indicates mastery of the chapter concepts.

11

Operational Calculations

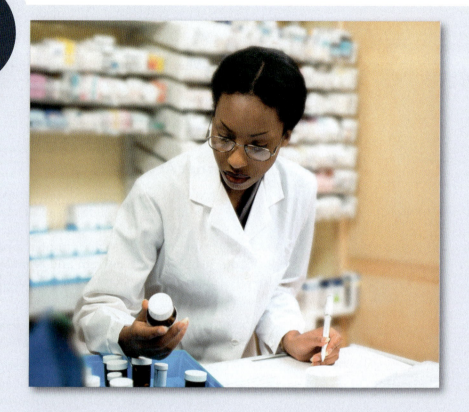

Learning Outcomes

When you have successfully completed Chapter 11, you will have mastered skills to be able to:

▸ Calculate overhead costs.

▸ Calculate profits.

▸ Calculate discount amounts.

▸ Calculate average wholesale price (AWP).

▸ Calculate inventory turnover rate.

▸ Calculate depreciation.

▸ Demonstrate understanding of capitation fee and AWP plus fee.

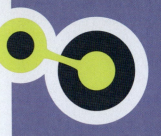

Introduction

As a pharmacy technician you need to be familiar with the aspects of the day-to-day operations of the pharmacy. The costs involved in running the pharmacy are many. While providing a service to the patients is important, the pharmacy must also make money in order to stay in business. In this chapter you will learn multiple operational calculations needed to run a profitable pharmacy.

Critical Thinking in the Pharmacy
What Is the Actual Cost?

You are the pharmacy technician working in a retail pharmacy. You are working in the pharmacy when the following prescription comes in: "Penicillin 250 mg, 1 PO QID for 10 days." The prescription selling price to the patient is $13.99. The patient has insurance. The insurance company will pay the AWP of 29 cents (or $0.29) per tablet of medication plus a $2.00 dispensing fee. The pharmacy's purchase price is 16 cents (or $0.16) per tablet of medication, and it charges a $3.00 dispensing fee.

When you have completed Chapter 11 you will be able to perform this calculation and determine the actual cost to the pharmacy to fill the prescription and if the pharmacy made a profit.

PTCB Correlations

When you have completed this chapter you will have the building block of knowledge needed to work with maintaining medications and inventory control systems.

- ▶ Knowledge of formulary or approved stock list (II-5).

- ▶ Knowledge of par and reorder levels and drug use (II-6).

- ▶ Knowledge of third-party reimbursement systems (III-31).

General Business Considerations

All businesses have costs associated with day-to-day operations. The pharmacy's income earned from sales must be higher than the operational costs associated with the business in order for the pharmacy to be profitable. In this section you will learn how to calculate overhead costs, profits, gross profits, net profits, and discounts.

Overhead

Overhead: All costs associated with business operations.

The pharmacy's **overhead** is all costs associated with the pharmacy's business operations. Employee salaries, rent, utility bills, insurance premiums, inventory/supplies, discounts, and sale items are all overhead costs. The total cost of the overhead is used to calculate the pharmacy's profit.

EXAMPLE ▶

Annual Overhead Costs

Employee salaries	$125,000.00
Rent	$24,000.00
Utilities	$12,000.00
Insurance	$6,000.00
Inventory/supplies	+$732,000.00
Annual overhead total	**$899,000.00**

Profits

Profit: The difference of overhead expenses from income earned from sales.

A **profit** is the difference between overhead expenses and income earned from sales. To calculate a profit you subtract the pharmacy's overhead costs from the income earned from sales.

EXAMPLE ▶

Annual sales	$1,548,370.00
Annual overhead costs	−$899,000.00
Annual profit	**$649,370.00**

Gross profit: The difference between the purchase price the pharmacy paid for products, such as medication, and the markup (the selling price).

Gross profit is the difference of the purchase price the pharmacy paid for products, for example medication, and markup price, which is the selling price. To calculate the gross profit you subtract the pharmacy's purchase price from the selling price.

EXAMPLE 1 ▶

Azithromycin 250 mg 6 tablets (Z-pak)

Selling price	$13.99
Purchase price	−$4.57
Gross profit	**$9.42**

EXAMPLE 2 ▶

The purchase price of Keflex® 500 mg is 55 cents per tablet and the selling price is $1.25 per tablet. Find the gross profit for a prescription of 20 tablets.

1. Find the purchase price. Multiply cost per tablet by number of tablets.

$$\$0.55 \times 20 = \$11.00$$

$$\text{Purchase price} = \$11.00$$

2. Find the selling price. Multiply cost per tablet by number of tablets.

$$\$1.25 \times 20 = \$25.00$$
$$\text{Selling price} = \$25.00$$

3. Subtract the purchase price from the selling price.

Selling price	$25.00
Purchase price	−$11.00
Gross profit	$13.00

The gross profit is $13.00.

Net profit: The difference of the selling price and the purchase price plus a dispensing fee.

Net profit is the difference between the selling price, and the purchase price plus a dispensing fee, which is used to offset the overhead costs used to fill prescriptions. The dispensing fee per prescription is determined by each pharmacy on the basis of the company's profit needs. It can be a set fee or a percentage. To determine the net profit, you subtract the purchase price and the dispensing fee from the selling price.

EXAMPLE 1 ▶ Azithromycin 250 mg 6 tablets (Z-pak)

Selling price	$13.99
Purchase price	−$4.57
Dispensing fee	−$4.00
Net profit	**$5.42**

EXAMPLE 2 ▶ The purchase price of Keflex® 500 mg is 55 cents per tablet and the selling price is $1.25 per tablet. There is a dispensing fee of $5.00 per prescription. Find the net profit for a prescription of 20 tablets.

1. Find the purchase price. Multiply cost per tablet by number of tablets.

$$\$0.55 \times 20 = \$11.00$$
$$\text{Purchase price} = \$11.00$$

2. Find the selling price. Multiply cost per tablet by number of tablets.

$$\$1.25 \times 20 = \$25.00$$
$$\text{Selling price} = \$25.00$$

3. Subtract the purchase price from the selling price.

Selling price	$25.00
Purchase price	−$11.00
Gross profit	$14.00

The gross profit is $13.00.

4. Subtract the dispensing fee from the gross profit.

Gross profit	$14.00
Dispensing fee	−$5.00
Net profit	$8.00

Discount: A reduced price from the normal selling price.

A **discount** is a reduced price from the normal selling price. Drug manufacturers may offer the pharmacy a discount for purchasing large quantities of certain medications. In turn, the pharmacy may also offer discounts to its customers. To determine a discounted price, you multiply the selling price by the discount percentage, which will give you discount amount, then you subtract the discount amount from the selling price.

EXAMPLE 1 ▶ The selling price for 1 bottle of 1000 tablets of medication is $50.00. For orders of 5 bottles or more the manufacturer offers a 10 percent discount. What is the discounted price for 1 bottle?

SOLUTION ▶ 1. Multiply the selling price by the discount percentage.

$$\$50.00 \times 10\% = \text{discount amount}$$
$$\$50.00 \times 0.10 = \$5.00$$

2. Subtract the discount amount from the selling price.

$$\begin{array}{r} \$50.00 \\ -\$5.00 \\ \hline \$45.00 \end{array}$$

The discounted price is $45.00.

EXAMPLE 2 ▶ The selling price for 1 bottle of 36 tablets of 81-mg aspirin is $2.49. Tuesday is senior discount day for all customers age 55 years and older. Customers age 55 years and older receive a 15 percent discount on Tuesdays. What is the discounted price?

SOLUTION ▶ 1. Multiply the selling price by the discount percentage.

$$\$2.49 \times 15\% = \text{discount amount}$$
$$\$2.49 \times 0.15 = \$0.37 \quad \text{or} \quad 37 \text{ cents}$$

2. Subtract the discount amount from the selling price.

$$\begin{array}{r} \$2.49 \\ -0.37 \text{ cents} \\ \hline \$2.12 \end{array}$$

The discounted price is $2.12.

Super Tech . . .

Open the CD-ROM that accompanies your textbook and select Chapter 11, Exercise 11-1. Review the animation and example problems, and then complete the practice problems. Continue to the next section of the book once you have mastered the information presented.

✓ Review and Practice 11-1 General Business Considerations

In Exercises 1–4, determine the overhead cost.

1. Employee salaries: 2 pharmacists at $65,000.00 each, 3 technicians at $25,000.00 each, rent at $24,000.00, utilities $5000.00, insurance $12,000.00 and inventory/supplies $475,000.00.

2. Employee salaries: 3 pharmacists at $75,000.00 each, 2 technicians at $26,500.00 each, rent at $18,000.00, utilities $3600.00, insurance $11,950.00 and inventory/supplies $357,495.00.

3. Employee salaries: 1 pharmacist at $70,000.00, 2 technicians at $22,500.00 each, rent at $15,000.00, utilities $2500.00, insurance $10,500.00 and inventory/supplies $225,750.00.

4. Employee salaries: 4 pharmacists at $72,000.00 each, 6 technicians at $27,500.00 each, rent at $28,000.00, utilities $7000.00, insurance $24,000.00 and inventory/supplies $525,000.00.

In Exercises 5–8, determine the annual profit using the overhead costs from Exercises 1–4.

5. Annual income from sales is $895,000.00. Using the answer in Exercise 1, determine the annual profit.

6. Annual income from sales is $695,000.00. Using the answer in Exercise 2, determine the annual profit.

7. Annual income from sales is $705,000.00. Using the answer in Exercise 3, determine the annual profit.

8. Annual income from sales is $1,710,500.00. Using the answer in Exercise 4, determine the annual profit.

In Exercises 9–12, determine the gross profit, then the net profit.

9. The selling price of 100 tablets of medication is $17.50 per bottle; the purchase price is $6.25.

   Gross profit _____

   Dispensing fee $3.50

   Net profit _____

10. The selling price per bottle of 500 capsules of medication is $27.00; the purchase price is $12.00.

    Gross profit _____

    Dispensing fee $5.00

    Net profit _____

11. The selling price per tablet of Motrin® 600 mg tablets is $1.15; the purchase price is 46 cents per tablet. Determine the gross and net profits for a 30-tablet prescription.

    Gross profit _____

    Dispensing fee $4.50

    Net profit _____

12. The selling price per tablet of penicillin 250 mg tablets is 85 cents; the purchase price is 13 cents per tablet. Determine the gross and net profits for a 40-tablet prescription.

    Gross profit _____

    Dispensing fee $3.50

    Net profit _____

In Exercises 13–15, determine the discounted price.

13. The selling price per bottle of 100 tablets of medication is $17.50; the manufacturer offers a 20 percent discount on orders of 25 bottles or more. What would the discounted price be on an order of 30 bottles?

14. The selling price per bottle of 500 capsules of medications $11.00; the manufacturer offers a 15 percent discount for orders of 20 bottles and a discount of 25 percent for orders of 50 bottles or more. What would the discounted price be on an order of 70 bottles?

15. The pharmacy has a sale offering a 20 percent discount on all store-brand cough drops. A 25-count bag sells for $1.99. What is the discounted price?

Inventory

A detailed list of all items for sale and their cost is called an **inventory.** The pharmacy must maintain an accurate inventory list—because of the nature of the business, it is extremely important to maintain adequate amounts of medications and supplies such as pill bottles, labels, and prescription leaflets. Keeping the inventory at optimal levels helps to ensure prescriptions are filled and that medications move off the shelf quickly.

To maintain a balanced profitable inventory, the value of inventory on hand should not exceed the cost of items sold during a specified time frame. Most pharmacies maintain inventory by using a method based on a number of days supply. Some may operate on a 7-day supply method, and others may operate on a 30-day supply method. Most pharmacies now maintain their inventory with computer programs that will automatically calculate profit and place orders. In this section you will learn how to calculate turnover rates and depreciation values.

Turnover

Turnover, simply stated, is the number of times an item is sold from inventory. When a pharmacy opens, there is an initial cost to stock it, and then there is a cost to maintain the stock based on the pharmacy's sales. For example, if the pharmacy's average current stock on hand is worth $200,000.00, that is the average inventory value. Then if the pharmacy spent $1,000,000.00 on maintaining its inventory over the past year, that is the annual inventory purchases. To determine the turnover rate you simply divide the annual inventory purchases by the average inventory value.

EXAMPLE ▶   Determine the turnover rate.

$$\frac{\text{Annual inventory purchases}}{\text{Average inventory value}} = \text{Turnover rate}$$

$$\frac{1,000,000.00}{200,000.00} = 5$$

$$\text{Turnover rate} = 5$$

Depreciation

Depreciation is a decrease in the value of an asset based on the age of the asset in relation to its estimated life. The depreciation value is calculated by using the value of the item when it is no longer usable or when it is considered disposable. An example would be a car that is 20 years old and is no longer drivable, but it has some value based on parts that could still possibly be used elsewhere, or sold for scrap.

Any property owned by the pharmacy is referred to as an asset. There are two types of assets: current assets and long-term assets. Any asset that will be converted into cash or consumed within one year is considered a **current asset.** Items that are not able to be converted into cash or consumed within a year, such as equipment and store buildings, are considered to be **long-term assets.** Over time, long-term assets lose their value from repeated use and basic age of the item. To determine the depreciation value of any given property, use the following formula:

$$\text{Annual depreciation} = \frac{\text{total cost-disposal value}}{\text{estimated life}}$$

EXAMPLE ▶ The pharmacy purchases a refrigerator to store medication for $700.00. The estimated life of the refrigerator is 8 years and the disposal value is $100.00. Determine the annual depreciation value.

$$\text{Annual depreciation value} = \frac{\$700.00 - \$100.00}{8} = \frac{\$600.00}{8}$$

$$\text{Annual depreciation value} = \$75.00$$

Super Tech . . .

Open the CD-ROM that accompanies your textbook and select Chapter 11, Exercise 11-2. Review the animation and example problems, and then complete the practice problems. Continue to the next section of the book once you have mastered the information presented.

✓ Review and Practice 11-2 Inventory

In Exercises 1–3, calculate the turnover rate.

1. The pharmacy's average inventory value is $275,000.00 and annual inventory purchases are $650,000.00.

2. The pharmacy's average inventory value is $36,000.00 and annual inventory purchases are $124,500.00.

3. The pharmacy's average inventory value is $125,000.00 and annual inventory purchases are $500,000.00.

In Exercises 4–6, calculate the depreciation value.

4. The pharmacy purchased a new cash register for $9750.00, the estimated life is 10 years, and the disposal value is $500.00.

5. The pharmacy purchased a new scale for $2000.00. The estimated life is 3 years, and the disposal value is $150.00.

6. The pharmacy purchased 4 new chairs for the waiting area at $80.00 per chair. The estimated life is 5 years, and the disposal value is $15.00.

Reimbursement Considerations

Pharmacies are often reimbursed for prescriptions by insurance companies. The pharmacy signs a contract with the insurance company and the reimbursement amounts are predetermined. The reimbursement amount may be based on a set price for specific medications, on the actual cost of a medication, or the average wholesale price of a medication. The pharmacy must submit a claim to the insurance company for reimbursement. Most claims are filed electronically by using an ICD-9 code (International Classification of Diseases) and the amount of reimbursement is paid per prescription according to the agreed upon contract.

Average Wholesale Price (AWP)

Average wholesale price (AWP):
The average price that pharmacies pay for medications purchased from a wholesaler, based on national averages.

The **average wholesale price (AWP)** is the average price that pharmacies pay for medications purchased from a wholesaler, based on national averages. The AWP is often used by insurance companies to calculate the amount a pharmacy is reimbursed for a prescription. Pharmacies often purchase larger quantities of fast-selling drugs from wholesalers to get a discount, bringing the cost of the medication below the AWP, in turn giving the pharmacy a higher net profit. For example, if the AWP for 500 tablets of a medication is $250.00, the price per tablet is 50 cents (or $0.50). The manufacturer offers the pharmacy a 20 percent discount for orders of 5 bottles or more. The pharmacy orders enough to receive the discount. The pharmacy now pays 40 cents per tablet instead of 50 cents per tablet. A patient brings in a prescription for 30 tablets and the insurance allows reimbursement of $15.00 for the medication, which is the AWP price of 50 cents per tablet × 30 tablets, and also pays a $3.00 dispensing fee. The total allowable reimbursement amount for this prescription is $18.00. The pharmacy paid $12.00 for the medication at the discounted rate of 0.40 cents per tablet × 30 tablets and charges a $3.00 dispensing fee per prescription, for a total of $15.00. The pharmacy made a net profit of $3.00.

EXAMPLE 1 ▶ The AWP is $75.00 per 100 capsules. The insurance company will pay AWP per capsules and a $2.00 dispensing fee. What is the AWP for 30 capsules?

1. Determine the AWP per capsule.

$$\frac{\$75.00}{100} = 0.75 \text{ cents/capsule}$$

2. Determine the AWP for 30 capsules.

$$00.75 \text{ } cents \times 30 = \$22.50$$
$$\text{AWP for 30 capsules} = \$22.50$$

EXAMPLE 2 ▶ The pharmacy orders 100 capsules of a medication from a wholesaler at 15 percent discount. The AWP is $75.00 per 100 capsules. The insurance company will pay AWP per 100 capsules and a $2.00 dispensing fee. Determine how much profit the pharmacy will make per capsule.

1. Determine the discounted price.

$$\$75.00 - 15\% \text{ of } \$75.00 = \text{discounted price}$$
$$\$75.00 \times \$0.15 = \$11.25 \text{ (amount of discount)}$$

AWP	$75.00
Amount of discount	−$11.25
Discounted price	$63.75

2. Determine the prices per capsule.

Reimbursement price = AWP $75.00 + $2.00 fee =
$77.00 ÷ 100 = $0.77 per capsule

Pharmacy's discounted price = $63.75 ÷ 100 =
$0.637/capsule = round to 64 cents

3. Determine profit per capsule

Reimbursement price	$0.77/capsule
Pharmacy's price	−$0.64/capsule
Profit/capsule	$0.13/capsule

Capitation fee

A **capitation fee** is a set amount of money that is paid monthly to the pharmacy for a patient by an insurance company, regardless of whether the patient receives no prescriptions during the month or receives multiple prescriptions. The pharmacy must fill all of the patient's prescriptions, even if the cost exceeds the monthly fee. For example, if the pharmacy agrees to a set fee of $250.00 per month, and that patient does not get any prescriptions filled in January, the pharmacy made $250.00 in January; however, if in February, the patient fills 5 prescriptions costing a total of $450.00, the pharmacy has lost $200.00 in February. But it is still ahead, as the total costs of prescriptions for the two months was $450.00 and the pharmacy received $500.00 from the insurance company.

EXAMPLE ▶

The pharmacy agrees to a monthly capitation fee of $300.00 for a patient.

The patient fills two prescriptions this month. One costs $125.00 and the other costs $82.50. Determine if the pharmacy made a profit.

1. Add the total costs of the prescriptions.

$125.00
+$82.50
$207.50

2. Subtract the total cost of the prescriptions from the monthly fee received by the pharmacy.

Fee paid to pharmacy	$300.00
Total cost of prescriptions	−$207.50
Profit to pharmacy	$92.50

Super Tech...

Open the CD-ROM that accompanies your textbook and select Chapter 11, Exercise 11-3. Review the animation and example problems, and then complete the practice problems. Continue to the next section of the book once you have mastered the information presented.

In Exercises 1–3, calculate the AWP

1. The AWP is $67.50 per 90 tablets. A patient has a prescription for 30 tablets. What is the AWP for the prescription?

2. The AWP is $87.63 for 1000 tablets; you dispense 120 tablets. What is the AWP of the tablets dispensed?

3. The pharmacy orders 200 capsules of a medication from a wholesaler at 10 percent discount. The AWP is $110.00 per 200 capsules. A patient has a prescription for 20 tablets. What is the AWP for the prescription?

In Exercises 4–6, determine if the pharmacy profits from the capitation fee.

4. The pharmacy agrees to a monthly capitation fee of $275.00 for a patient.

   The patient fills two prescriptions this month. One costs $112.00 and the other costs $57.20. Determine if the pharmacy made a profit on this patient's capitation fee.

5. The pharmacy agrees to a monthly capitation fee of $275.00 for another patient. The other patient filled 5 prescriptions, each costing $65.00. Determine if the pharmacy made a profit on this patient's capitation fee.

6. The pharmacy received 2 capitation fees of $275.00 each, and filled a total of 7 prescriptions for two patients. Use the costs of the prescriptions in Exercises 4 and 5 to determine if the pharmacy made a profit.

Calculating Correct Costs and Correct Change

In retail pharmacies it is the pharmacy technicians' responsibility to collect payment for prescriptions. We rely on the high level of electronic technology available today, such as a cash register that displays how much change to give the patient; however, it may not always be available or may malfunction. In the event the pharmacy has a power outage, the pharmacy may very well remain open to provide patients their medication, especially in an emergency situation, such as natural disasters, or inclement weather. Let's review some basic math skills that will assist you in manually calculating correct costs and correct change. You should calculate the cents first, up to the next dollar, and then calculate the dollars to the amount that patient gave you. For example, if the total cost of a single prescription is $3.95 and the patient gives you $5.00, you need to give 5 cents (a nickel) to equal the next dollar amount of $4.00 and $1.00 (1 dollar bill) to equal the total amount the patient gave you of $5.00.

EXAMPLE 1 ▶ Determine the total correct cost of the prescription(s) and the correct change to be given.

1. Add the total costs of the prescription(s).

$125.00
+$82.50
$207.50

2. Subtract the total cost of the prescriptions from the amount given to you from the patient.

Patient gives $210.00
Total cost of prescriptions   −$207.50

Calculate the cents due to the patient.

$208.00 − $207.50 = $0.50   or   50 cents

Calculate the dollars due to the patient.

$210.00 − $208.00 = $2.00

Add the dollar and cents amounts.

$2.00
+0.50
2.50

Change due to patient: $2.50

EXAMPLE 2 ▶ Determine the total correct cost of the prescription(s) and the correct change to be given.

1. Add the total costs of the prescription(s).

$14.75
+$24.00
$38.75

2. Subtract the total cost of the prescriptions from the amount given to you from the patient.

Patient gives $50.00
Total cost of prescriptions   −$38.75

Calculate the cents due to the patient.

$39.00 − $38.75 = $0.25   or   25 cents

Calculate the dollars due to the patient.

$50.00 − $39.00 = $11.00

Add the dollar and cents amounts.

$11.00
+$0.25
$11.25

Change due to patient: $11.25.

Super Tech . . .

Open the CD-ROM that accompanies your textbook and select Chapter 11, Exercise 11-4. Review the animation and example problems, and then complete the practice problems. Continue to the next section of the book once you have mastered the information presented.

Review and Practice 11-4 Calculating Correct Costs and Correct Change

In Exercises 1–5 determine the correct change to be given.

1. Total costs of the prescription(s), $12.76, and amount given by patient $15.00.

2. Total costs of the prescription(s), $49.51, and amount given by patient $60.00.

3. Total costs of the prescription(s), $214.34, and amount given by patient $215.00.

4. Total costs of the prescription(s), $72.62, and amount given by patient $80.00.

5. Total costs of the prescription(s), $191.34, and amount given by patient $200.00.

Chapter 11 Review

Test Your Knowledge

Multiple Choice

Select the best answer and write the letter on the line.

_____ 1. The number of times an item is sold from inventory.
A. Depreciation
B. Overhead
C. Profit
D. Turnover

_____ 2. All costs associated with the pharmacy's operation.
A. Depreciation
B. Overhead
C. Profit
D. Turnover

_____ 3. A decrease in the value of an asset based on the age of the asset.
A. Depreciation
B. Overhead
C. Profit
D. Turnover

_____ 4. The difference between overhead expenses and the income earned from sales.
A. Depreciation
B. Overhead
C. Profit
D. Turnover

Practice Your Knowledge

In Exercises 5–8, determine the overhead cost.

5. Employee salaries: 2 pharmacists at $55,000.00 each, 3 technicians at $30,000.00 each, rent at $14,000.00, utilities $3000.00, insurance $12,000.00, and inventory/supplies $375,000.00.

6. Employee salaries: 3 pharmacists at $65,000.00 each, 2 technicians at $24,500.00 each, rent at $28,000.00, utilities $4600.00, insurance $8000.00, and inventory/supplies $457,495.00.

7. Employee salaries: 1 pharmacist at $80,000.00 and 2 technicians at $26,500.00 each, rent at $15,000.00, utilities $2500.00, insurance $10,500.00, and inventory/supplies $325,000.00.

8. Employee salaries: 4 pharmacists at $67,000.00 each, 6 technicians at $24,500.00 each, rent at $28,000.00, utilities $6000.00, insurance $24,000.00, and inventory/supplies $425,000.00.

In Exercises 9–12 determine the annual profit using the overhead from Exercises 5–8.

9. Annual income from sales is $650,000.00. Using the answer in Exercise 5 determine the annual profit.

10. Annual income from sales is $875,000.00. Using the answer in Exercise 6, determine the annual profit.

11. Annual income from sales is $727,000.00. Using the answer in Exercise 7, determine the annual profit.

12. Annual income from sales is $943,000.00. Using the answer in Exercise 8, determine the annual profit.

In Exercises 13–16 determine the gross profit, then the net profit.

13. The selling price of 200 tablets of medication is $37.50 per bottle; the purchase price is $18.79.

    Gross profit _____

    Dispensing fee $3.50

    Net profit _____

14. The selling price per bottle of 300 capsules of medication is $19.00; the purchase price is $12.00.

    Gross profit_____

    Dispensing fee $3.00

    Net profit _____

15. The selling price per tablet of medication tablets is $1.15; the purchase price is 46 cents per tablet. Determine the gross and net profits for a 60-tablet prescription.

    Gross profit _____

    Dispensing fee $4.50

    Net profit _____

16. The selling price per tablet of medication is 65 cents; the purchase price is 19 cents per tablet. Determine the gross and net profits for a 40-tablet prescription.

    Gross profit _____

    Dispensing fee $2.50

    Net profit _____

In Exercises 17–19, determine the discounted price.

17. The selling price per bottle of 200 tablets of medication is $27.50; the manufacturer offers a 20 percent discount on orders of 10 bottles or more. What would the discount be on an order of 20 bottles?

18. The selling price per bottle of 1000 capsules of medications $17.75; the manufacturer offers a 10 percent discount for orders of 10 bottles and a discount of 15 percent for orders of 20 bottles or more. What would the discount be on an order of 25 bottles?

19. The pharmacy has a sale offering a 25 percent discount on store brand facial tissue. A 120-count box sells for $2.19. What is the discounted price?

In Exercises 20–22, calculate the turnover rate.

20. The pharmacy's average inventory value is $325,000.00 and annual inventory purchases are $975,000.00.

21. The pharmacy's average inventory value is $22,000.00 and annual inventory purchases are $143,000.00.

22. The pharmacy's average inventory value is $25,000.00 and annual inventory purchases are $60,000.00.

In Exercises 23–25, calculate the depreciation value.

23. The pharmacy purchased a new computer for $2375.00. The estimated life is 4 years, and the disposal value is $200.00.

24. The pharmacy purchased a new phone system for $15,000.00. The estimated life is 10 years, and the disposal value is $750.00.

25. The pharmacy purchased a new sign for outside the building for $4750.00. The estimated life is 5 years, and the disposal value is $125.00.

In Exercises 26–28, calculate the AWP.

26. The AWP is $39.57 per 200 tablets. A patient has a prescription for 34 tablets. What is the AWP for the prescription?

27. The AWP is $63.87 for 500 tablets. You dispense 180 tablets. What is the AWP of the tablets dispensed?

28. The pharmacy orders 500 capsules of a medication from a wholesaler at 15 percent discount. The AWP is $96.72 per 100 capsules. A patient has a prescription for 90 tablets. What is the AWP for the prescription.

In Exercises 29–30, determine if the pharmacy profits from the capitation fee.

29. The pharmacy agrees to a monthly capitation fee of $325.00 for a patient. The patient fills four prescriptions this month. The costs are $72.25, $13.99, $184.25 and $54.51. Determine if the pharmacy made a profit on this patient's capitation fee.

30. The pharmacy agrees to a monthly capitation fee of $250.00 for a patient. The patient filled 3 prescriptions, each costing $45.00. Determine if the pharmacy made a profit on this patient's capitation fee.

In Exercises 31–34, determine the correct change to be given.

31. Total costs of the prescription(s) $42.51, and amount given by patient $45.00.

32. Total costs of the prescription(s) $294.51, and amount given by patient $300.00.

33. Total costs of the prescription(s) $17.83, and amount given by patient $25.00.

34. Total costs of the prescription(s) $136.17, and amount given by patient $150.00.

Apply Your Knowledge

What Is the Actual Cost?

You are the pharmacy technician working in a retail pharmacy. You are working in the pharmacy when the following prescription comes in: "Penicillin 250 mg, 1 PO QID for 10 days." The prescription selling price to the patient is $13.99. The patient has insurance. The insurance company will pay the AWP of 29 cents per tablet of medication plus a $2.00 dispensing fee. The pharmacy purchase price is 16 cents per tablet of medication and charges a $3.00 dispensing fee.

Answer the following questions:

1. How many tablets need to be dispensed to fill the prescription?

   _____

2. What is the AWP for the prescription?

   _____

3. What is the actual cost to the pharmacy to fill this prescription?

   _____

4. Did the pharmacy make a profit?

   _____

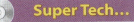

Super Tech...

Open the CD-ROM that accompanies your textbook and complete a final review of Chapter 11. For a final evaluation, take the chapter test and email or print your results for your instructor. A score of 95 percent or above indicates mastery of the chapter concepts.

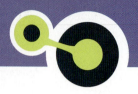

Comprehensive Evaluation

The following test will help you check your dosage calculation skills. Throughout the book you have learned a variety of methods for calculating dosages. In these questions, you should use the methods with which you are most comfortable and competent. Since medication errors are serious, mastery is considered when all problems are calculated correctly.

In Exercises 1–4, determine the percent strength of mixtures.

1. An intravenous (IV) bag contains 200 mL of dextrose 5 percent (a 5 percent drug solution). How many grams of dextrose are in the bag?

2. How many grams of dextrose will a patient receive from a 100-mL bag of dextrose 10 percent (a 10 percent solution of dextrose)?

3. How many grams of dextrose will a patient receive from 20 mL of a 5 percent solution?

4. A full 1000-mL bag of a 10 percent drug solution contains how many grams of the drug?

In Exercises 5–8 interpret the prescription, refer to prescription A.

5. How much Amoxil® should the pharmacy technician dispense?

6. How much Amoxil® should the patient take at one time?

7. How many times can this prescription be refilled?

8. How often should the patient take Amoxil®?

Alan Capsella, MD
Westtown Medical Clinic
989-555-1234

Name _Mark Ward_   Date _April 10, 2012_

Address _____

Rx: _Amoxil – oral susp_

QUANTITY: _100 mL_

SIG: _i tsp po q8h_

Refills: _0_

_MD398475_   _Alan Capsella MD_
Prescriber ID #

Prescription A

In Exercises 9–12, refer to label A.

9. What is the generic name of the drug?

10. At what temperature should the drug be stored?

11. What is the dosage strength?

12. If an adult took twice the usual adult dose, how long would the container last?

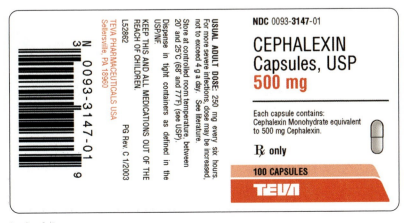

Label A

In Exercises 13 and 14, refer to label B.

13. How much fluid is used to reconstitute the entire container of suspension?

14. If the dosage prescribed for a child is 250 mg, how many doses are in the container?

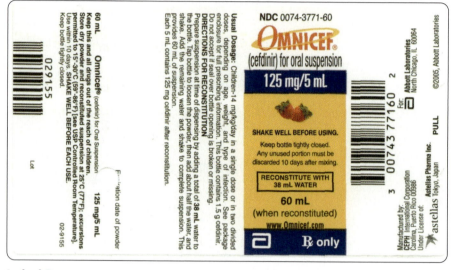

Label B

In Exercises 15 and 16, refer to labels C and D.

15. Using the diluent provided, how much fluid is used to reconstitute the entire vial for sub-Q use?

16. When it is reconstituted, how many international units are in 0.2 mg?

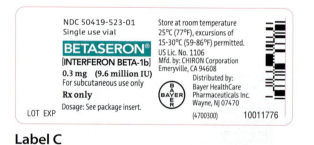

Label C

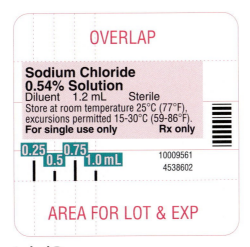

Label D

In Exercises 17–32, calculate the amount to be administered.

17. Ordered: Zoloft® 75 mg PO qd
    On hand: Zoloft® 50-mg scored tablets

18. Ordered: Zovirax® 0.2 g PO q4h 5×/day
    On hand: Zovirax® suspension 200 mg/5 mL

19. Ordered: Nitroglycerin gr 1/200 SL stat
    On hand: Nitroglycerin 0.3-mg tablets

20. Ordered: Morphine sulfate gr ¼ sub-Q q4h prn/pain
    On hand: Morphine sulfate 10 mg/mL vial

21. Ordered: Claforan® 0.6 g IM 30 min pre-op
    On hand: Claforan® 300 mg/mL when reconstituted

22. Ordered: Sandostatin® 0.3 mg sub-Q tid
    On hand: Sandostatin® 200 mcg/mL multidose vial

23. The patient is 14 years old and weighs 97 lb.

    Ordered: Agenerase® sol 17 mg/kg PO tid
    On hand: Agenerase® oral solution, 15 mg/mL

24. The patient is 10 years old and weighs 62 lb.

    Ordered: Vancocin® 10 mg/kg IV q6h
    On hand: Vancocin® 500 mg/100 mL

25. Ordered: Follistim® 200 IU sub-Q qd
    On hand: Follistim® reconstituted to 225 IU/mL

26. The patient is 7 years old and weighs 49 lb.

    Ordered: Zinacef® 20 mg/kg IM q6h
    On hand: Zinacef® 220 mg/mL when reconstituted

In Exercises 27 and 28, determine the estimated days supply.

27. If the patient gets all the refills permitted, how long will the medication last the patient if taken correctly? Refer to prescription B.

28. How long will the medication last the patient if taken correctly? Refer to prescription C.

Alan Capsella, MD
Total Care Clinic
989-555-1234

Name _B. Talbott_   Date _May 10, 2012_

Address _____

Rx: _Norvasc 5 mg_

QUANTITY: _#30_

SIG: _i po_

Refills: _2_

_____MD239485_____   _Cynthia Buckwalter MD_
Prescriber ID #

Prescription B

Ellen Trent, MD
Westtown Medical Clinic
989-555-1234

Name _Arthur Simons_   Date _July 2, 2012_

Address _____

Rx: _Doxycycline 100 mg_

QUANTITY: _#20_

SIG: _cap i po BID pc_

Refills: _0_

_____MD123456_____   _E Trent MD_
Prescriber ID #

Prescription C

In Exercises 29 and 30, determine how many drops are needed for the prescription and what amount to dispense. (Use the conversion factor of 20 drops/mL.)

29. Ordered: 2 gtts AU tid for 10 days.
    On hand: Refer to Label E.

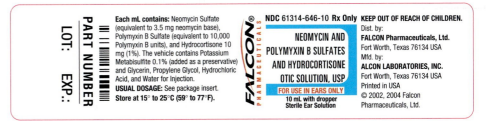

Label E

How many drops are needed? _____

How many milliliters are needed? _____

What amount will be dispensed? _____

30. Ordered: 2 gtts OS qid for 10 days.
    On hand: Refer to Label F.

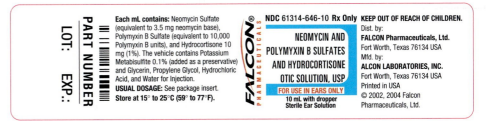

Label F

How many drops are needed? _____

How many mL's are needed? _____

What amount will be dispensed? _____

In Exercises 31–35, find the flow rate.

31. Ordered: 1000 mL RL over 8 hours, using an infusion pump.

32. Ordered: 600 mL D5W over 4 h, 15 gtt/mL tubing.

33. Find the flow rate for an adult who weighs 147 lb.

    Ordered: Garamycin® 1.2 mg/kg IV q8h over 45 min.
    On hand: Garamycin® injectable, 2-mL vial with 40 mg/mL, and 15 gtt/mL tubing; the injection is diluted with 68 mL of D5W.

34. Find the flow rate for a child who weighs 68 lb.

    Ordered: Zofran® 0.1 mg/kg IV over 4 min.
    On hand: Zofran®, premixed with 32 mg in 5 percent dextrose, 50 mL, and 10 gtt/mg tubing.

35. Find the flow rate for an adult who weighs 134 lb.

  Ordered: Ciprofloxacin 10 mg/kg in 150 mL 5 percent DW over 60 min. q12h.
  On hand: Refer to label M. Tubing is 20 gtt/mL.

In Exercises 36–38 convert the following weights to kilograms and determine the correct dose based on the follow order: Penicillin 5 mg/kg

36. 44 lb.

  Weight in kilograms _____

  Dose _____

37. 154 lb

  Weight in kilograms _____

  Dose _____

38. 79 lb

  Weight in kilograms _____

  Dose _____

In Exercises 39 and 40, prepare a dilution from a concentration using the alligation method

39. How would you prepare 500 mL of 50 percent ethanol from 90 percent ethanol? (You will use water as a diluent.)

40. How would you prepare 100 mL of 5 percent iodine from 10 percent and 2 percent iodine solutions?

In Exercises 41 and 42 write a recipe for percent solids and solids

41. Write a recipe for preparing 100 g of 10 percent zinc oxide from zinc oxide powder and petroleum jelly.

42. Write a recipe for preparing 100 mL of 2 percent lidocaine solution.

In Exercises 43–46, use Clark's or Young's Rule to calculate the correct dose.

43. A 7-year-old child needs a dose of medication; the average adult dose is 500 mg.

44. A 2-year-old child needs a dose of medication; the average adult dose is 175 mg.

45. A child who weighs 45 lb needs a dose of medication; the average adult dose is 300 mg.

46. A child who weighs 30 lb needs a dose of medication; the average adult dose is 250 mg.

In Exercises 47–50, perform the following business calculations.

47. Determine overhead costs.

    Employee salaries: 1 pharmacist at $75,000.00, 2 technicians at $27,500.00, rent at $32,000.00, utilities $6000.00, insurance $10,000.00 and inventory/supplies $375,000.00.

48. Determine the gross profit, then the net profit.

    The selling price of 100 tablets of medication is $27.50 per bottle; the purchase price is $11.75

    Gross profit _____

    Dispensing fee $4.50

    Net profit _____

49. The AWP is $176.50 per 100 tablets. A patient has a prescription for 30 tablets. What is the AWP for the prescription?

50. Determine the total correct cost of the prescriptions and the correct change to be given.

    Costs of the prescriptions: $12.42, $9.00, and $16.50.

    What is the total cost of the prescriptions? _____

    Dollar amount given to you by the patient is $50.02.

    What is the correct change to be given to the patient? _____

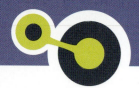

Appendix A

Common Look/Alike and Sound/Alike Medications

As a pharmacy technician, you should perform accurate and safe calculations to prevent medication errors. In addition, be aware of the medication you select. Many medications look alike or sound alike and can be a cause for medication errors as well. Be careful when selecting any medication off the shelf, but take extra caution when working with look/alike and sound/alike medications.

Accupril®	AcipHex® Accolate® Accutane® Altace® Aricept® Monopril®
Acetaminophen and codeine	Acetaminophen and hydrocodone Acetaminophen and oxycodone
AcipHex®	Accupril® Adipex-P® Aricept® Vioxx®
Actos®	Actonel®
Acyclovir	Acetazolamide Famciclovir
Adderal®l	Inderal®
Advair®	Advicor®
Albuterol	Acebutolol
Allegra	Adalat® CC Allegra-D® Asacol® Viagra®
Allegra-D®	Allegra® AlleRx-D
Allopurinol	Apresoline
Alprazolam	Clonazepam Diazepam Lorazepam

Altace®	Accupril® Amaryl® Artane® Norvasc®
Amaryl®	Altace® Avandia® Reminyl Symmetrel®
Ambien®	Amen Ativan® Coumadin®
Amiodarone	Trazodone® Amantadine Amlodipine Amrinone (former nomenclature for Inamrinone)
Amitriptyline	Aminophylline Imipramine Nortriptyline
Amoxicillin	Amoxi® Ampicillin Atarax® Augmentin®
Amoxil®	Amoxicillin
Aricept®	Accupril® AcipHex® Anzemet®
Atacand®	Antacid Avandia®
Atarax®	Ativan®
Atenolol	Metoprolol
Augmentin®	Amoxicillin Ampicillin
Avandia®	Amaryl® Atacand® Avelox® Coumadin® Prandin®
Avapro®	Anaprox® Avelox®
Avelox®	Avandia® Avapro® Cerebyx®
Bactrim®	Biaxin®
Bactrim® DS	Bancap HC
Benadryl®	Benazepril Bentyl®

Benazepril	Benadryl® Benzonatate Donepezil Lisinopril
Benzonatate	Benazepril Benztropine
Biaxin®	Bactrim®
Bisoprolol	Bisacodyl® Fosinopril
Bupropion	Buspirone
Butalbital, acetaminophen, and caffeine	Butalbital, aspirin, and caffeine
Capoten®	Catapres®
Captopril	Carvedilol
Cardizem® CD	Cardizem® SR
Cartia XT® (diltiazem in U.S.)	Diltia XT® Procardia XL® Cartia (aspirin in New Zealand)
Cataflam®	Catapres®
Cefaclor	Cephalexin
Ceftin®	Cefzil® Rocephin®
Cefzil®	Cefol Ceftin® Kefzol
Celebrex®	Celexa®
Celexa®	Zyprexa®
Cephalexin	Cefaclor
Chlorhexidine	Chlorpromazine
Ciprofloxacin	Cephalexin Levofloxacin Ofloxacin
Claritin®	Claritin-D®
Clomiphene	Clomipramine
Clonazepam	Alprazolam Clonidine Clorazepate Diazepam Lorazepam
Clonidine	Colchicine Cardizem® Klonopin®
Cosopt®	Trusopt®

Coumadin®	Avandia® Cardura® Cordarone® Ambien®
Cozaar®	Corgard Hyzaar® Zocor®
Cyclobenzaprine	Cetirizine Cyproheptadine
Danazol	Dantrium®
Danocrine®	Dantrium®
Darvocet®	Percocet
Darvocet-N®	Darvon® Darvon-N®
Depakene®	Depakote
Depakote®	Senokot
Depakote® (delayed release)	Depakote® ER (extended release)
Detrol®	Datril Dextrostat®
Diazepam	Alprazolam Clonazepam Ditropan® Ditropan XL® Lorazepam Midazolam
Dicyclomine	Demeclocycline Diphenhydramine Doxycycline
Diflucan®	Dilantin® Diprivan®
Digoxin	Doxepin
Dilantin®	Diflucan®
Diovan®	Darvon® Zyban®
Diphenhydramine	Dicyclomine Dipyridamole
Ditropan®	Diazepam Diprivan®
Docusate® calcium	Docusate® sodium
Doxazosin	Terazosin Donepezil
Doxepin	Digoxin Doxycycline
Doxycycline	Dicloxacillin Dicyclomine Doxepin

Effexor®	Effexor® XR
Elidel®	Eligard®
Enalapril	Eldepryl® Lisinopril®
Erythromycin	Azithromycin
Esomeprazole	Omeprazole
Estradiol	Ethinyl estradiol Risperdal®
Estratest®	Estratab Estratest® HS
Famotidine	Fluoxetine Furosemide
Fioricet®	Fiorinal®
Flomax®	Flonase® Flovent® Fosamax® Volmax
Flovent®	Atrovent® Flomax® Flonase®
Fluocinolone	Fluocinonide
Fluoxetine	Fluphenazine Fluvoxamine Famotidine Fluvastatin Furosemide Paroxetine
FML Forte	FML S.O.P.
Folinic Acid	Folic acid
Fosinopril	Bisoprolol Furosemide Lisinopril Minoxidil
Furosemide	Famotidine Fluoxetine Fosinopril Torsemide
Glucophage® XR	Glucotrol® XL Glucophage®
Glucotrol®	Glucotrol® XL Glyburide
Glyburide	Glipizide
Haldol®	Halcion®
Humalog®	Humalog® Mix
Humalog, insulin human	Humulin®, insulin human

Humulin® 70/30	Humulin® N Humulin® R
Humulin® N	Humulin® 70/30 Humulin® R Humulin® U Novolin® N Humulin® L
Hydralazine	Hydroxyzine
Hydrochlorothiazide	Hydralazine Hydroxychloroquine
Hydrocortisone	Cortisone Hydralazine Hydrocodone
Hydroxychloroquine	Hydrochlorothiazide
Hydroxyzine	Hydralazine Hydroxyurea
Hyzaar®	Cozaar®
Inderal® LA	Imdur®
Indocin®	Imodium®
Isosorbide mononitrate	Isosorbide dinitrate
K-Lor®	K-Dur® K-Lyte®
Lamictal®	Labetolol Lamisil® Lomotil® Ludiomil®
Lamisil®	Lamicel® Lamictal® Lomotil®
Lanoxin®	Levothyroxine Inapsine® Lasix® Lomotil® Levoxyl® Levsin® Lonox® Lovenox® Xanax®
Lantus®, insulin human	Lente, insulin human
Levaquin®	Heparin Lovenox® Tequin®
Levothyroxine	Lanoxin® Leucovorin Liothyronine
Levoxyl®	Lanoxin® Luvox

Lexapro®	Loxapine
Lipitor®	Zocor®
Lisinopril	Benazepril Enalapril Fosinopril Quinapril Risperdal
Lomotil®	Lamictal® Lamisil Lanoxin Lasix
Loratadine	Losartan
Lorazepam	Alprazolam Clonazepam Diazepam Loperamide Midazolam Temazepam
Lortab®	Lorabid
Lovastatin	Lotensin
Medroxyprogesterone	Methylprednisolone Metolazone
Metformin	Metronidazole
Methotrexate	Methohexital Metolazone
Methylprednisolone	Medroxyprogesterone Prednisone
Metoclopramide	Metolazone Metoprolol Metronidazole
Metoprolol	Atenolol Metoclopramide Metolazone Metronidazole Misoprostol
MetroGel®	MetroGel-Vaginal
Metronidazole	Metformin Methazolamide Metoclopramide Metoprolol Miconazole
Miacalcin®	Micatin
MiraLax®	Mirapex
Mobic®	Moban
Morphine	Hydromorphone Meperidine

Naprosyn®	Naprelan Niaspan
Nasacort®	Azmacort
Neurontin®	Neoral® Noroxin®
Niaspan®	Naprosyn® Niacin
Nifedipine	Felodipine Nicardipine Nimodipine
Nitroglycerin	Glycerin
NitroQuick®	Nitro-Dur®
Nortriptyline	Amitriptyline Desipramine Norpramin®
Norvasc®	Altace® Navane® Nolvadex® Norflex® Vasotec®
Omeprazole	Esomeprazole
Ortho Tri-Cyclen®	Ortho-Cyclen® Tri-Levlen®
Oxybutynin	OxyContin®
Oxycodone	Oxazepam OxyContin®
OxyContin®	MS Contin® Oxybutynin Oxycodone
Paroxetine	Fluoxetine Paclitaxel Pyridoxine
Paxil®	Paclitaxel Plavix® Taxol®
Penicillin	Penicillamine
Percocet®	Percodan®
Phenazopyridine	Promethazine
Phenobarbital	Pentobarbital
Phenytoin	Fosphenytoin Phenylephrine
Plavix®	Elavil® Paxil®

Plendil	Pindolol Pletal® Prilosec® Prinivil®
Potassium chloride	Potassium acetate Potassium citrate Sodium chloride
Pravachol®	Prevacid® Prinivil® Propranolol
Pravastatin	Atorvastatin
Prednisone	Methylprednisolone Potassium Prednisolone Prilosec® Primidone Pseudoephedrine
Premarin®	Prempro® Prevacid® Primaxin® Provera®
Premphase®	Prempro®
Prempro®	Premarin® Premphase®
Prevacid®	Prinivil® Pepcid® Pravachol® Premarin® Prilosec®
Prinivil®	Plendi® Pravachol® Prevacid® Prilose® Prinzide® Proventil®
Promethazine	Phenazopyridine Prochlorperazine
Promethazine with codeine	Promethazine VC with codeine
Proscar®	Procan SR ProSom® Prozac®Provera®
Protonix®	Lotronex®
Pulmicort®	Pulmozyme®
Quinine	Quinidine
Ranitidine	Amantadine Rimantadine Felodipine

Rifampin	Rifabutin
Risperdal®	Estradiol Lisinopril Pediapred® Requip® Reserpine Risperidone Restoril®
Risperidone	Reserpine Risperdal® Risedronate Ropinirole
Robitussin® AC	Robitussin® DAC
Serevent® Diskus®	Serevent®
Seroquel®	Serentil® Serzone Symmetrel® Sinequan® Sertraline
Singulair®	Sinequan®
Soma® Compound	Soma®
Synthroid®	Symmetrel®
Tamoxifen	Tamiflu® Tamsulosin
Temazepam	Flurazepam Lorazepam Oxazepam
Terazosin	Prazosin Doxazosin
Tetracycline	Tetradecyl Sulfate
Timoptic®	Timoptic-XE®
Tizanidine	Nizatidine Tiagabine
Tobrex®	TobraDex®
Topamax®	Toprol-XL®
Topiramate	Torsemide
Toprol-XL®	Tegretol®-XR Topamax®
Tramadol	Toradol® Trandolapril Trazodone Voltaren®
Trazodone	Amiodarone Tramadol
Trileptal®	Tegretol®

Ultracet® (acetaminophen/ tramadol hydrochloride in U.S.)	Ultracef® (cefadroxil in other countries)
Valtrex	Valcyte®
Vancenase AQ	Vanceril® DS
Vanceril®	Vancenase
Vanceril® DS	Vancenase AQ
Verapamil	Verelan®
Viagra®	Allegra®
Vicodin®	Vicodin® ES
Vioxx®	AciPhex® Vicodin® Zyvox®
Wellbutrin®	Wellbutrin® SR
Xalatan®	Xalcom™ (latanoprost/timolol in other countries)
Xanax®	Lanoxin® Zanaflex® Zantac® Zyrtec®
Zantac®	Xanax® Zofran® Zyrtec®
Zithromax®	Zinacef®
Zocor®	Cozaar® Lipitor® Yocon Zestril® Ziac® Zoloft®
Zoloft®	Zocor® Zyloprim®
Zyprexa®	Celexa® Zaroxolyn® Zyprexa® Zydis® Zyrtec®
Zyrtec®	Xanax® Zestril® Zyprexa®

Information obtained from *USP Quality Review*, no. 79, April 2004.

Appendix B

Answer Key—Review and Practice Problems
Chapter 1

Review and Practice

1-1 Arabic Numbers and Roman Numerals

1. 17 1.7 $\frac{1}{7}$

2. 35 3.5 $\frac{3}{5}$

3. 23 2.3 $\frac{2}{3}$

4. 56 5.6 $\frac{5}{6}$

5. 6

6. 12

7. 9

8. 14

9. 24

10. 18

11. $5\frac{1}{2}$

12. $9\frac{1}{2}$

13. $11\frac{1}{2}$

14. 25

15. 19

16. $8\frac{1}{2}$

17. $4 + 17 = 21$

18. $12 + 14 = 26$

19. $8 + 3 = 11$

20. $5 + 5 = 10$

21. $23 - 7 = 16$

22. $16 - 9 = 7$

23. $21 - 3 = 18$

24. $30 - 5 = 25$

1-2 Fractions and Mixed Numbers

1. 17

2. 8

3. 100

4. 1

5. $\frac{3}{16}$

6. $\frac{4}{15}$

7. $\frac{3}{4}$

8. a. = b. < c. >

9. $7\frac{1}{6}$

10. $5\frac{2}{3}$

11. 5

12. $1\frac{3}{5}$

13. $\frac{20}{7}$

14. $\frac{80}{9}$

15. $\frac{11}{10}$

16. $\frac{33}{8}$

1-3 Reducing Fractions to Lowest Terms

1. $\frac{5}{6}$

2. $\frac{1}{2}$

3. $\frac{1}{3}$

4. $\frac{1}{2}$

5. $\frac{1}{10}$

6. $\frac{11}{20}$

7. $\frac{4}{5}$

8. $\frac{6}{17}$

9. $\frac{7}{9}$

10. $\frac{7}{10}$

1-4 Finding Common Denominators

1. LCD: 21 $\quad \dfrac{7}{21}$ and $\dfrac{3}{21}$

2. LCD: 40 $\quad \dfrac{8}{40}$ and $\dfrac{5}{40}$

3. LCD: 200 $\quad \dfrac{8}{200}$ and $\dfrac{5}{200}$

4. LCD: 72 $\quad \dfrac{3}{72}$ and $\dfrac{2}{72}$

5. LCD: 12 $\quad \dfrac{6}{12}$ and $\dfrac{1}{12}$

1-5 Adding Fractions

1. $\dfrac{1}{2}$

2. $\dfrac{4}{7}$

3. $\dfrac{2}{7}$

4. $\dfrac{2}{3}$

5. $\dfrac{13}{24}$

6. $\dfrac{12}{25}$

7. $1\dfrac{5}{24}$

8. $1\dfrac{11}{18}$

9. $2\dfrac{4}{5}$

10. $3\dfrac{8}{11}$

1-6 Subtracting Fractions

1. $\dfrac{1}{5}$

2. $\dfrac{1}{5}$

3. $3\dfrac{1}{3}$

4. $\dfrac{3}{7}$

5. $\dfrac{7}{18}$

6. $\dfrac{7}{12}$

7. $1\dfrac{5}{8}$

8. $2\dfrac{1}{8}$

9. $5\dfrac{1}{2}$

10. $3\dfrac{3}{4}$

1-7 Multiplying Fractions

1. $\dfrac{1}{48}$

2. $\dfrac{6}{35}$

3. $\dfrac{3}{8}$

4. $\dfrac{1}{9}$

5. $\dfrac{1}{6}$

6. $\dfrac{1}{6}$

7. 1

8. $\dfrac{9}{56}$

9. $\dfrac{2}{5}$

10. $\dfrac{7}{24}$

1-8 Dividing Fractions

1. $\dfrac{28}{45}$

2. $\dfrac{15}{44}$

3. $\dfrac{3}{4}$

4. $\dfrac{2}{9}$

5. $2\dfrac{2}{5}$

6. $1\dfrac{7}{15}$

7. $1\dfrac{1}{2}$

8. 1

9. $2\dfrac{5}{8}$

10. $\dfrac{1}{2}$

1-9 Decimals

1. 0.2

2. 0.17

3. 6.5

4. 7.19

5. 0.003

6. >

7. >

8. <

9. >

10. <

11. >

12. >

13. <

14. <

15. >

1-10 Rounding Decimals

1. 14.3	4. 0.2	7. 4.01	10. 20
2. 3.5	5. 9.29	8. 2.21	11. 2
3. 0.9	6. 55.17	9. 11	12. 51

1-11 Adding and Subtracting Decimals

1. 10.82	4. 26.512	7. 13.8	9. 14.25
2. 165.12	5. 2.51	8. 0.82	10. 14.625
3. 13.66	6. 5.57		

1-12 Converting Decimals into Fractions

1. $1\dfrac{1}{5}$ 2. $98\dfrac{3}{5}$ 3. $\dfrac{3}{10}$ 4. $\dfrac{221}{500}$ 5. $5\dfrac{3}{100}$

1-13 Converting Fractions into Decimals

1. 0.4   2. 0.35   3. 0.75   4. 0.5   5. 0.333

1-14 Multiplying Decimals

1. 60.68   2. 9.031   3. 1.26   4. 0.1216   5. 0.275   6. 0.0108

1-15 Dividing Decimals

1. 2   2. 27   3. 127   4. 2   5. 2.5   6. 0.4

Chapter 2

2-1 Percents

1. 0.14	6. 3	11. 6 percent	15. 17 percent
2. 0.3	7. 404 percent	12. 1.3 percent	16. 56 percent
3. 0.02	8. 230 percent	13. 75 percent	17. 110 percent
4. 0.09	9. 70 percent	14. 80 percent	18. 225 percent
5. 1.03	10. 33 percent		

2-2 Ratios

1. $\dfrac{3}{4}$	6. $\dfrac{1}{250}$	12. 0.13	18. 41 percent
2. $\dfrac{4}{9}$	7. 2:3	13. 0.75	19. 7:50
3. $1\dfrac{2}{3}$	8. 6:7	14. 0.4	20. 13:20
4. $\dfrac{10}{1}$	9. 5:4	15. 25 percent	21. 4:1
5. $\dfrac{1}{20}$	10. 7:3	16. 4 percent	22. 7:4
	11. 0.25	17. 22 percent	

2-3 Ratio Strengths

1. 1 g : 20 mL
2. 1 g : 20 mL
3. 5 mg : 1 capsule
4. 40 mg : 1 tablet
5. 1 mg : 5 mL
6. 1 mg : 10 mL
7. 1 g : 5 mL
8. 500 mg : 1 capsule
9. 1 mg : 2 mL
10. 250 mg : 1 tablet

2-4 Proportions

1. $\frac{4}{5} = \frac{8}{10}$
2. $\frac{5}{12} = \frac{10}{24}$
3. $\frac{1}{10} = \frac{100}{1000}$
4. $\frac{2}{3} = \frac{20}{30}$
5. 3 : 4 :: 75 : 100
6. 1 : 5 :: 3 : 15
7. 8 : 4 :: 2 : 1
8. 8 : 7 :: 24 : 21

2-5 Cross-Multiplying

1. Not true
2. True
3. True
4. Not true
5. 1
6. 25
7. 24
8. 150

2-6 Means and Extremes

1. True
2. Not true
3. Not true
4. True
5. 16
6. 8
7. 100
8. 20

2-7 Strength of Mixtures

1. 5 g
2. 6 g
3. 10 g
4. 1 g
5. 50 percent

Chapter 3

3-1 Metric System

1. d
2. d
3. c
4. d
5. b
6. c
7. d
8. b
9. b
10. a
11. 4.5 mL
12. 0.62 g
13. 0.75 mL
14. 0.7 m
15. 12 L
16. 0.75 kg
17. 157 kg
18. 7.75 L
19. 93 mcg
20. 0.08 mg

3-2 Converting within the Metric System

1. 7000 mg
2. 1.2 g
3. 0.023 kg
4. 8000 g
5. 8010 mL
6. 0.1 L
7. 3600 mL
8. 5.233 g
9. 0.5 L
10. 3250 g
11. 250 mcg
12. 462,000 mcg
13. 0.25 mg
14. 0.075 mg
15. 60,000 mcg
16. 500,000 mcg
17. 0.008 g
18. 0.02 g

3-3 Other Systems of Measurements

1. m or ♏
2. dr or ℨ
3. gr
4. oz or ℥
5. gtt
6. tsp or t
7. tbs or T
8. pt
9. mEq
10. U
11. gr vii or gr $\overline{\text{vii}}$
12. ℨ v or ℨ $\bar{\text{v}}$
13. 3 oz ℥ or iii or ℥ $\overline{\text{iii}}$
14. 8 oz or ℥ viii or ℥ $\overline{\text{viii}}$
15. gr 14 or gr $\overline{\text{xiv}}$
16. gr 17 or gr $\overline{\text{xvii}}$
17. $\frac{1}{2}$ tsp
18. $\frac{1}{2}$ tbs
19. gr ss
20. $\frac{1}{2}$ oz or ℥ ss

3-4 Converting among Metric, Apothecary, and Household Systems

1. 4 tsp (using Table 3-7)
2. 25 tsp
3. 24 tsp
4. 8 oz
5. gr $\frac{1}{4}$
6. 900 mg
7. gr $\frac{1}{6}$
8. gr 37ss
9. 92.4 lb
10. 20 kg
11. 10 mL
12. 143 lb
13. 85 kg
14. $2\frac{2}{3}$ tbs (using Table 3-7)
15. 960 mL

3-5 Temperature

1. 93.2°F
2. 105.8°F
3. 35°C
4. 38.9°C
5. 7.4°C
6. 100°C
7. 77°F
8. 212°F
9. 15°C
10. 152.6°F

3-6 Time

1. 0235
2. 0757
3. 0008
4. 0055
5. 1349
6. 1514
7. 2354
8. 2219
9. 1859
10. 0426
11. 12:11 a.m.
12. 12:36 a.m.
13. 3:25 a.m.
14. 8:49 a.m.
15. 1:13 p.m.
16. 3:27 p.m.
17. 9:45 p.m.
18. 11:59 p.m.
19. 8:37 p.m.
20. 6:18 p.m.

Chapter 4

4-1 The Rights of Drug Administration

1. D   2. F   3. A   4. G   5. B   6. C   7. E

4-2 Abbreviations

1. immediately   _____ stat _____
2. twice a day   _____ bid _____
3. hour of sleep, at bedtime   _____ hs _____

4. after meals ———— p.c. ————

5. when necessary, when required, as needed ———— prn ————

6. every morning ———— qam ————

7. daily ———— qd ————

8. 4 times a day ———— qid ————

9. 3 times a day ———— tid ————

10. before meals ———— a.c. ————

11. right ear ———— A.D.

12. both ears ———— A.U. ————

13. left ear ———— A.S. ————

14. right eye ———— O.D. ————

15. both eyes ———— O.U. ————

16. left eye ———— O.S. ————

17. discontinue ———— d.c. ————

18. dispense ———— disp————

19. one and one-half ———— i_ss ————

20. no known drug allergies ———— NKDA ————

21. nothing by mouth ———— NPO ————

22. after ———— P ————

23. every ———— Q ————

24. without ———— s̄ ————

25. write on label ———— sig. s ————

26. as directed ———— ud ————

27. teaspoon ———— tsp ————

28. tablespoon ———— tbs ————

29. capsule ———— cap ————

30. compound ———— comp ————

31. dilute ———— dil. ————

32. enteric-coated ———— EC ————

33. elixir ———— elix. ————

34. extract ———— ext. ————

35. fluid ———— fl ————

36. drop, drops ———— gtt, gtts ————

37. hypodermic ———— H ————

38. long-acting ———— LA ————

39. liquid _____ liq _____

40. metered-dose inhaler _____ MDI _____

41. solution _____ sol, soln. _____

42. slow-release _____ SR _____

43. suppository _____ supp. _____

44. suspension _____ susp. _____

45. syrup _____ syr, syp. _____

46. syringe _____ syr _____

47. tablet _____ tab _____

48. tincture _____ tr, tinct, tinc. _____

49. ointment _____ ung, oint _____

50. by mouth; orally _____ PO _____

51. Rectally _____ R _____

52. Subcutaneous, beneath the skin _____ Sub-q _____

53. Sublingually, under the tongue _____ SL _____

54. Topical, applied to the skin surface _____ top _____

55. Intramuscular _____ IM _____

4-3 Interpreting Physicians' Orders and Prescriptions

1. The card is complete.

2. 90

3. Three times a day

4. 50 mg

5. 180 days or approximately 6 months

6. The strength of the oral suspension is not listed.

7. 100 mL; however, the pharmacy technician still needs to know the solution strength.

8. One teaspoon (i tsp)

9. It cannot be refilled.

10. Every 8 h (q8h)

11. Prescription C does not include adequate information to determine the dose. Norvasc® comes in strengths of 2.5, 5, and 10 mg per tablet. It is unknown which strength to use. The frequency of dosing is missing and should read "daily" to ensure proper dosing. The form of the medication is also missing.

12. 30; however, the pharmacy technician still needs to know the proper dosage.

13. One; 1 po, but the frequency of dosing needs to be clarified.

14. This prescription can be refilled 2 times.

15. It is not possible to determine how long it will last since the number per day is not written.

4-4 Controlled Substances

1. **Yes**

   $1 + 2 + 2 = 5$

   $7 + 5 + 4 = 16$

   $16 \times 2 = 32$

   $32 + 5 = 37$

2. **Yes**

   $9 + 1 + 8 = 18$

   $3 + 4 + 6 = 13$

   $13 \times 2 = 26$

   $26 + 18 = 44$

3. **No**

   $5 + 3 + 6 = 14$

   $4 + 2 + 7 = 13$

   $13 \times 2 = 26$

   $26 + 14 = 40$

4. **No**

   $6 + 1 + 9 = 16$

   $7 + 8 + 4 = 19$

   $19 \times 2 = 38$

   $38 + 16 = 54$

5. **No**

   $1 + 5 + 4 = 10$

   $3 + 2 + 6 = 11$

   $11 \times 2 = 22$

   $22 + 10 = 32$

4-5 Detecting Errors and Forged or Altered Prescriptions

1. B   2. C   3. D   4. A   5. F   6. E

Chapter 5

5-1 Drug Labels and Package Inserts

1. Provera®

2. Medroxyprogesterone acetate

3. Multiple doses (500 tablets)

4. Pharmacia-Upjohn Co. (a division of Pfizer, Inc)

5. 10 mg/tablet

6. 20–25°C (68–77°F); store at controlled room temperature.

7. Fluoxetine

8. Prozac®

9. 20 mg/capsule

10. Eli Lilly and Co.

11. 0777-3105-02

12. Dispense in tight, light-resistant container, keep tightly closed, store at controlled room temperature 59–86°F (15–30°C).

13. Tigan®

14. King Pharmaceuticals

15. 300 mg/capsule

16. Multiple doses (100 capsules)

17. 25°C (77°F)

18. Dispense in tight, child-resistant container.

19. Cefprozil

20. Oral

21. See package insert.

22. 125 mg/5 mL

23. 2 teaspoons

24. 7.5 days

25. Nitroglycerin tablets

26. Nitrostat®

27. Sublingual

28. 20–25°C (68–77°F) (see USP); dispense in original, unopened container.

29. 100

30. 0.4 mg/tab (1/150 gr/tab)

31. Amoxicillin and clavulanate potassium

32. With 170 mL of water in two parts

33. 2/3 of the water

34. 600 mg/5 mL Amoxicillin and 42.9 mg per 5 mL Clavulanate Potassium

35. Keep tightly closed. Shake well before using. Store reconstituted suspension under refrigeration. Discard unused suspension after 10 days.

36. 20

37. Zyrtec®

38. Cetirizine HCl

39. 5 mg per tab

40. 0069-0732-66

41. Orally. The label states that the medication is a tablet.

42. 100 tablets divided by 30 per prescription equals 3 with 10 tablets left over.

43. Pfizer Labs

5-2 *Reading Drug Labels*

1. 57664-397-99
2. 500 mg per tablet
3. Yes
4. 100
5. Levoxyl®
6. King Pharmaceuticals
7. 50 mcg/tablet
8. 100
9. Morphine sulfate controlled-release
10. 100
11. 30 mg/capsule
12. No
13. 59 mL of water
14. 125 mg/5 mL
15. 75 mL
16. 14 days

5-3 *Parenteral Drugs*

1. 50,000 units
2. For intramuscular use
3. Reconstituting with 9.8 mL of sodium chloride injection containing 2 percent procaine hydrochloride will result in 5000 units per mL.
4. Discard after 14 days.
5. 500 mg, 100 mg/mL when reconstituted with 4.8 mL of sterile water for injection
6. 0069-3150-83
7. Azithromycin
8. for IV infusion only
9. Store below 86°F. After reconstitution, solution should be refrigerated. Discard after 7 days.
10. 250000 Units/mL, 500000 Units/mL or 1000000 Units/mL depending on how it is reconstituted.
11. For intravenous infusion only
12. 0049-0530-28
13. rDNA origin
14. 100 units/mL
15. Lilly
16. 100 doses
17. 150 mg/mL
18. Medroxyprogesterone acetate
19. Single-dose vial
20. Pharmacia-Upjohn Co. (a division of Pfizer Inc.)

5-4 Drugs Administered by Other Routes

1. Becaplermin
2. 0.01 percent of the gel
3. For topical use only
4. 2–8°C (36–46°F), DO NOT FREEZE.
5. Transdermally
6. 50458-036-05
7. 100 mcg/h for 72 h
8. 5
9. For oral inhalation only
10. Flunisolide
11. 100 metered inhalations
12. No, label reads for oral inhalation only

5-5 Package Inserts

1. Description
   Clinical pharmacology
   Indications and usage
   Contraindications
   Warnings
   Precautions
   Adverse reactions
   Overdosage
   Dosage and administration
   Preparation for administration

2. Manufacturer supply chemical and physical description of the drug
   Description of the actions of the drug
   Medical conditions in which the drug is safe and effective; instructions for use
   Conditions and situations under which the drug should not be administered
   Information about serious, possibly fatal, side effects
   Information about drug interactions and other conditions that may cause unwanted side effects
   Less serious, anticipated side effects that can be caused by the drug
   Effects of overdoses and instructions for treatment
   Recommended dosages under various and recommendations for administration routes
   Directions for reconstituting or diluting the drug, if necessary
   Information on dosage strengths and forms of the drug available

3. Aricept® (donepezil hydrochloride) is a reversible of the drug inhibitor of the enzyme acetylcholinesterase, known chemically as ($\pm$)-2, 3-dihydro-5, 5-dimethoxy-2-[[1-(phenylmethyl)-4 -piperidinyl]methyl]-1H-inden-1-one hydrochloride.

   Current theories on the pathogenesis of the cognitive signs and symptoms of Alzheimer's disease attribute some of them to a deficiency of cholinergic neurotransmission.
   Aricept® is indicated for the treatment of mild to moderate dementia of the Alzheimer's type.

Aricept® is contraindicated in patients with known hypersensitivity to donepezil hydrochloride or to piperidine derivatives.

Gastrointestinal conditions: Through their primary action, cholinesterase inhibitors may be expected to increase gastric acid secretion due to increased cholinergic activity.

Use with anticholinergics: Because of their mechanism of action, cholinesterase inhibitors have the potential to interfere with the activity of anticholinergic medications.

These include nausea, diarrhea, insomnia, vomiting, muscle cramps, fatigue, and anorexia. These adverse events were often of mild intensity and transient, resolving during continued Aricept® treatment without the need for dose modification.

As in any case of overdose, general supportive measures should be utilized. Overdosage with cholinesterase inhibitors can result in cholinergic crisis characterized by severe nausea, vomiting, salivation, sweating, bradycardia, hypotension, respiratory depression, collapse, and convulsions.

The dosages of Aricept® shown to be effective in controlled clinical trials are 5 mg and 10 mg administered once per day.

Aricept® should be taken in the evening, just prior to retiring. Aricept® can be taken with or without food.

Aricept® is supplied as film-coated, round tablets containing either 5 mg or 10 mg of donepezil hydrochloride.

Chapter 6

6-1 Doses and Dosages

1. Desired dose: 250 mg, 4
2. Desired dose: 500 mg, 2
3. Desired dose: 30 mg, 1
4. Desired dose: 250 mg, 3
5. Desired dose: 150 mcg, 1
6. Desired dose: 1 tsp, 4, if necessary
7. Desired dose: 10 cc, 4 to 6, as needed
8. Desired dose: 1000 mg, 1
9. Desired dose: 15 mg, 2, if necessary
10. Desired dose: 50 mcg, 1
11. Desired dose: 88 mcg, 1
12. Desired dose: 500 mg, 1
13. Desired dose: 0.25 mg, 1
14. Desired dose: 7.5 mL, 4
15. Desired dose: $1\frac{1}{2}$ tsp, 6
16. Desired dose: 137 mcg, 1
17. Desired dose: 0.25 mg, 1
18. Desired dose: 1000 mg, 1

6-2 Calculating the Amount to Dispense

1. Amount to dispense: 2 tablets
   Drug order: Take 2 tablets Thorazine® (20 mg) by mouth 3 times a day.

2. Amount to dispense: 10 mL
   Drug order: Take 10 mL (2 teaspoons) Zantac® by mouth 2 times a day.

3. Amount to dispense: 10 mL
   Drug order: Take 10 mL (2 teaspoons) Ceclor® by mouth daily.

4. Amount to dispense: 2 tablets
Drug order: Take 2 tablets (0.6mg) Nitroglycerin under tongue immediately.

5. Amount to dispense: 5 mL
Drug order: Take 5 mL (1 teaspoon) Amoxicillin by mouth 3 times daily.

6. Amount to dispense: 2 tablets
Drug order: Take 2 tablets (108 mg) Tricor® by mouth daily.

7. Amount to dispense: 2 capsules
Drug order: Take 2 capsules (20 mg) Procardia® by mouth 3 times a day.

8. Amount to dispense: 2 tablets
Drug order: Take 2 tablets (15mg) moexipril hydrochloric by mouth everyday with meals.

9. Amount to dispense: 2 tablets
Drug order: Take 2 tablets (0.3mg) Synthroid® by mouth every day.

10. Amount to dispense: 2 tablets
Drug order: Take 2 tablets (0.2g) Wellbutrin® by mouth 2 times a day.

11. Amount to dispense: 10 mL
Drug order: Take 10 mL (2 teaspoons) Keflex® by mouth every 12 hours.

12. Amount to dispense: 1.5 mL
Drug order: Inject 1.5 mL Decadron® intramuscularly 4 times per day.

13. Amount to dispense: $\frac{1}{2}$ tablet
Drug order: Take a half tablet (100 mg) Ketoconazole by mouth 2 times a day.

14. Amount to dispense: 3.75 mL
Drug order: Take 3.75 mL (¾ teaspoon) Erythromycin by mouth 2 times a day.

6-3 Estimated Days Supply

1. 60 days   2. 10 days   3. 30 days   4. 14 days   5. 30 days

Chapter 7

7-1 Tablets and Capsules

1. 1 tablet, 90 days
2. 1 tablet, 30 days
3. 1 tablet, 10 days
4. $1\frac{1}{2}$ tablets
5. $1\frac{1}{2}$ tablets
6. 2 tablets
7. $2\frac{1}{2}$ tablets
8. $1\frac{1}{2}$ tablets
9. $1\frac{1}{2}$ tablets
10. 3 tablets

7-2 Liquid Medications

1. 4 mL
2. 7.5 mL
3. 5 mL
4. 0.78125 mL = 0.8 mL
5. 10 mL, 5 days
6. 30 mL, 15 days
7. 20 mL, 10 days
8. 20 mL, 7 days

7-3 Parenteral Dosages

1. Administer 2.5 mL.

2. Administer 2 mL.

3. Administer 0.3 mL.

4. Administer 0.5 mL.

5. Administer 0.8 mL.

6. Administer 1 mL.

7. Administer 0.8 mL.

8. Administer 0.5 mL.

9. Administer: 2.5 mL   Syringe: standard syringe

10. Administer: 2 mL   Syringe: standard syringe

11. Administer: 2 mL   Syringe: standard syringe

12. Administer: 0.4 mL   Syringe: 0.5-mL tuberculin syringe

13. Administer: 0.3 mL   Syringe: 0.5 mL tuberculin syringe

14. Administer: 0.8 mL   Syringe: 1-mL tuberculin syringe

15. Administer: 0.88 mL   Syringe: 1-mL tuberculin syringe

7-4 Reconstituting Medications

1. 17.5 mL of sterile diluent

2. 20 mg/1 mL

3. Sterile water or bacteriostatic water for injection

4. 0.75 mL

7-5 Other Medication Routes

1. 5 mL

2. 0.5 mL

3. 1.25 mL

4. 2 suppositories

5. One 10-mg and one 5-mg suppository

6. $\frac{1}{2}$ suppository. Check manufacturer's directions to verify that suppository can be divided before administration.

7. 2.5 mL = 50 drops, patient needs 48 drops, 4 drops for 12 days

8. One TTS-3 patch and one TTS-2 patch

9. One 0.1 mg/day patch with one 0.05 mg/day patch, or two 0.75 mg/day patches

10. One 0.2 mg/h patch with one 0.1 mg/h patch

11. 8.33 days, 1 drop in each eye 6 times a day = 12 drops a day, $100 \div 12 = 8.33$

12. 15 days, 0.5 mL per 4 times per day = 2 mL per day, 30 ÷ 2 =15

13. 30 days, 1 per day, 30 ÷ 1 = 30

14. 2 days, 1 two time a day, 4 ÷ 2 = 2

Chapter 8

8-1 IV Solutions

1. Hypertonic
2. Hypotonic
3. Isotonic
4. KVO fluids
5. Replacement fluids
6. Maintenance fluids
7. Therapeutic fluids

8-2 Calculating Flow Rates

1. 167 mL/h
2. 150 mL/h
3. 125 mL/h
4. 100 mL/h
5. 125 mL/h
6. 83 mL/h
7. 94 mL/h
8. 100 mL/h
9. 75 mL/h
10. 83 mL/h
11. 14 gtt/min
12. 8 gtt/min
13. 31 gtt/min
14. 14 gtt/min
15. 50 gtt/min
16. 16 gtt/min
17. 21 gtt/min
18. 50 gtt/min
19. 50 gtt/min
20. 50 gtt/min
21. 28 gtt/min
22. 23 gtt/min

8-3 Infusion Time and Volume

1. 12 h 3 min
2. 4 h
3. 24 h, 12 min
4. 5 h
5. $2\frac{1}{2}$ h or 2 h 30 min
6. The infusion will be finished at 0800 the next day.
7. The infusion will be finished the next day at 11:30 a.m.
8. The infusion will be finished at 0100 the next day.
9. The infusion will be finished at 4 a.m. the next day.
10. The infusion will be finished at 2255, or 10:55 p.m.
11. 187.5 mL
12. 800 mL
13. 1500 mL
14. 150 mL

8-4 Intermittent IV Infusions

1. 250 mL/h
2. 63 gtt/min
3. 150 mL/h
4. 25 gtt/min

Chapter 9

9-1 Compounds

1.

0.9% sodium chloride	
NaCl	4.5 g
Water	QSAD 500 mL

2.

2% lidocaine	
Lidocaine	1 g
Water	QSAD 50 mL

3.

3% hydrocortisone ointment	
Hydrocortisone	3 g
Petroleum jelly	97 g

9-2 Alligations

1. 12 percent dextrose water =

   20 percent dextrose 466.7 mL

   5 percent dextrose QSAD 1000 mL, or 533.3 mL of 5 percent dextrose

2. 30 percent ethyl alcohol =

   95 percent ethyl alcohol 473.7 mL

   Water qsad 1500 mL or 1026.30 of water

3. 20 percent iodine =

   25 percent iodine 67 mL

   10 percent iodine QSAD 100 mL, or 33 mL of 10 percent iodine

9-3 Preparing a Dilution from Concentrate

1.

1% hydrocortisone cream	
2.5% hydrocortisone cream	20 g Cream base
Water	QSAD 50 g

2.

40% dextrose	
80% dextrose	125 mL
Water	QSAD 250 mL

3.

30% ethyl alcohol	
95% ethyl alcohol	473.7 mL
Water	QSAD 1500 mL

4.

100 mL 20% Iodine	
25% Iodine	66.7 mL
10% Iodine	33.3 mL

9-4 Insulin

1. 1 vial
2. 1 vial
3. 2 vials
4. 6 vials

5. 2 vials
6. 2 vials
7. 2 vials

8. 5 vials
9. 3 vials
10. 1 vial

Chapter 10

10-1 Pharmacokinetics—How Drugs Are Used by the Body

1. Biotransformation   2. Absorption   3. Elimination   4. Distribution

10-2 Pediatric and Geriatric Dosing

1. 30 kg
2. 35 kg

3. 24.55 kg
4. 16.82 kg

5. 69.09 kg
6. 91.82 kg

7. Two doses of 5 mg, or 10 mg/day, are within a safe range.
   Amount to dispense: 0.5 mL

8. The order is above the appropriate starting dosage for a patient of this weight. Consult the physician.

9. The order of 225 mg per dose is above the maximum safe dose for a child with a severe infection. Consult the prescribing physician.

10. The ordered dose of 30 mg is within a safe range.
    Amount to dispense 1.2 mL

10-3 Pediatric Specific Dosage Calculations

1. 300 mg   2. 60 mg   3. 150 mg   4. 75 mg

10-4 Dosage Based on Body Surface Area (BSA)

1. 0.57 m^2
2. 0.58 m^2
3. 0.25 m^2
4. 0.37 m^2
5. $1.0 = 1 \text{ m}^2$

6. 0.69 m^2
7. 0.36 m^2
8. 0.42 m^2
9. 144 mcg
10. 0.26 mg

11. 14.65 mcg
12. 0.18 mg
13. 14.7 mL/dose
14. 1.7 mL/dose
15. 1.1 mL

Chapter 11

11-1 *General Business Considerations*

1. $721,000.00
2. $669,045.00
3. $368,750.00
4. $1,037,000.00
5. $174,000.00
6. $25,955.00
7. $336,250.00
8. $673,500.00
9. $11.25, $7.75
10. $15.00, $10.00
11. $20.70, $16.20
12. $28.80, $25.30
13. $420.00
14. $557.50
15. $1.59

11-2 *Inventory*

1. 2.36
2. 3.46
3. 4
4. $925.00/year
5. $616.67/year
6. $52.00/year

11-3 *Reimbursement Considerations*

1. $22.50
2. $10.52
3. $11.00
4. Yes. Profit of $105.80
5. No. Loss of $50.00
6. Yes. Profit of $55.80

11-4 *Calculating Correct Costs and Correct Change*

1. $2.24
2. $10.49
3. $0.66
4. $7.38
5. $8.66

Glossary

absorption Movement of a drug from the site where it is given into the bloodstream.

alligation One method for calculating dilutions.

amount to dispense The volume of liquid number or solid dosage units that contain the desired dose.

average wholesale price (AWP) The average price that pharmacies pay for medications purchased from a wholesaler based on national averages.

B

biotransformation Chemical changes of a drug in the body.

C

capitation fee A set amount of money that is paid monthly to the pharmacy for a patient by an insurance company, regardless of whether the patient does not receive any prescription during the month or receives multiple prescriptions.

caplet Oval-shaped pill similar to a tablet but having a coating for easy swallowing.

capsule Oval-shaped gelatin shell, usually in two pieces, that contains powder or granules.

centi The metric prefix that indicates one-hundredth of the basic unit.

Clark's Rule Calculation that uses the weight of the child to determine the desired dose of medication.

common denominator Any number that is a common multiple of all the denominators in the fractions of your expression.

compound Two or more chemicals mixed together to make a specific mixture or solution.

controlled substance A drug that has the potential for addiction, abuse, or chemical dependency.

cross-multiplying Multiplying the numerator of the first fraction by the denominator of the second fraction and the numerator of the second fraction by the denominator of the first fraction.

current asset Any asset that will be converted into cash or consumed within one year.

D

denominator The number listed below the fraction bar or the bottom number of your fraction; represents the whole.

depreciation A decrease in the value of an asset based on the age of the asset in relation to its estimated life.

desired dose The amount of the drug that the patient is to take a single time.

dilution A solution created from an already prepared concentrated solution.

discount A reduction in price from the normal selling price.

distribution Movement of a drug from the bloodstream into other body tissues and fluids.

dosage ordered The amount of drug the physician has ordered and the frequency that it should be taken or given.

dosage strength The amount of drug per dosage unit.

dose on hand Amount of drug contained in each dosage unit.

dose unit The unit by which the drug will be measured when taken by or given to the patent.

dram Common unit of volume in the apothecary system.

E

elimination The process in which a drug leaves the body.

enteric-coated Medications that dissolve only in the alkaline environment of the small intestines.

estimated days supply How long the medication will last the patient if taken correctly.

equivalent fractions Two fractions written differently that have the same value.

F

Facts and Comparisons A comprehensive drug information reference available in print, online, or on a PDA; updated on a monthly basis.

Final volume/final strength The amount and strength of a prepared mixture from dilutions or concentrations.

fraction proportion Mathematical statement that indicates two fractions are equal.

G

gelcap Medication, usually liquid in a gelatin shell; not designed to be opened.

generic name A drug's official name.

geriatric Typically considered anyone over the age of 65.

grain The basic unit of weight in the apothecary system.

gram The basic unit of measurement for weight in the metric system.

gross profit The difference between the purchase price the pharmacy paid for products, for example, medication, and the markup (selling) price.

H

heparin lock An infusion port attached to an already inserted catheter for IV access; flushed with heparin.

hypertonic Fluids that draw fluids from cells and tissues across the cell membrane into the bloodstream, such as 3 percent saline.

hypotonic Fluids that move across the cell membrane into surrounding cells and tissues, such as $\frac{1}{2}$ NS ((0.45% Sodium Chloride) and 0.3% Sodium Chloride (NaCl).

I

inhalant Medication administered directly to the lungs, usually through a metered-dose inhaler or nebulizer.

insulin A pancreatic hormone that stimulates glucose metabolism.

international unit The amount of medication needed to produce a certain effect, standardized by international agreement.

intradermal (ID) Medication administered between the layers of the skin by injection.

intramuscular (IM) Medication administered into a muscle by injection.

intravenous (IV) Medication administered delivered directly into the bloodstream through a vein.

inventory A detailed list of all items for sale and their cost.

isotonic Fluids that do not affect the fluid balance of the surrounding cells or tissues, such as D5W, NS, and lactated Ringer's.

K

kilo The metric prefix that indicates the basic unit multiplied by 1000.

KVO fluids Fluids prescribed to keep the veins open that provide access to the vascular system for emergency situations.

L

least common denominator (LCD) This is the smallest number that is a common multiple of the denominators in a group of fractions.

liter The basic unit for measurement of volume in the metric system.

long-term asset Items that cannot be converted into cash or consumed within a year, such as equipment and store buildings.

M

maintenance fluids Fluids that maintain the fluid and electrolyte balance for patients.

means and extremes For the equation $A:B::C:D$, B and C are the means (middle) and A and D are the extremes (ends).

medication administration record (MAR) A record that contains a list of medications ordered for a patient and space to document the administration of those medications.

meter The basic unit of length in the metric system.

micro The metric prefix that indicates one-millionth of the basic unit.

milli The metric prefix that indicates one-thousandth of the basic unit.

milliequivalents A unit of measure based on the chemical combining power of the substance; one-thousandth of an equivalent of a chemical.

minim Common unit of volume in the apothecary system.

mixed number A fraction that is greater than 1 and written as a whole number and a fraction.

N

National Formulary (NF) A book of public pharmacopeia standards.

NDC (National Drug Code) number A specific identification number on the drug product.

net profit The difference between the selling price and the purchase price plus a dispensing fee.

nomogram A special chart used to determine a patient's body surface area (BSA).

numerator The number on the top of the fraction bar; represents parts of the whole.

O

ounce Common unit of volume in the apothecary system.

overhead All costs associated with business operations.

P

package insert Paper insert that provides complete and authoritative information about a medication.

parenteral Medication administered by a route other than oral; medications that are delivered outside the digestive tract; most often referred to as injections.

pediatric Patients under the age of 18 years.

percent Means per 100, or divided by 100.

pharmacokinetics The study of what happens to a drug after it is administered to a patient.

***Physicians' Desk Reference* (PDR)** A compilation of information from package inserts of medications; reprinted every year.

prescriptions A written or computerized form for medication orders; used in outpatient settings.

prime number A whole number other than 1 that can be evenly divided only by itself and 1.

profit The difference between overhead expenses and income earned from sales.

proportion A mathematical statement that two ratios are equal.

Q

QSAD Abbreviation of a Latin phrase meaning "a sufficient quantity to adjust the dimensions to . . . "; used in preparing solutions.

R

ratio Expression of the relationship of a part to the whole.

ratio proportion Mathematical statement that indicates two ratios are equal.

ratio strength The amount of drug in a solution or the amount of drug in a solid dosage form such as a tablet or capsule; dosage strength.

reconstitute Process of adding liquid to a powder medication.

rectal Medication administered through the rectum, usually a suppository.

Remington: *The Science and Practice of Pharmacy* A comprehensive reference book with 10 sections providing essential information on the practice of pharmacy; published every five years.

replacement fluids Fluids that replace electrolytes or fluids lost from dehydration, hemorrhage, vomitting, or diarrhea.

route Method by which a medication is to be delivered to a patient.

S

saline lock An infusion port attached to an already inserted catheter for IV access; flushed with saline

scored Medication tablets having indented lines indicating where they may be broken or divided.

secondary line Also known as piggyback; line used to add medications or other additives to an existing IV or infusion port.

solute Chemicals dissolved in a solvent, making a solution; drug or substance being dissolved in a solution.

solution The combined mixture of solvent or diluent.

solvent or diluent Liquid used to dissolve other chemicals, making a solution.

spansules Special capsule that contains coated granules to delay the release of the medication.

strength of mixtures Are used to indicate the concentration of ingredients in mixtures such as solutions, lotions, creams, and ointments.

subcutaneously (sub-Q) Medication administered under the skin by injection.

sustained-release Medication that releases slowly into the bloodstream over several hours.

T

tablet A solid disk or cylinder that contains a drug plus inactive ingredients.

therapeutic fluids IV fluids that deliver medication to patients.

topical Medication applied to the skin.

trade name The name of the drug owned by a specific company, also referred to as *brand name* or *proprietary name*.

transdermal Medication administered through the skin, typically via a patch.

turnover The number of times an item is sold from inventory.

U

U-100 Common concentration of insulin; meaning that 100 units of insulin is contained in 1 mL of solution.

unit The amount of a medication required to produce a certain effect.

***United States Pharmacopeia* (USP)** The official public standards-setting authority for all prescription and over-the-counter medicines, dietary supplements, and other health care products manufactured and sold in the United States.

V

vaginal Medication administered through the vagina, in suppository, cream, or tablet form.

Y

Young's Rule Calculation that uses the age of the child to determine the desired dose of medication.

Credits

Index

MATH FORMULAS

The Fraction Proportion Method

$$\frac{dosage\ unit}{dose\ on\ hand} = \frac{amount\ to\ administer}{desired\ dose} \quad \textbf{Or} \quad \frac{Q}{H} = \frac{A}{D}$$

The Ratio Proportion Method

dosage unit : dose on hand :: amount to dispense : desired dose

Or

$$Q : H :: A : D$$

The Formula Method

$$\frac{desired\ dose}{dose\ on\ hand} \times dosage\ unit = amount\ to\ administer \quad \textbf{Or} \quad \frac{D}{H} \times Q = A$$

COMMON APPROXIMATIONS

1 milliliter (mL) = 15 to 20 drops (gtt) (droppers vary)
5 milliliter (mL) = 1 teaspoon (tsp)
15 milliliter (mL) = 1 tablespoon (tbsp)
30 milliliter (mL) = 1 ounce (oz)
1 kilogram (kg) = 2.2 pounds (lbs)
1 tablespoon (tbsp) = 3 teaspoon (tsp)
1 ounce (oz) = 2 tablespoons (tbsp)
1 cup (c) = 8 ounces (oz)
1 pint (pt) = 2 cups (c) = 16 ounces (oz)
1 grain (gr) = 60 or 65 milligrams (mg)

COMMON ABBREVIATIONS USED IN PHARMACY

Form of Medication			
Abbreviation	**Meaning**	**Abbreviation**	**Meaning**
cap, caps	capsule	MDI	metered-dose inhaler
comp	compound	sol, soln.	solution
dil.	dilute	SR	slow-release
EC	enteric-coated	supp.	suppository
elix.	elixir	susp.	suspension
ext.	extract	syr, syp.	syrup
fld., fl	fluid	syr	syringe
gt, gtt	drop, drops	tab	tablet
H	hypodermic	tr, tinct, tinc.	tincture
LA	long-acting	ung, oint	ointment
liq	liquid		
Where to Administer			
Abbreviation	**Meaning**	**Abbreviation**	**Meaning**
ad, A.D., AD*	right ear	od, O.D., OD	right eye
as, A.S., AS*	left ear	os, O.S., OS	left eye
au, A.U., AU*	both ears	ou, O.U., OU	both eyes

*Indicates a "Do not use" or "undesirable" abbreviation according to JCAHO.

DETERMINE THE TOTAL AMOUNT OF LIQUID MEDICATION TO DISPENSE

1 oz = 30 mL	5 oz = 150 mL	9 oz = 270 mL
2 oz = 60 mL	6 oz = 180 mL	10 oz = 300 mL
3 oz = 90 mL.	7 oz = 210 mL	11 oz = 330 mL
4 oz = 120 mL	8 oz = 240 mL	12 oz = 360 mL

1 tsp/5 mL bid/q12h (10 mL/day) for 10 days = 100 mL = 3.33 oz

1 tsp/5 mL tid/q8h (15 mL/day) for 10 days = 150 mL = 5 oz

1 tsp/5 mL qid/q6h (20 mL/day) for 10 days = 200 mL = 6.66 oz

1 tsp/5 mL q4h/six times a day (30 mL/day) for 10 days = 300 mL = 10 oz

2 tsp/10 mL bid/q12h (20 mL/day) for 10 days = 200 mL = 6.66 oz

2 tsp/10 mL tid/q8h (30 mL/day) for 10 days = 300 mL = 10 oz

2 tsp/10 mL qid/q6h (40 mL/day) for 10 days = 400 mL = 13.33 oz

2 tsp/10 mL q4h/six times a day (60 mL/day) for 10 days = 600 mL = 20 oz

METRIC-TO-METRIC EQUIVALENTS

Metric Weight Measure

1 kilogram (kg) = 1000 grams (g)
1 gram (g) = 0.001 kilogram (kg)
1 gram (g) = 1000 milligrams (mg)
1 milligram (mg) = 0.001 gram (g)
1 milligram (mg) = 1000 micrograms (mcg)
1 microgram (mcg) = 0.001 milligram (mg)

Metric Fluid Measure

1 liter (L) = 1000 milliliters (mL)
1 milliliter (mL) = 0.001 liter (L)
1 milliliter (mL) = 1 cubic centimeter (CC)

ALLIGATION

The concentration of the higher concentrated solution		Parts of the higher concentrated solution needed **
	The desired concentration needed	
The concentration of the less concentrated solution*		Parts of the **lesser** concentrated solution needed ***

* When you are diluting with water, the less concentrated solution has a concentration of ZERO.

** The difference between the concentration needed and the concentration of the LESSER concentrated solution. (The **diagonal** difference)

*** The difference between the concentration needed and the concentration of the HIGHER concentrated solution. (The **diagonal** difference)

DETERMINE THE TOTAL NUMBER OF TABLETS/CAPSULES TO DISPENSE

1 tab/cap daily for 1 month = 30 tab/cap ($\frac{1}{2}$ tab daily = 15 tablets)

1 tab/cap bid/q12h for 1 month = 60 tab/cap ($\frac{1}{2}$ tab bid/q12h = 30 tablets)

1 tab/cap tid/q8h for 1 month = 90 tab/cap ($\frac{1}{2}$ tab tid/q8h = 45 tablets)

1 tab/cap qid/q6h for 1 month = 120 tab/cap ($\frac{1}{2}$ tab qid/q6h = 60 tablets)

1 tab/cap daily for 3 months = 90 tab/cap ($\frac{1}{2}$ tab daily = 45 tablets)

1 tab/cap bid/q12h for 3 months = 180 tab/cap ($\frac{1}{2}$ tab bid/q12h = 90 tablets)

1 tab/cap tid/q8h for 3 months = 270 tab/cap ($\frac{1}{2}$ tab tid/q8h = 135 tablets)

1 tab/cap qid/q6h for 3 months = 360 tab/cap ($\frac{1}{2}$ tab qid/q6h = 180 tablets)

COMMON ABBREVIATIONS USED IN PHARMACY

Frequency			
Abbreviation	**Meaning**	**Abbreviation**	**Meaning**
a.c., ac, AC, a̅c̅	before meals	qam, q.a.m.	every morning
ad. lib, ad lib	as desired, freely	qpm, o.n., q.n.	every night
b.i.d., bid, BID	twice a day	q.d.,* qd*	daily
b.i.w.	twice a week	q.h., qh	every hour
h, hr	hour	q. ____ hrs, q ____ h	every _____ hours
h.s.,* hs,* HS*	hour of sleep, at bedtime	qhs, q.h.s.	every night, at bedtime
LOS	length of stay	q.i.d., qid, QID	4 times a day
min	minute	q.o.d.,* qod*	every other day
non rep	do not repeat	rep	repeat
n, noc, noct	night	SOS, s.o.s.	once if necessary, as necessary
qd*	every day	stat	immediately
p.c., pc, PC, p̅c̅	after meals	t.i.d., tid, TID	3 times a day
p.r.n., prn, PRN	when necessary, when required, as needed	t.i.w.*	3 times a week

*Indicates a "Do not use" or "undesirable" abbreviation according to JCAHO.